# Handbook of TOTAL PARENTERAL NUTRITION

**JOHN P. GRANT, M.D.**

Director, Nutritional Support Service
Assistant Professor of Surgery
Duke University Medical Center
Durham, North Carolina

W. B. SAUNDERS COMPANY • PHILADELPHIA • LONDON • TORONTO

W. B. Saunders Company:   West Washington Square
Philadelphia, Pa.   19105

1 St. Anne's Road
Eastbourne, East Sussex BN21 3UN, England

1 Goldthorne Avenue
Toronto, Ontario M8Z 5T9, Canada

**Library of Congress Cataloging in Publication Data**

Grant, John Palmer, 1942–

Handbook of total parenteral nutrition.

Includes index.

1. Parenteral feeding.    I. Title.

RM224.G72     615.8'55     79–64592

ISBN 0–7216–4210–1

Handbook of Total Parenteral Nutrition          ISBN  0-7216-4210-1

Last digit is the print number:   9    8    7    6    5    4    3

*To*
*my loving wife and children:*

LUCY, MARGARET and ANDREW

# FOREWORD

During the past 15 years knowledge and experience in clinical nutrition have increased exponentially and in unprecedented fashion. This has largely been the result of the reproducible demonstration that sufficient nutrient substrates can be administered parenterally to support normal growth and development in neonates, infants, and children and to maintain or improve nutritional status and body composition in adults under a wide variety of clinical pathophysiologic conditions. Once the obvious relevance of maintaining optimal nutrition in critically ill patients had been appreciated by clinicians and scientists of many disciplines throughout the world, a great wave of activity in this vital area of clinical biochemistry followed. Concomitantly, there has been a virtual explosion in the availability of new techniques, solutions, infusion apparatus, and myriad related products for the safe and efficacious administration of total parenteral nutrition. In point of fact, it has been almost impossible to keep abreast of the many practical applications and clinically documented developments in this constantly changing area of endeavor, much less the plethora of basic advances being made daily in this seemingly limitless frontier. Accordingly, it has been frustrating at times for the novice to acquire the knowledge necessary to use total parenteral nutrition (TPN) with confidence and competence.

Dr. John P. Grant has undertaken the awesome task of attempting to summarize the current status of the art and science in this handbook. He has succeeded brilliantly in presenting not only a most equitable and comprehensive review of the literature but also valuable insight into his personal experiences and those of his team at Duke University Medical Center. Certainly a handbook of this nature is long overdue and will be an asset to the library of anyone with an interest in clinical nutrition.

This book, well written throughout its 11 chapters, covers the salient features of parenteral nutrition, beginning with an historical perspective and ending with discussions of the vitamin and trace element requirements and deficiencies related to total parenteral nutrition. Principles of patient selection, catheter insertion and long-term maintenance, preparation and administration of solutions, and recognition and management of all potential complications are presented successfully and succinctly. The text is complemented aptly by 24 tables, 83 figures, and almost 1000 references. Those of us with an interest in total parenteral nutrition and those who will develop such an interest and who will acquire an expertise in total parenteral nutrition owe the author a great debt of gratitude for his efforts on our behalf.

STANLEY J. DUDRICK, M.D.
*Houston, Texas*

# PREFACE

Since introduction of techniques for intravenous nutrition in 1968 by Dudrick, Vars, and Rhoads, indications for its use and application to the hospitalized and home patient have greatly increased. With this growing experience, there has been a rapid accumulation of new metabolic and technical information, knowledge of which is now essential for the safe delivery of parenteral nutrition. In recognition of the growing need for highly specialized nutritional support, many medical centers have formed Nutritional Support Services consisting of physicians, nurses, pharmacists, dieticians, and physical therapists. Although specialized nutritional support teams are highly advantageous, especially in the larger medical centers, they are by no means necessary for safe and efficacious administration of parenteral nutrition. All that is required is a highly motivated, conscientious, and well-informed core of individuals, which may consist of only one physician and a nurse, pharmacist, dietician, or physical therapist.

It is the purpose of this monograph to summarize the many advances which have been made in intravenous nutrition over the past 10 years with emphasis on that new body of knowledge specifically related to safe and efficacious administration of intravenous support. The work is flavored in all sections by my experience in research and clinical application of total parenteral nutrition since 1969. To a great extent it reflects the experience at Duke University Medical Center since 1975, when a Nutritional Support Service was established. The initial impetus to undertake this monograph arose from constant questions concerning administration of parenteral nutrition from students, residents in training, practicing physicians, nurses, pharmacists, and dieticians. There was an apparent need for a reference source which presented a workable "cook book" approach to parenteral nutrition as well as a review of pertinent past and ongoing research material to answer specific questions and to guide further investigation for the nutritional enthusiast. This monograph is intended to begin to fulfill that need. It is hoped that the individual with little or no prior experience in total parenteral nutrition will gain a level of expertise that will permit him to identify patients requiring intensive nutritional support, initiate a support program, and avoid as much as possible technical, metabolic, and septic complications. It is hoped that individuals with a sound background in total parenteral nutrition will find in this work new "tricks of the trade" that I have found quite helpful in my practice. For these individuals an exhaustive list of references with each chapter has been included for more in-depth review. The last two chapters concerning requirements for vitamin and trace element supplementation during total parenteral nutrition may offer further stimulus for thought to the trained parenteral nutritionist, as many more questions are raised in these chapters than are answered.

The monograph is organized in a progressive manner beginning with initial patient evaluation and continuing through catheter insertion, catheter maintenance, solution formulation, solution administration, and recognition and avoidance of various metabolic and technical complications. Chapters have been inserted on the history of parenteral nutrition, the organization of a nutritional support service, and basic human metabolism as related to parenteral nutrition and are recommended to the reader.

In a field that is changing rapidly, it is impossible to publish an entirely current monograph. However, an attempt has been made to reference all pertinent literature up to and including October, 1979. The reader must be cautioned that any drug products, recommended dosages, and therapeutic procedures mentioned within this manual are subject to change with time and he is advised to refer to continuing publications for new information as it becomes available.

JOHN P. GRANT, M.D.

# CONTENTS

# Chapter 1

# HISTORY OF PARENTERAL NUTRITION

The beginnings of parenteral nutrition can be traced to the middle and latter parts of the seventeenth century when Sir Christopher Wren, Robert Boyle, Caspar Scotus, and Courten injected various substances intravenously into animals. Opium, wine, and oil were given and the researchers predicted that similar solutions could be safely injected into the bloodstream of man. It was not until 1831, however, that a substance was successfully infused into man. In that year a Scottish physician, Latta, injected a salt solution into patients stricken with cholera.[1] Claude Bernard demonstrated in 1843 that sugar solutions could be safely given to animals. Menzel and Perco, after extensive animal experiments, administered fat by subcutaneous injection to an emaciated patient suffering from Pott's disease in 1869.[2] Several attempts at intravenous infusion of fresh cow's milk into man for both intravascular volume expansion and nutritional support were reported by Thomas, Hodder, and Howe in 1878 with surprisingly good results.[3] Eighteen years later, in 1896, Biedl and Kraus successfully administered a glucose solution intravenously to man.[4]

As techniques of intravenous infusion were refined, interest in human metabolic processes and nutritional support grew rapidly. A new era of metabolic research began around the turn of this century with many researchers seeking the development of total intravenous nutritional support. The importance of protein administration for nitrogen balance, weight gain, and general well-being was demonstrated as early as 1852 by Bidder and Schmidt[5] and confirmed by Voit in 1866.[6] Intravenous administration of crude protein solutions, however, resulted in strong allergic reactions. Abderhalden and Rona[7] experimented with rectal instillation of protein in animals in 1904 and concluded that they had achieved nitrogen absorption and utilization. In 1906 they applied the same technique to a boy who could not eat and again claimed nitrogen equilibrium.[8] In 1913 Henriques and Anderson[9] hydrolyzed casein to form a non-allergenic, amino acid, di- and tripeptide solution and successfully infused the mixture intravenously to nourish a goat. Similar success was achieved in animals by Elman in 1937.[10] Two years later he and Weiner[11] infused a solution of 2 per cent casein hydrolysate and 8 per cent dextrose into a patient, with no adverse reactions. A variety of protein hydrolysates have since been studied; including hydrolysates of lactalbumin, bovine serum protein, human serum albumin, meat, fibrin, and casein. In 1940 Schohl and Blackfan[12] infused a mixture of synthetic crystalline amino acids into infants. Refinements in crystalline amino acid solutions have since increased their metabolic usefulness by supplying L-isomers[13] and defining more optimal ratios of essential to total amino acids.

Infused protein and amino acids are also utilized extensively for energy production when adequate caloric support is not given. Various substances, including fructose, sorbitol, xylitol, glycerol, and alcohol, have been administered as caloric sources

1

to decrease protein catabolism. Fat emulsions derived from castor oil and cotton seed oil appeared to be ideal solutions because of their high caloric value and low osmolarity; however, intravenous administration of these substances resulted in fever, low back pain, non-specific coagulation defects, liver infiltration by ceroid pigment, and jaundice.[14] Because of these untoward reactions, the Food and Drug Administration banned use of fat emulsions in the United States in 1964. Continuing investigations in Europe, however, led to a new fat emulsion derived from soybean oil. No significant side effects were observed, and the fat appeared to be readily utilized.[15] These findings, along with data from selected research centers in the United States,[16] led to the recent FDA approval for parenteral use of a soybean oil fat emulsion, Intralipid* and a safflower oil emulsion, Liposyn.†

None of the above caloric sources, however, has been found superior to the low-cost, abundant, and metabolically efficient substance dextrose. In 1944 Helfrick and Abelson[17] supported a five-month-old infant for five days by providing through an ankle vein a solution of 50 per cent glucose and 10 per cent casein hydrolysate alternated with a homogenized 10 per cent olive oil-lecithin emulsion. Although marked thrombophlebitis occurred, the infant's general nutritional status greatly improved. Dennis et al.[18, 19] met with variable success in attempting to maintain nutrition by administering 15 to 20 per cent dextrose with blood and blood products through peripheral central venous lines. In 1949 Meng and Early[20] and Rhode et al.[21] reported maintenance of normal nutrition in dogs with infusion of hypertonic dextrose and protein solutions through catheters placed in the central venous system. In 1960 Rhoads[22] experimented with large-volume infusions of 10 per cent dextrose and hydrolyzed proteins, maintaining fluid balance with generous use of diuretics.

The perfection of a technique for placement of intravenous catheters in the superior vena cava via the subclavian vein made possible administration of hypertonic dextrose and protein solutions over prolonged periods without phlebitis and thrombosis. In 1968 and 1969 Dudrick et al.[23, 24] demonstrated that solutions of 20 to 25 per cent dextrose and 4 per cent to 5 per cent amino acids could be administered through such catheters with minimal side effects. Daily caloric needs, essential nitrogenous building blocks, and necessary electrolytes, minerals, and vitamins could be provided easily. Their work renewed interest in the metabolic needs of seriously ill, catabolic patients and in the role of nutrition in their management. Ongoing studies continue to demonstrate the utility of parenteral nutrition in the treatment of a wide range of diseases.

Since 1970 numerous publications have reported research in human metabolism utilizing intravenous nutrition. Several books review this research for the interested reader.[25–30] In this monograph, emphasis will be placed on the techniques of providing parenteral nutrition to the adult patient. Patient selection, catheter placement and care, solution preparation and administration, and recognition and management of complications will be dealt with in detail. Introductory chapters on trace element and vitamin requirements and metabolism are included in recognition of the significant role they will certainly play in future research on nutritional support.

*Cutter Laboratories, Inc., Berkeley, Calif. 94710.
†Abbott Laboratories, North Chicago, Ill. 60064.

## REFERENCES

1. Wilkinson, A. W.: Historical background of intravenous feeding. Nutr. Dieta, 5:295–297, 1963.
2. Menzel, A., and Perco, H.: Uber die Resorption von Nahrungs mitteln vom Unterhautzellgewebe aus. Wien. Med. Wochenschr., 19:517–525, 1869.
3. Thomas, T. G.: The intravenous injection of milk as a substitute for the transfusion of blood. N.Y. Med. J., 28:449–465, 1878.
4. Biedle, A., and Krause, R. Quoted in Elman, R.: Parenteral Alimentation in Surgery with Special Reference to Proteins and Amino-Acids. New York, Hoeber Medical Books (Harper & Row, Publishers, Inc), 1947.
5. Bidder, F., and Schmidt, C.: Die Verdauungssaefte und der Stoffwechsel. Leipsig, 1852.
6. Voit, C.: Untersuchungen uber die Ausschie-

dungswege der stickstoffhaltigen zersel-
zungs — produkte aus dem thierischen Organismus. Z. Biol., 2:189–195, 1866.

7. Abderhalden, E., and Rona, P.: Futterungsver-
suche mit durch Pankreatin, durch Pepsin-
salzsaure plus Pankreatin und durch Saure
hydrolysiertem Casein. Hoppe Seyler's Z.
Physiol. Chem., 42:528–531, 1904.

8. Abderhalden, E., Frank, F., and Schittenhelm, A.:
Uber die Verwertung von tief afgebautem
Eiweiss im menschlichen Organismus.
Hoppe Seyler's Z. Physiol. Chem., 63:215–
221, 1909.

9. Henriques, V., and Anderson, A. C.: Uber paren-
terale Ernahrung durch intravenose Injektion.
Hoppe Seyler's Z. Physiol. Chem., 88:357–
369, 1913.

10. Elman, R.: Amino-acid content of the blood following intravenous injection of hydrolyzed
casein. Proc. Soc. Exp. Biol. Med., 37:437–445,
1937.

11. Elman, R., and Weiner, D. O.: Intravenous alimentation with special reference to protein
(amino acid) metabolism. J.A.M.A., 112:796–
802, 1939.

12. Schohl, A. T., and Blackfan, K. D.: Intravenous
administration of crystalline amino acids to
infants. J. Nutr., 20:305–316, 1940.

13. Peaston, M. J. T.: A comparison of hydrolyzed L-
and synthesized DL-amino acids for complete
parenteral nutrition. Clin. Pharmacol. Ther.,
9:61–66, 1967.

14. Lehr, H. L., Rosenthal, O., Rawnsley, H. M.,
Rhoads, J. E., and Sen, M. B.: Clinical experience with intravenous fat emulsions. Metabolism, 6:666–672, 1957.

15. Edgren, B., and Wretlind, A.: Ernahrungsphysio-
logische und pharmakologische Gesicht-
spunkte der Verwendung von Aminosauren
und Fett in der intravenosen Ernahrung.
Wien. Med. Wochenschr., 117:32–41, 1967.

16. Hansen, L. M., Hardie, W. R., and Hidalgo, J.: Fat
emulsion for intravenous administration:
Clinical experience with Intralipid 10%. Ann.
Surg., 184:80–88, 1976.

17. Helfrick, F. W., and Abelson, N. M.: Intravenous
feeding of a complete diet in a child: Report of
a case. J. Pediatr., 25:400–403, 1944.

18. Dennis, C.: Preoperative and postoperative care
for the bad-risk patient. Minn. Med., 27:538–
543, 1944.

19. Dennis, C., Eddy, F. D., Frykman, H. M.,
McCarthy, A. M., and Westover, D.: The response to vagotomy in idiopathic ulcerative
colitis and regional enteritis. Ann. Surg.,
128:479–496, 1948.

20. Meng, H. C., and Early, F.: Study of complete
parenteral alimentation in dogs. J. Lab. Clin.
Med., 34:1121–1132, 1949.

21. Rhode, C. M., Parkins, W. M., and Vars, H. M.:
Nitrogen balances of dogs continuously infused with 50 per cent glucose and protein
preparations. Am. J. Physiol., 159:415–425,
1949.

22. Rhoads, J. E.: Diuretics as an adjuvant in dispos-
ing of extra water employed as a vehicle in
parenteral hyperalimentation. Fed. Proc.,
21:389, 1962.

23. Dudrick, S. J., Wilmore, D. W., Vars, H. M., and
Rhoads, J. E.: Long-term total parenteral nutrition with growth, development and positive nitrogen balance. Surgery, 64:134–142,
1968.

24. Dudrick, S. J., Wilmore, D. W., Vars, H. M., and
Rhoads, J. E.: Can intravenous feeding as the
sole means of nutrition support growth in the
child and restore weight loss in an adult? An
affirmative answer. Ann. Surg., 169:974–984,
1969.

25. American College of Surgeons, Committee on Pre-
and Postoperative Care: Manual of Surgical
Nutrition. Philadelphia, W.B. Saunders Company, 1975.

26. Lee, H. A. (ed.): Parenteral nutrition in Acute
Metabolic Illness. New York, Academic Press,
Inc., 1974.

27. Wilkinson, A.: Parenteral Nutrition, Edinburgh,
Churchill Livingstone, 1972.

28. Ghadimi, H.: Total Parenteral Nutrition. New
York, John Wiley & Sons, Inc., 1975.

29. Johnston, I. D. A. (ed.): Advances in Parenteral
Nutrition. Lancaster, England, Medical &
Technical Publishing Co. Ltd., 1978.

30. Richards, J. R., and Kinney, J. M. (eds.). Nutritional Aspects of Care in the Critically Ill.
Edinburgh, Churchill Livingstone, 1977.

# Chapter 2

# A  TEAM  APPROACH

Parenteral nutrition has become increasingly complex. To administer parenteral nutrition effectively and safely, it is necessary to possess a basic understanding of nutrition, biochemistry, physiology, bacteriology, epidemiology, pharmacology, and psychology. Although intravenous nutrition can be lifesaving in many situations, careless use, through inadequate understanding or poor supervision, can result in devastating complications, including septicemia, metabolic imbalances, and death. To maximize benefits and minimize complications, many medical centers have developed a team approach to parenteral nutrition. Solution preparation, catheter insertion, dressing care, and patient management are performed by well-trained individuals.

Duke University Medical Center has developed a Nutritional Support Service under the Department of Surgery, incorporating physicians, clinical pharmacists, a nurse-clinician, a dietician, members of the intravenous line team (I.V. team), physical therapists, and the nursing staffs of the various wards. Their individual responsibilities are outlined below.

*Physicians.*   The director of the Nutritional Support Service is a surgical staff physician. He is responsible for the development and implementation of guidelines for the use of metabolic and nutritional support techniques and procedures. His duties also include supervision of nutritional research. The director oversees the activity of the entire team and periodically reviews statistical data to assure optimal results. He is directly responsible for senior surgical residents, who rotate through the service for two-month periods. These residents consult on all potential candidates

for nutritional support. When intravenous nutrition is indicated, they place a central line under controlled conditions and, with the pharmacist-clinician, review the metabolic data and write parenteral nutrition fluid orders. They make rounds daily on all patients and are available 24 hours a day for management of complications. Both the director and senior surgical resident conduct in-service training programs for the hospital nursing staff and are involved in the medical school education program.

An infectious disease physician is available upon request to review practices of the parenteral nutrition team. When an infectious complication is detected, he assists in the evaluation of possible etiology and offers suggestions for improvements in the protocol. His service is of particular value during parenteral nutrition for severely infected, septic patients.

*Clinical Pharmacists.*   Duke has established two positions for clinical pharmacists who devote full time to the parenteral nutrition team. They have a special interest in the clinical application of pharmacology and contribute necessary expertise in complex drug-nutrient interactions. They monitor patients closely, make rounds daily with the senior surgical resident, collect and record metabolic data, and assist in writing daily fluid orders. It is their responsibility to assure correct formulation of nutritional fluids under strictly controlled aseptic conditions and to monitor quality control data closely. They are also available to assist in the insertion of subclavian catheters and may evaluate candidates for parenteral nutrition.

*Nurse-Research Clinician.*   A registered nurse functions as a central figure in patient relations and in the conduct of clinical research. The nurse, who makes daily rounds with the senior surgical resident and the pharmacist-clinician, interprets the team goals and activities for the patient and answers questions he may have. The nurse sees all patients returning for outpatient visits and assists in the care of patients on home parenteral nutrition. The nurse is also the liaison between the team and the nursing staff and is responsible for in-service education programs.

In addition to patient care responsibilities, the nurse-clinician maintains all permanent records, periodically reviews all aspects of the team's performance, and prepares a quarterly statistical report on technical and metabolic complications and therapeutic results. The nurse maintains a reference library on nutrition, which is open to medical students and the house staff. Finally, the nurse has specific duties in all research projects conducted by the Nutritional Support Service. These duties include seeing that research protocols are thoroughly understood and followed by personnel who care for study patients, collecting appropriate metabolic data, and assisting in data interpretation.

*Dietician.* A dietician who is interested in active patient care and knowledgeable in special dietary formulas and tube feeding programs is essential to the parenteral nutrition team. All consultations for the team are first referred to the dietician, who performs an initial nutritional assessment that includes evaluations of visceral and somatic proteins, fat depots, dietary intake, and metabolic requirements. These assessments are then reviewed by the senior surgical resident, and a decision is made from the three alternatives available: pursuing further nutritional assessment, initiating oral or enteral nutritional support, or beginning parenteral nutrition. If oral or enteral nutritional support is indicated, the dietician assumes full responsibility for its delivery. Another responsibility of the dietician is the periodic nutritional assessment of every patient receiving nutritional support. This allows for continual monitoring of therapeutic results. The dietician is also helpful in weaning patients from parenteral nutrition when various malabsorption problems or food intolerances are present.

The dietician meets daily with the director of the Nutritional Support Service and makes rounds daily on all patients receiving oral or enteral nutritional support.

*IV Team.* The hospital intravenous line team (IV team), composed of registered nurses, is charged with the responsibility of changing subclavian dressings on a regular basis. It is our policy to change dressings every Monday, Wednesday, and Friday, with daily checks and additional changes as needed. A strict protocol for changing dressings is followed, as discussed in Chapter 5. The IV team is also available to assist in catheter placement.

*Physical Therapist.* While physical therapy has occasionally been employed as an adjunct to nutritional support, the role of mobilization and daily activity in the care of the malnourished patient is still poorly defined. There is evidence, however, that regular exercise benefits the malnourished patient by enhancing utilization of nutrients and promoting synthesis of lean body mass. Muscle work exerts an effect parallel to, but independent of, insulin in the transport of some sugars across the cell barrier.[1, 2] Further, it has been shown that the rate of amino acid transport in skeletal muscle increases with muscle work and is related to protein synthesis during work-induced muscle hypertrophy.

Clinical studies of normal adult men immobilized in spica casts for six to seven weeks have shown increased nitrogen excretion and loss of muscles mass and strength in spite of a dietary intake that maintained nitrogen balance during control and recovery periods.[3] The nitrogen losses were reduced if the patient was placed in an oscillating bed during the study period.[4] Patients in oscillating beds demonstrated a more rapid recovery of metabolic and physiologic functions than the first group. Other studies have shown that a hypercaloric diet given to non-exercised patients may lead to increased fat deposition rather than increased lean body mass.

In addition to the metabolic benefits of exercise, there are general benefits for bedridden patients, particularly with respect to maintenance of the circulatory and respiratory systems. A daily routine of light exercise and mobilization can minimize complications of orthostatic hypotension, thrombophlebitis, and pneumonia. There are also psychologic benefits in that exercise is one of the more easily understood aspects of nutritional support. Exercise gives the patient an opportunity to participate actively in his care and provides positive feedback as increases in strength allow more independence. The interest shown in improving the patient's strength and energy and the welcome change in environment if the patient can go to the physical therapy department instill a new attitude of hope, enthusiasm, and cooperation in the often depressed patient. This response may carry over into other areas of his treatment.

The physical therapist visits all patients prior to and during nutritional support. A dynamic skeletal muscle and respiratory muscle evaluation is performed (see Chapter 3 concerning nutritional evaluation) and an individualized exercise program is developed for each patient for maximal activity. The exercise program consists of daily light exercise and functional activities, especially ambulation. Also included are breathing exercises based on results of respiratory testing. The exercise program is performed for brief periods three or four times daily, with care being taken not to induce fatigue. Some patients become more motivated as their nutritional status improves and can be instructed in an independent exercise program that does not require daily visits from the physical therapist.

If personnel resources are limited and a physical therapist is not available to see every patient, the physical therapist should serve as a consultant in establishing an exercise program that can be administered by other hospital staff members. The investment of staff time and energy in implementing some type of exercise program for the malnourished patient enhances the overall rehabilitation effort and often results in the return of an independently functioning individual concurrent with nutritional recovery.

*Nursing Staff.* Nurses perform primary patient surveillance. It is their responsibility to monitor vital signs, keep accurate records of fluid balance, and assure constant infusion of the parenteral or enteral nutrition solution, maintaining sterility at all times. They must be familiar with early symptoms of possible complications so that the physician can be alerted. The importance of the nurse's role cannot be overemphasized. The nurse is the vital link between the nutrition team and the patient. Inadequate knowledge, lack of concern, or neglect on the nurse's part can result in serious complications regardless of the efforts of the remaining team members.

The team approach has become recognized as an indispensable part of medical care for many diseases. It has been used effectively in treating renal transplant patients, patients receiving chemotherapy for metastatic malignant diseases, patients needing open heart surgery, and children with various types of leukemia. Nutritional support requires a similar team approach. The team outlined above works well at Duke University Medical Center but is only one example for institutions considering establishment of similar teams. The team members may vary, but it is vital to have a small number of highly interested people involved in the administration of parenteral nutrition. Whether one utilizes technicians, nurses, pharmacists, or house staff physicians, the goal should be the same: maximal benefit from intravenous nutrition with minimal complications.

## REFERENCES

1. Goldberg, A. L.: Protein turnover in skeletal muscle. I. Protein catabolism during work-induced hypertrophy and growth induced by growth hormone. J. Biol. Chem., 244:3217–3222, 1969.
2. Goldberg, A. L., and Goodman, H. M.: Amino acid transport during work-induced growth of skeletal muscle. Am. J. Physiol., 216:1111–1115, 1969.
3. Dietrick, J. E., Whedon, G. D., and Shorr, E.: Effects of immobilization upon various metabolic and physiologic functions of normal men. Am. J. Med., 4:3–36, 1948.
4. Whedon, G. D., Deitrick, J. E., and Shorr, E.: Modification of the effects of immobilization upon metabolic and physiologic functions of normal men by use of an oscillating bed. Am. J. Med., 6:684–711, 1949.

# Chapter 3

# PATIENT SELECTION

The administration of parenteral nutrition should be considered whenever adequate nutrition cannot be maintained through the gastrointestinal tract. It should not be considered if the gastrointestinal tract is capable of absorbing nutrients taken orally or infused through a nasogastric tube except when the patient might benefit from bowel rest. In general, parenteral nutrition should not be initiated unless it is anticipated that intravenous support will be required for at least five days, although preliminary data indicate as little as 72 hours preoperatively may be beneficial for malnourished patients.[1] An exception to this restriction is in the treatment of malnourished or stressed patients for whom nutritional support is urgent but whose gastrointestinal function is questionable. With these and other selected patients it is advisable to begin parenteral and enteral nutritional support simultaneously. As soon as the enteral diet is tolerated at the necessary protein-calorie load, the patient should be weaned from the parenteral infusion. In many patients, combined therapy may be necessary for only a few days. In others it may be necessary for several days or weeks, during which time intestinal adaptation to the osmotic load and volume of the enteral diet may occur and the optimal dietary formula may be found without progressive nutritional depletion.

Concomitant infections elsewhere in the body, diabetes, and obesity are not in themselves contraindications to parenteral nutrition. It is recognized that these conditions increase the risk of septic complications during parenteral nutrition, but, with proper care, the incidence of infectious complications should be only 4 to 5 per cent or less, with little morbidity.[2] Patients with either localized infection or generalized septicemia demonstrate a marked hypermetabolic response as great as that seen with trauma or stress. Therefore, instead of being a contraindication to parenteral nutrition, infection is a relative indication.

Diabetic patients usually present no special problems with respect to glucose tolerance. Hyperglycemia can be easily controlled by addition of regular insulin (up to 350 units of insulin per 250 grams of glucose) to the parenteral nutrition solution (see Chapter 7 concerning insulin). Further, the improved glucose tolerance that may occur with administration of glucose[3, 4] and the increased insulin release due to amino acid infusion (leucine in particular) decrease exogenous insulin requirements.

Moderate to marked obesity does not lessen the need for parenteral nutrition. Fatty tissue is poorly mobilized because of the hyperinsulinemia associated with the insulin resistance of stress (insulin is a potent inhibitor of peripheral fat mobilization).[5, 6] Administration of 5 per cent dextrose solutions also stimulates insulin secretion, further inhibiting peripheral fat mobilization.[7, 8] Consequently, during starvation and stress obese patients have protein catabolism and nitrogen losses similar to those of thinner patients and require similar nutritional support.

A partial list of indications for parenteral nutrition is given in Table 3–1. Experi-

**Table 3–1** INDICATIONS FOR PAREN-
TERAL NUTRITION

1. Protein-calorie malnutrition

   Anorexia nervosa
   Chronic vomiting
   Chronic diarrhea
   Malabsorption syndromes
   Prolonged ileus or gastrointestinal obstruction

2. Short bowel syndrome
3. Acute pancreatitis and pancreatic fistulas
4. Enterocutaneous fistulas
5. Inflammatory bowel disease
6. Malignant diseases
7. Renal failure
8. Hepatic failure
9. Hypercatabolic states
10. Burns
11. Trauma

mental and clinical data relating to parenteral nutrition in some of these disease
states will be presented below.

## PROTEIN-CALORIE MALNUTRITION

Several studies of hospitalized patients
have reported frequent occurrence of malnutrition, based on serum albumin concentrations, hypovitaminemia, and anthropometric measurements.[9-13] Bistrian et al.[11]
reported as many as half of the patients
evaluated in an urban municipal hospital
showed signs of moderate or greater protein-calorie malnutrition. Patients not only
exhibit pre-existing malnutrition but often
become more malnourished during hospi-
talization. Attention is frequently focused
on diagnosis and the institution of medical
or surgical therapy, while the nutritional
status of the patient is overlooked. A patient with an acute exacerbation of chronic
ulcer disease, progressively severe gastric
outlet obstruction, and a 15 to 20 per cent
weight loss due to poor dietary intake may
undergo an upper gastrointestinal x-ray examination, saline load test, gastric acid
analysis, and gastroduodenoscopy. Performance of these tests may require four to
seven days of restricted dietary intake.
Three to five additional days of nasogastric
suction may be recommended to reduce py-
loric edema or to prepare the patient for
surgery. Postoperatively, five to seven days

or more of nasogastric suction may be required before the gastroenterostomy functions adequately. In all, two to three weeks
of restricted dietary intake may follow pre-
existing malnutrition. A patient with partially obstructing colonic carcinoma and a
recent weight loss of 10 to 20 per cent may
undergo bowel preparation for a barium
enema and proctoscopy or colonoscopy. In
preparation for partial colectomy he may be
placed on a clear-liquid diet and be given
laxatives for three to five more days. Following surgery, an oral diet may not be
resumed for five to seven days.

It is not uncommon to receive a consul-
tation requesting nutritional support for a
chronically ill, severely depleted patient, in
whom all therapeutic modalities have
failed. Often the patient's physician will
say that little else can be done medically
and will ask whether parenteral nutrition
has anything to offer. The neglect of progressive nutritional depletion is unfortu-
nate, especially since the correlation of starvation with morbidity and mortality has
been long known.[14-17] Mild malnutrition is
associated with an increased incidence of
clean-wound infections[18, 19] and postoperative ileus. In addition, a progressive increase in respiratory infections and insufficiency is seen with malnutrition. This is
due, in part, to deterioration of respiratory
muscle function and also to depression of
the immune defense system. Doekel et al.[20]
have proposed another possible contributing factor. They found that a balanced diet
restricted to 500 calories a day for ten days
significantly reduced ventilatory responses
to hypoxia in healthy volunteers. Such depressed responses, they proposed, could
contribute to the hypoxia and respiratory
failure often seen in patients with malnutrition. Moderate malnutrition further contributes to patient morbidity[21, 22] by markedly impairing collagen synthesis,[23, 24]
adversely affecting wound healing,[25-27] and
depressing the immune response, which
leads to decreased infection resistance (see
later parts of this section). With marked
malnutrition (acute loss of 30 to 35 per cent
body weight) complications become so severe that a 90 to 95 per cent mortality is not
uncommon.

The following section will outline comprehensive, yet clinically useful, techniques for nutritional assessment. All patients who have suffered moderate nutritional depletion, as described below, or who are hypercatabolic are candidates for nutritional support. No patient, unless suffering from a terminal illness, should deteriorate or expire from complications of malnutrition or starvation while undergoing evaluation or therapy.

## NUTRITIONAL ASSESSMENT

Protein-calorie malnutrition has been divided into three major classifications, based on pathogenesis and clinical findings, with the following International Classification of Diseases (ICDA) codes: marasmus (268.0), kwashiorkor-like (267), and mixed or other disorders (269.9). Marasmus is seen in cases in which prolonged starvation has occurred, although the diet contains an acceptable protein-calorie ratio. The patient develops adipose and skeletal muscle atrophy and weight loss and may also exhibit depression of skin test reactivity to recall antigens. Kwashiorkor, on the other hand, is usually associated with a diet containing ample calories, derived mainly, if not entirely, from carbohydrate, but little or no protein. Patients are often of normal weight or slightly overweight. Extracellular water spaces are markedly expanded with salt retention, pitting edema, ascites, and anasarca. Visceral protein stores are depleted, with depressed concentrations of serum albumin, transferrin, thyroxin-binding prealbumin, and retinol-binding protein. Total lymphocyte counts may be significantly depressed, and skin test reactivity to common antigens may be absent. Skeletal muscle mass is usually normal or only slightly depressed.

Not uncommonly, malnourished hospitalized patients demonstrate signs of both types of protein-calorie depletion, a condition called marasmic-kwashiorkor. It is important to determine the nature and severity of protein-calorie depletion so that appropriate nutritional support can be given. Various forms have been devised to record nutritional assessment data. The form in use at Duke University Medical Center is shown in Figure 3–1. Table 3–2 indicates a range of values for Figure 3–1 associated with various degrees of malnutrition.

*Dietary Adequacy.* The first step in nutritional assessment is comparison of dietary caloric intake with estimated caloric expenditure. The patient's caloric intake is estimated as accurately as possible from counts of dietary calories, including any additional carbohydrate calories from intravenous fluids. Caloric expenditure can be estimated from various formulas or measured directly from oxygen consumption.

To estimate caloric expenditure with formulas, one must first determine the basal energy expenditure (BEE), which is the predicted caloric expenditure of a specific patient in a resting, fasting, unstressed state, a state seldom encountered clinically. Either formula below can be used in this determination:[28]

(1) Men = $66 + (13.7 \times W) + (5 \times H) - (6.8 \times A)$ (kcal/day)
Women = $655 + (9.6 \times W) + (1.7 \times H) - (4.7 \times A)$ (kcal/day)

(W = Weight in kg, H = Height in cm, A = Age in years)

(2) Body surface area (sq m) × Basal metabolic rate × 24 hours (kcal/days)

(See Figures 6–1 and 6–2 for calculation of body surface area and determination of basal metabolic rate.)

To derive the actual energy expenditure of a patient, one must add caloric requirements for stress and fever to the predicted BEE. The caloric needs due to stress can be estimated either from total urinary nitrogen excretion or from clinical impressions. If the metabolic activity factor (MAF), which reflects the degree of stress as computed in Figure 3–2, is multiplied by the basal energy expenditure, the derived value is the estimated actual energy expenditure of a patient over 24 hours. Additional caloric requirements due to fever can be calculated

Age _____ Sex _____ Height _____ cm  Wrist Circumference _____ cm  Diagnosis:

Height/Wrist _____  Ideal Weight _____ kg  Usual Weight _____ kg

_____ frame  Body Surface Area _____ m²  Basal Energy Expenditure _____ kcal/day

| PARAMETERS | Date: VALUE | IMPAIRMENT Adequate | Mild | Moderate | Severe | Date: VALUE | IMPAIRMENT Adequate | Mild | Moderate | Severe | Date: VALUE | IMPAIRMENT Adequate | Mild | Moderate | Severe |
|---|---|---|---|---|---|---|---|---|---|---|---|---|---|---|---|
|  | wt |  |  |  |  | wt |  |  |  |  | wt |  |  |  |  |
| FAT RESERVE | mm |  |  |  |  | mm |  |  |  |  | mm |  |  |  |  |
| SOMATIC PROTEIN |  |  |  |  |  |  |  |  |  |  |  |  |  |  |  |
| Arm Muscle Area | cm² |  |  |  |  | cm² |  |  |  |  | cm² |  |  |  |  |
| Wt. as % Ideal | % |  |  |  |  | % |  |  |  |  | % |  |  |  |  |
| Wt. as % Usual | % |  |  |  |  | % |  |  |  |  | % |  |  |  |  |
| Creatinine Excretion Index | % |  |  |  |  | % |  |  |  |  | % |  |  |  |  |
| VISCERAL PROTEIN |  |  |  |  |  |  |  |  |  |  |  |  |  |  |  |
| Albumin | gm% |  |  |  |  | gm% |  |  |  |  | gm% |  |  |  |  |
| Transferrin | mg% |  |  |  |  | mg% |  |  |  |  | mg% |  |  |  |  |
| Prealbumin | mg% |  |  |  |  | mg% |  |  |  |  | mg% |  |  |  |  |
| IMMUNE COMPETENCE |  |  |  |  |  |  |  |  |  |  |  |  |  |  |  |
| Total Lymphocyte Count | mm³ |  |  |  |  | mm³ |  |  |  |  | mm³ |  |  |  |  |
| Cell Mediated Immunity | Reactive | | | | Anergic | Reactive | | | | Anergic | Reactive | | | | Anergic |
| MUSCLE FUNCTION |  | Adequate | Mild | Moderate | Severe |  | Adequate | Mild | Moderate | Severe |  | Adequate | Mild | Moderate | Severe |
| Respiratory |  |  |  |  |  |  |  |  |  |  |  |  |  |  |  |
| Skeletal |  |  |  |  |  |  |  |  |  |  |  |  |  |  |  |
| METABOLIC DATA |  |  |  |  |  |  |  |  |  |  |  |  |  |  |  |
| Nitrogen Excretion |  |  |  |  |  |  |  |  |  |  |  |  |  |  |  |
| Nitrogen Balance |  |  |  |  |  |  |  |  |  |  |  |  |  |  |  |
| Respiratory Quotient |  |  |  |  |  |  |  |  |  |  |  |  |  |  |  |
| Actual Energy Expenditure (Calculated/Measured) |  |  |  |  |  |  |  |  |  |  |  |  |  |  |  |

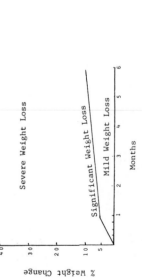

Severe Weight Loss

Significant Weight Loss

Mild Weight Loss

% Weight Change

Months

**Figure 3-1**  Standard nutritional assessment form.

**Table 3-2** RANGE OF VALUES USED IN DETERMINING DEGREE OF MALNUTRITION

| | IMPAIRMENT | | |
|---|---|---|---|
| | *Mild* | *Moderate* | *Severe* |
| Fat reserves (triceps skinfold) | 40 to 50th percentile | 30 to 39th percentile | <30th percentile |
| Somatic protein | 40 to 50th percentile | 30 to 39th percentile | <30th percentile |
| Arm muscle area, sq cm | 80 to 90% | 70 to 79% | <70% |
| Wt as % ideal | 85 to 95% | 75 to 84% | <75% |
| Wt as % usual* | 60 to 80% | 40 to 59% | <40% |
| Creatinine excretion index | | | |
| Visceral protein | | | |
| Albumin, grams per 100 ml | 2.8 to 3.4 | 2.1 to 2.7 | <2.1 |
| Transferrin, mg per 100 ml | 150 to 200 | 100 to 149 | <100 |
| Prealbumin, mg per 100 ml | 10 to 15 | 5 to 10 | <5 |
| Immune competence | | | |
| Total lymphocyte count | 1200 to 2000 | 800 to 1199 | <800 |
| Cell-mediated immunity | Reactive | Reactive | Anergic |

*Influenced by rate of loss (see per cent weight change graph).

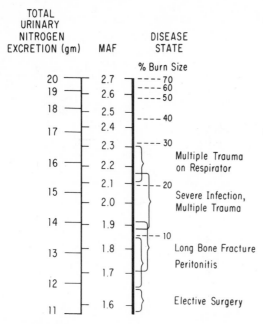

```
TOTAL
URINARY
NITROGEN                    DISEASE
EXCRETION (gm)    MAF       STATE

                           % Burn Size
   20  ─┬─    2.7    ────70
   19  ─┤     2.6    ────60
                     ────50
   18  ─┤     2.5
                     ────40
   17  ─┤     2.4
              2.3    ────30
   16  ─┤     2.2           Multiple Trauma
                            on Respirator
              2.1
   15  ─┤     2.0    ──20    Severe Infection,
                            Multiple Trauma
   14  ─┤     1.9
                     ──10
   13  ─┤     1.8           Long Bone Fracture

              1.7          Peritonitis
   12  ─┤
                           Elective Surgery
   11  ─┴─    1.6
```

**Figure 3–2** Determination of metabolic activity factor (MAF).

from: Calories = 12 per cent BEE per degree above 37° C per day (kcal). This final estimate of actual caloric requirement should be adequate for the establishment and maintenance of positive nitrogen balance and weight gain. Calories required for maintenance of existing body weight and neutral nitrogen balance can be estimated by reducing the actual energy expenditure by 25 per cent.

Actual calorie expenditure can be calculated from the measurement of oxygen consumption by either a closed-circuit or open-circuit technique.[29, 30] The closed-circuit technique utilizes a displacement spirometer with a carbon dioxide absorber (Fig. 3–3A). The tank is filled with either room air or oxygen, and the patient breathes from the spirometer through a mouthpiece or face mask. The volume decrease in the spirometer over a measured period of time is recorded and represents oxygen utilization. Oxygen utilization is then converted to caloric expenditure as follows:

Caloric expenditure (kcal/sq m/hour) =

$$\frac{O_2 \text{ consumption (liters/hour)} \times \text{kcal equivalent}}{\text{Body surface area}}$$

Where $O_2$ consumption = volume $O_2$ in spirometer × [273 ÷ (273 + temperature in Celsius)] × [(barometric pressure − vapor pressure) ÷ 760] × [60 minutes ÷ minutes of study]; and kcal equivalent = 3.9 + (1.1 × respiratory quotient, measured or estimated).

In the open-circuit technique, the patient breathes room air, and expired gases are collected in a Douglas bag over a measured period of time (Fig. 3–3B). $O_2$ consumption and $CO_2$ production are calculated:

$$(1) \quad \frac{O_2 \text{ consumption}}{\text{Unit time}}, (\dot{V}O_2) =$$

$$\frac{20.9 - \text{Bag } O_2 \text{ concentration}}{} \times \frac{\text{Volume gas expired}}{\text{Unit time}}$$

$$(2) \quad \frac{CO_2 \text{ production}}{\text{Unit time}}, (\dot{V}CO_2) =$$

$$\text{Bag } CO_2 \text{ concentration} \times \frac{\text{Volume gas expired}}{\text{Unit time}}$$

Corrections are made to standard temperature and barometric pressure and dry gas, and caloric expenditure is calculated:

Caloric expenditure = $3.9 \, \dot{V}O_2 + 11.1 \, \dot{V}CO_2$

If urinary nitrogen excretion is known the formula expands to:[31]

Caloric expenditure = $3.94 \, \dot{V}O_2 +$
$1.11 \, \dot{V}CO_2 - 2.17$ urinary nitrogen

Possible sources of error for both techniques include a non-steady state, excessive protein catabolism, and wide fluctuations in the respiratory quotient. From a plot of caloric intake versus energy expenditure, the adequacy of caloric intake on the day of the test can be obtained.

In addition to calculating caloric balance, it is also important to determine nitrogen balance as an estimate of the net flux of lean body mass. A 24-hour urine collection can be assayed for total nitrogen content by the micro-Kjeldahl method. Nitrogen balance is then calculated from the formula:

$$N_{bal} = \frac{\text{Protein intake}}{6.25} - \text{TUN}^a -$$

$$5 \text{ mg N/kg}^b - 12 \text{ mg N/kg}^c$$

## A. Closed circuit oxygen consumption technique

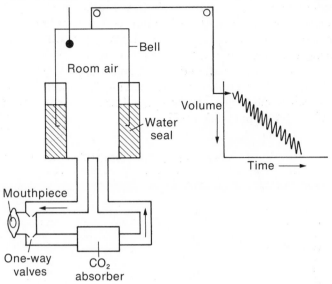

**Figure 3–3** Techniques for determination of oxygen consumption.

## B. Open circuit oxygen consumption technique

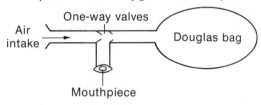

a = Total urinary nitrogen excreted over 24 hours
b = Insensible nitrogen losses
c = Nitrogen losses from the gastrointestinal tract

If the micro-Kjeldahl nitrogen assay is unavailable, a fairly accurate estimate of total urinary nitrogen losses can be obtained by adding 2 grams nitrogen to the total urinary urea nitrogen.[32] If proteinuria is present, an additional factor (grams proteinuria per 24 hours ÷ 6.25) should be added. The severity of catabolism can be estimated from nitrogen balance. A positive balance signifies an anabolic state. A negative balance indicates a catabolic state, with 5 to 10 grams/day representing mild, 10 to 15 grams/day moderate, and 15 grams or more/day severe catabolism.[28]

*Lean Body Mass.* Depletion of lean body mass is a characteristic finding in patients with marasmus. To maintain vital organ function, the body resorts to proteolysis early in starvation, with many of the released amino acids being channeled into gluconeogenesis. Although all body protein sources are utilized, skeletal muscle appears to be most vulnerable (see Chapter 6).

*Body composition studies* by multiple isotope dilution techniques provide the most accurate method for characterization of body weight in terms of body fat, extracellular supporting components, and the body cell mass.[33–37] Shizgal et al.[33, 35, 36] utilized such studies before and during parenteral nutrition to estimate patients' caloric and nitrogen requirements for anabolism. They stated that changes in body composition parameters were more sensitive than nitrogen balance studies alone. They found a significant correlation between the state of nutrition and the size of the extracellular supporting component, as reflected by total body exchangeable sodium ($Na_e$), and body cell mass, as reflected by total body exchangeable potassium ($K_e$). Increases in the ratio $Na_e/K_e$ were associated with malnutrition, and decreases in that ratio with body cell mass repletion. From measurements of total body water, using tritiated water, and total exchangeable sodium, using sodium-22, one can calculate lean body mass (LBM = TBW ÷ 0.73), body fat (BF = body weight − LBM), body cell mass (BCM = 0.00833 × exchangeable potassium, where exchangeable potassium is calculated from TBW and sodium-22 data), and extracellular mass (ECM = LBM − BCM).[38]

The isotope dilution assay just described is ideal for body compartment assessment in the clinical setting because the isotopes used are inexpensive and relative-

**Table 3–3**   IDEAL WEIGHT (kg) FOR HEIGHT, ADULTS*

| | MALES | | | FEMALES | | |
|---|---|---|---|---|---|---|
| cm | Small Frame | Medium Frame | Large Frame | Small Frame | Medium Frame | Large Frame |
| 142 | | | | 41.8 | 45.0 | 49.5 |
| 143 | | | | 42.3 | 45.3 | 49.8 |
| 144 | | | | 42.8 | 45.6 | 50.1 |
| 145 | | | | 43.2 | 45.9 | 50.5 |
| 146 | | | | 43.7 | 46.6 | 51.2 |
| 147 | | | | 44.1 | 47.3 | 51.8 |
| 148 | | | | 44.6 | 47.7 | 52.3 |
| 149 | | | | 45.1 | 48.1 | 52.8 |
| 150 | | | | 45.5 | 48.6 | 53.2 |
| 151 | | | | 46.2 | 49.3 | 54.0 |
| 152 | | | | 46.8 | 50.0 | 54.5 |
| 153 | | | | 47.3 | 50.5 | 55.0 |
| 154 | | | | 47.8 | 51.0 | 55.5 |
| 155 | 50.0 | 53.6 | 58.2 | 48.2 | 51.4 | 55.9 |
| 156 | 50.7 | 54.3 | 58.8 | 48.9 | 52.3 | 56.8 |
| 157 | 51.4 | 55.0 | 59.5 | 49.5 | 53.2 | 57.7 |
| 158 | 51.8 | 55.5 | 60.0 | 50.0 | 53.6 | 58.3 |
| 159 | 52.2 | 56.0 | 60.5 | 50.5 | 54.0 | 58.9 |
| 160 | 52.7 | 56.4 | 60.9 | 50.9 | 54.5 | 59.5 |
| 161 | 53.2 | 56.8 | 61.5 | 51.5 | 55.3 | 60.1 |
| 162 | 53.7 | 57.2 | 62.1 | 52.1 | 56.1 | 60.7 |
| 163 | 54.1 | 57.7 | 62.7 | 52.7 | 56.8 | 61.4 |
| 164 | 55.0 | 58.5 | 63.4 | 53.6 | 57.7 | 62.3 |
| 165 | 55.9 | 59.5 | 64.1 | 54.5 | 58.6 | 63.2 |
| 166 | 56.5 | 60.1 | 64.8 | 55.1 | 59.2 | 63.8 |
| 167 | 57.1 | 60.7 | 65.6 | 55.7 | 59.8 | 64.4 |
| 168 | 57.7 | 61.4 | 66.4 | 56.4 | 60.5 | 65.0 |
| 169 | 58.6 | 62.3 | 67.5 | 57.3 | 61.4 | 65.9 |
| 170 | 59.5 | 63.2 | 68.6 | 58.2 | 62.2 | 66.8 |
| 171 | 60.1 | 63.8 | 69.2 | 58.8 | 62.8 | 67.4 |
| 172 | 60.7 | 64.4 | 69.8 | 59.4 | 63.4 | 68.0 |
| 173 | 61.4 | 65.0 | 70.5 | 60.0 | 64.1 | 68.6 |
| 174 | 62.3 | 65.9 | 71.4 | 60.9 | 65.0 | 69.8 |
| 175 | 63.2 | 66.8 | 72.3 | 61.8 | 65.9 | 70.9 |
| 176 | 63.8 | 67.5 | 72.9 | 62.4 | 66.5 | 71.7 |
| 177 | 64.4 | 68.2 | 73.5 | 63.0 | 67.1 | 72.5 |
| 178 | 65.0 | 69.0 | 74.1 | 63.6 | 67.7 | 73.2 |
| 179 | 65.9 | 69.9 | 75.3 | 64.5 | 68.6 | 74.1 |
| 180 | 66.8 | 70.9 | 76.4 | 65.5 | 69.5 | 75.0 |
| 181 | 67.4 | 71.7 | 77.1 | 66.1 | 70.1 | 75.6 |
| 182 | 68.0 | 72.5 | 77.8 | 66.7 | 70.7 | 76.2 |
| 183 | 68.6 | 73.2 | 78.6 | 67.3 | 71.4 | 76.8 |
| 184 | 69.8 | 74.1 | 79.8 | | | |
| 185 | 70.9 | 75.0 | 80.9 | | | |
| 186 | 71.5 | 75.8 | 81.7 | | | |
| 187 | 72.1 | 76.6 | 82.5 | | | |
| 188 | 72.7 | 77.3 | 83.2 | | | |
| 189 | 73.3 | 78.0 | 83.8 | | | |
| 190 | 73.9 | 78.7 | 84.4 | | | |
| 191 | 74.5 | 79.5 | 85.0 | | | |

*These tables correct the 1969 Metropolitan Life Insurance Co. standards to height without shoes and nude weight.[192]

ly stable (half-life of $^3$H is 12.4 years and of $^{22}$Na 2.6 years). Total radiation exposure from one study has been estimated as approximately 257 mRem, which is less than a standard upper gastrointestinal x-ray study.[35] This technique, however, is seldom available in clinical practice, and other clinically useful but less accurate estimates of body composition have been developed.

*Per cent ideal body weight* has been used to assess both long- and short-term nutritional depletion. Ideal body weight (IBW) is determined from 1969 Metropolitan Life Insurance tables, which have been adjusted to height without shoes and nude weight (Table 3–3). The midpoints of the frame ranges are used. Body frame size has previously been determined by clinical impression, as no accepted standards have been developed. In a study of more than 100 male and 100 female adult patients at Duke University Medical Center, we related body frame size to a height-wrist circumference ratio (r). We recorded height without shoes and wrist circumference measured just distal to the styloid process at the wrist crease on the right arm.

$$r = \frac{\text{Height (cm)}}{\text{Wrist circumference (cm)}}$$

Frame size can be determined as follows:

| *Males* | *Females* |
|---|---|
| r > 10.4 small | r > 11.0 small |
| r = 9.6–10.4 medium | r = 10.1–11.0 medium |
| r < 9.6 large | r < 10.1 large |

The ideal weight is obtained from Table 3–3 by entering the appropriate frame size at the patient's height. Weight as a per cent of ideal is calculated from the formula:

$$\% \text{IBW} = \frac{\text{Actual weight}}{\text{IBW}} \times 100$$

A weight of 80 to 90 per cent of ideal is classified as mild weight loss, 70 to 80 per cent as moderate, and less than 70 per cent as severe weight loss characteristic of marasmus (see Table 3–2).

It must be understood that some patients will normally weigh more or less than the ideal weight for their height. Caution must be taken when using per cent ideal body weight as an indicator of malnutrition. This ratio will significantly overestimate malnutrition in the ectomorphic patient, while in the obese patient, malnutrition may be overlooked. A better parameter for nutritional assessment is weight as per cent of usual body weight (see below). All estimates of malnutrition based on body weight underestimate actual nutritional depletion because of the increase in extracellular fluid volume associated with starvation.[33, 34]

*Per cent usual body weight* is a more accurate indicator of recent or chronic nutritional deprivation than is weight as a per cent of ideal. It indicates changes from what is normal for the patient, whereas per cent of ideal only gives a value for what the patient should weigh according to population standards. The patient's usual or pre-illness weight must be obtained. If the patient is unable to help, a family member should be asked or the patient's old medical record consulted. Per cent usual body weight can then be determined by:

Per cent usual body weight =

$$\frac{\text{Actual weight}}{\text{Usual weight}} \times 100$$

A weight 85 to 95 per cent of usual is classified as mild depletion, 75 to 84 per cent as moderate, and less than 75 per cent of usual weight as severe (see Table 3–2).

*Recent weight change* is determined by relating per cent weight loss from a patient's usual weight or pre-illness weight to the time period over which the loss occurred (Fig. 3–4). This comparison gives even more significance to weight loss and indicates the severity of a patient's stress.

*The Creatinine excretion index* serves as another indirect measurement of lean body mass. Creatinine is derived from constant breakdown of creatine, an energy depot molecule synthesized by the liver and present mostly within skeletal muscle. Creatinine is excreted unaltered in the urine. The

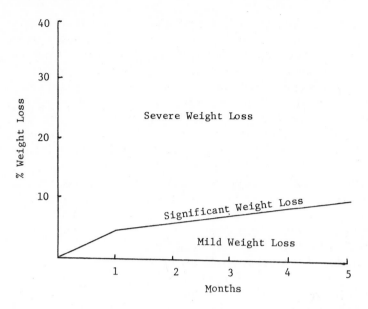

**Figure 3–4** Evaluation of recent weight loss. The severity of recent weight loss is determined by plotting per cent loss from normal weight against the length of time over which the weight was lost. (Blackburn, G. L. et al.: Nutritional and metabolic assessment of the hospitalized patient. J. Parenteral Enteral Nutr., *1*:11–22, 1977.)

production of creatinine and the creatinine excretion index decrease during malnourished states in proportion to skeletal muscle depletion. If renal function is normal, men should excrete 23 mg creatinine per kilogram ideal body weight per day and women 18 mg creatinine/kg/day.[39] A 24-hour urine collection is assayed for total creatinine, and the creatinine excretion index calculated:

Creatinine excretion index =

$$\frac{\text{Actual 24-hour creatinine excretion}}{\text{Predicted 24-hour creatinine excretion}} \times 100$$

Creatinine excretion index values of 60 to 80 per cent represent mild somatic protein depletion, 40 to 50 per cent moderate, and less than 40 per cent severe (see Table 3–2).[40]

Normal tables for predicted urinary creatinine excretion were established for a population of healthy young adults. Normal values have not been determined for the elderly, and it is known that creatinine excretion does decrease with age. Also, the usefulness of the index in evaluating traumatized and critically ill or septic patients has not yet been established. Comparing a patient's creatinine excretion to the expected excretion of an ideal subject of the same height may misrepresent the degree of malnutrition in normally muscular or

ectomorphic patients. Clinical judgment is therefore important in the interpretation of the creatinine excretion index.

*Upper arm circumference* is a combination of muscle mass, bone size, and subcutaneous fat deposits. Diminished arm circumference occurs with both acute and chronic wasting. The measurement is taken midway between the acromion and olecranon process with an insert-type or metal tape measure. The tape should encompass the perimeter of the arm but not cinch the skin. Measurements should be taken on the right arm while it is hanging relaxed at the side. Table 3–4 lists percentiles of arm circumference for each sex at different ages.[41]

The *Triceps skin-fold thickness* is an indirect estimate of body fat stores. As these stores change slowly with malnutrition, a decrease in triceps skin-fold thickness reflects chronically inadequate nutritional intake. The triceps skin-fold thickness measurement should be done on the right arm while the patient is sitting with the arm dangling at the side. As an alternative the patient may lie in bed with the arm folded comfortably across the chest. Subsequent measurement should be performed in the same position as the initial one.

Again the distance between the acromion and olecranon process is measured, and a point halfway between is marked on

**Table 3–4  ARM CIRCUMFERENCE PERCENTILES (mm)**

| Age | 10th | 20th | 30th | 40th | 50th | 60th | 70th | 80th | 90th |
|---|---|---|---|---|---|---|---|---|---|
| | | | | | MALES | | | | |
| 10 | 175 | 183 | 189 | 194 | 200 | 208 | 216 | 224 | 241 |
| 11 | 182 | 189 | 195 | 202 | 208 | 217 | 226 | 235 | 258 |
| 12 | 189 | 197 | 203 | 210 | 216 | 227 | 237 | 248 | 257 |
| 13 | 192 | 203 | 212 | 221 | 230 | 241 | 253 | 264 | 284 |
| 14 | 204 | 216 | 221 | 234 | 243 | 253 | 263 | 274 | 300 |
| 15 | 211 | 225 | 234 | 244 | 253 | 267 | 281 | 295 | 311 |
| 16 | 224 | 236 | 245 | 253 | 262 | 273 | 284 | 294 | 318 |
| 17 | 234 | 243 | 254 | 264 | 275 | 284 | 293 | 302 | 316 |
| 21 | 257 | 268 | 276 | 284 | 292 | 303 | 314 | 324 | 342 |
| 30 | 270 | 284 | 293 | 301 | 310 | 320 | 329 | 339 | 355 |
| 40 | 270 | 284 | 294 | 303 | 312 | 321 | 331 | 340 | 358 |
| | | | | | FEMALES | | | | |
| 10 | 176 | 184 | 190 | 197 | 203 | 212 | 222 | 231 | 250 |
| 11 | 180 | 189 | 196 | 203 | 210 | 222 | 233 | 245 | 266 |
| 12 | 190 | 199 | 206 | 213 | 220 | 230 | 240 | 251 | 266 |
| 13 | 195 | 208 | 215 | 222 | 230 | 241 | 253 | 264 | 282 |
| 14 | 207 | 218 | 225 | 232 | 240 | 252 | 265 | 278 | 295 |
| 15 | 210 | 220 | 228 | 237 | 245 | 255 | 266 | 276 | 296 |
| 16 | 218 | 228 | 235 | 242 | 249 | 260 | 270 | 281 | 304 |
| 17 | 216 | 228 | 235 | 242 | 250 | 262 | 273 | 285 | 310 |
| 21 | 224 | 237 | 244 | 252 | 260 | 270 | 281 | 292 | 313 |
| 30 | 236 | 248 | 257 | 266 | 275 | 289 | 303 | 317 | 342 |
| 40 | 241 | 255 | 265 | 276 | 286 | 301 | 317 | 332 | 357 |

Modified from tables by Frisancho, A. R.: Triceps skin fold and upper arm muscle size norms for assessment of nutritional status. Am. J. Clin. Nutr., 27:1052–1058, 1974.

**Table 3-5**  TRICEPS  SKIN-FOLD  THICKNESS  PERCENTILES (mm)

| Age | 10th | 20th | 30th | 40th | 50th | 60th | 70th | 80th | 90th |
|---|---|---|---|---|---|---|---|---|---|
| | | | | | MALES | | | | |
| 10 | 5.5 | 6.5 | 7.7 | 8.8 | 10 | 11.7 | 13.4 | 15.1 | 19 |
| 11 | 6.5 | 7.4 | 8.3 | 9.1 | 10 | 12 | 14 | 16 | 21 |
| 12 | 6.0 | 7.6 | 8.7 | 9.8 | 11 | 13.3 | 15.6 | 17.8 | 22.5 |
| 13 | 5.5 | 6.6 | 7.7 | 8.8 | 10 | 12.3 | 14.6 | 16.8 | 21.5 |
| 14 | 5.5 | 6.6 | 7.7 | 8.8 | 10 | 12 | 14 | 16 | 20.5 |
| 15 | 5.0 | 6.4 | 7.3 | 8.1 | 9 | 11.8 | 14.7 | 17.6 | 22.5 |
| 16 | 4.5 | 5.6 | 6.7 | 7.8 | 9 | 12.1 | 15.3 | 18.4 | 23.5 |
| 17 | 4.5 | 5.4 | 6.3 | 7.1 | 8 | 9.7 | 11.4 | 13.1 | 17 |
| 21 | 4.5 | 5.7 | 7.1 | 8.6 | 10 | 12.3 | 14.6 | 16.8 | 21.5 |
| 30 | 5.0 | 6.7 | 8.1 | 9.6 | 11 | 13.8 | 16.7 | 19.6 | 24.5 |
| 40 | 5.0 | 6.8 | 8.6 | 10.3 | 12 | 14.8 | 17.7 | 20.6 | 25 |
| | | | | | FEMALES | | | | |
| 10 | 7.0 | 8.6 | 9.7 | 10.8 | 12 | 14 | 16 | 18 | 21.5 |
| 11 | 7.5 | 8.6 | 9.7 | 10.8 | 12 | 14.3 | 16.6 | 18.8 | 24.5 |
| 12 | 7.5 | 9.6 | 10.7 | 11.8 | 13 | 15 | 17 | 19 | 22.5 |
| 13 | 8.0 | 9.7 | 11.1 | 12.6 | 14 | 16.6 | 19.1 | 21.7 | 26.5 |
| 14 | 9.0 | 10.7 | 12.1 | 13.6 | 15 | 17 | 19 | 21 | 25 |
| 15 | 9.5 | 11.7 | 13.1 | 14.6 | 16 | 18.3 | 20.6 | 22.8 | 27 |
| 16 | 9.0 | 10.7 | 12.1 | 13.6 | 15 | 17.3 | 19.6 | 21.8 | 25 |
| 17 | 10.5 | 12.6 | 13.7 | 14.8 | 16 | 18.8 | 21.7 | 24.6 | 28.5 |
| 21 | 10.5 | 12.7 | 14.1 | 15.6 | 17 | 19.3 | 21.6 | 23.8 | 28 |
| 30 | 10.5 | 13 | 15 | 17 | 19 | 21.8 | 24.7 | 27.6 | 31.5 |
| 40 | 12 | 15.1 | 17.4 | 19.7 | 22 | 24.8 | 27.7 | 30.6 | 35.5 |

Modified from tables by Frisancho, A. R.: Triceps skin fold and upper arm muscle size norms for assessment of nutritional status. Am. J. Clin. Nutr., 27:1052–1058, 1974.

the posterior aspect of the arm. The skin is gently pinched slightly below the midpoint and its thickness measured at the midpoint with a Lange Skinfold Caliper (this instrument applies a pressure of 10 grams/sq mm of contact surface). To standardize the measurement, the calipers should be applied for three seconds before the thickness is recorded. The patient's triceps skin-fold thickness percentile is then determined from Table 3–5 by entering the skin-fold thickness value at the appropriate patient age.[41] The degree of triceps fat pad depletion is then recorded: thirty-fifth to fortieth percentile, mild; twenty-fifth to thirty-fourth percentile, moderate; and twenty-fourth percentile and lower, severe depletion (see Table 3–2).

At this time there are no standards for patients older than 44. Caution must therefore be exercised in applying these standards to the elderly patient. Several investigators have advocated taking multiple skin-fold thickness measurements at various body sites. They propose that the sum reflects more accurately the total body fat depot. The clinical usefulness of multiple measurements is currently under investigation.

From the mid-humerus arm circumference and the triceps skin-fold thickness, the *arm muscle area* can be derived from a nomogram (Fig. 3–5).[42] This value is the best anthropometric indicator of the skeletal muscle protein mass. The arm muscle area is derived from Figure 3–5 by placing a straight edge between the arm circumference and the triceps skin-fold thickness and reading the muscle area at the point of intersection with the middle line. To obtain the upper arm muscle area percentile, enter the arm muscle area at the patient's age in Table 3–6.[41] The degree of impairment is determined as follows: thirty-fifth to fortieth percentile, mild; twenty-fifth to thirty-fourth percentile, moderate; and twenty-fourth percentile and lower, severe muscle depletion. As with the triceps skin-fold thickness, there are no standards for patients older than 44, and caution must be exercised in interpreting this measurement for elderly persons.

In addition to estimating body composition to discover nutritional status, it is important to determine the rate of change occurring in the lean body mass. The rate of *skeletal muscle turnover* can be estimated from measurement of urinary excretion of 3-methylhistidine.[43] This amino acid is an end-product of actin and myosin degradation and is neither further broken down nor reutilized by the body in the synthesis of new muscle. The excretion of this amino acid, therefore, serves as an index for normal muscle turnover and also additional muscle turnover secondary to proteolysis. Measurement of 3-methylhistidine, however, requires an amino acid analyzer, which is not always available. Another more readily available study is determination of urinary urea nitrogen excretion. Amino acids released by proteolysis of skeletal muscle are utilized by the liver in gluconeogenesis with the production of urea. Increased excretion of urea nitrogen therefore reflects increased protein metabolism. Excretion of 3 to 8 grams urea nitrogen a day while the patient is taking in no protein or amino acids represents mild skeletal muscle turnover; 8 to 13 is moderate, and greater than 13 is severe.

*Muscle Function.* Of equal, if not greater, importance to the estimation of body mass is an estimation of *muscle function.* There are two muscle groups of greatest concern: the respiratory muscles, because weakness increases complications of respiratory infections and insufficiency, and the muscles of the extremities, whose function strongly affects patient activity. Routine pulmonary function tests, including that for arterial blood gases, primarily measure airway resistance, pulmonary compliance, and gas exchange. Of all pulmonary function tests, maximal minute ventilation best reflects normal and accessory respiratory muscle function, although increased airway resistance and decreased patient compliance significantly affect results.

In a study of more than 50 hospitalized patients at Duke University Medical Center we found that a simple instrument that measures maximal state inspiratory and ex-

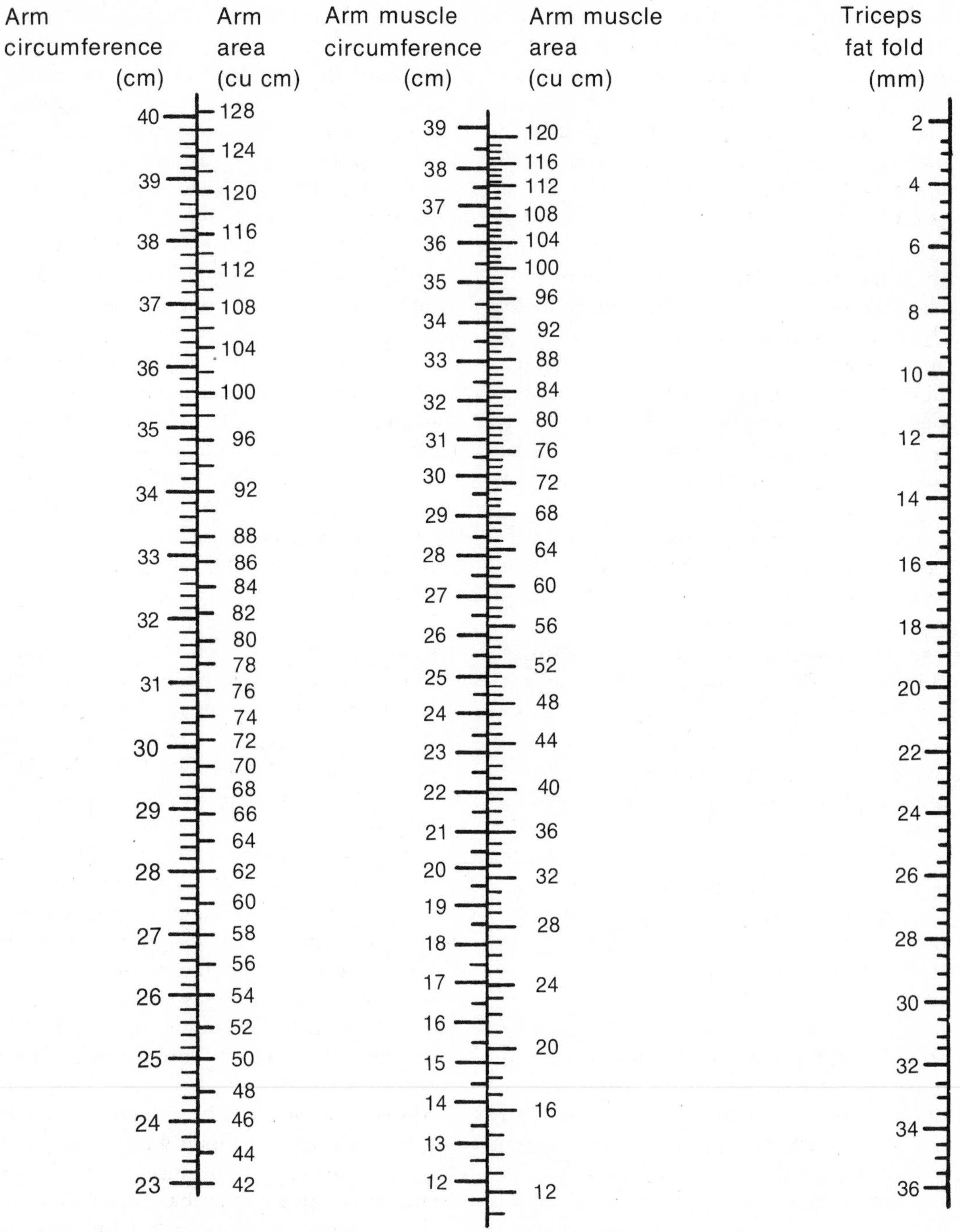

| Arm circumference (cm) | Arm area (cu cm) | Arm muscle circumference (cm) | Arm muscle area (cu cm) | Triceps fat fold (mm) |
|---|---|---|---|---|

To obtain muscle circumference:
1. Lay ruler between value of arm circumference and fat fold
2. Read off muscle circumference on middle line

To obtain tissue areas:
1. The arm area and muscle area are alongside their respective circumferences
2. Fat area = arm area − muscle area

**Figure 3–5** Nomogram for calculation of arm muscle area. (Gurney, J. M., and Jelliffe, D. B.: Arm anthropometry in nutritional assessment: Nomogram for rapid calculation of muscle circumference and cross-sectional muscle and fat areas. Am. J. Clin. Nutr., 26:912–915, 1973.)

**Table 3-6  ARM MUSCLE AREA PERCENTILES (sq cm)**

MALES

| Age | 10th | 20th | 30th | 40th | 50th | 60th | 70th | 80th | 90th |
|---|---|---|---|---|---|---|---|---|---|
| 10 | 17.2 | 18.9 | 20.1 | 21.2 | 22.4 | 23.8 | 25.3 | 26.8 | 30.0 |
| 11 | 18.9 | 20.5 | 21.7 | 22.9 | 24.1 | 25.8 | 27.4 | 29.2 | 32.7 |
| 12 | 20.0 | 21.9 | 23.3 | 24.7 | 26.0 | 28.3 | 30.6 | 32.9 | 36.5 |
| 13 | 21.4 | 23.8 | 25.9 | 28.0 | 30.1 | 32.9 | 35.8 | 38.6 | 43.3 |
| 14 | 24.4 | 27.7 | 30.3 | 32.9 | 35.4 | 37.8 | 40.1 | 42.4 | 49.8 |
| 15 | 25.5 | 28.9 | 32.2 | 35.4 | 38.7 | 42.1 | 45.5 | 48.9 | 54.4 |
| 16 | 30.4 | 34.5 | 37.0 | 39.4 | 41.8 | 45.2 | 48.6 | 51.9 | 58.1 |
| 17 | 35.6 | 38.9 | 41.8 | 44.8 | 47.7 | 50.7 | 53.7 | 56.8 | 62.7 |
| 21 | 40.1 | 44.2 | 47.2 | 50.2 | 53.2 | 56.6 | 60.1 | 63.6 | 69.7 |
| 30 | 42.4 | 48.0 | 51.3 | 54.7 | 58.0 | 61.2 | 64.4 | 67.5 | 74.2 |
| 40 | 42.5 | 47.4 | 51.0 | 54.6 | 58.2 | 62.1 | 66.0 | 70.0 | 76.1 |

FEMALES

| Age | 10th | 20th | 30th | 40th | 50th | 60th | 70th | 80th | 90th |
|---|---|---|---|---|---|---|---|---|---|
| 10 | 16.3 | 17.8 | 18.9 | 20.0 | 21.2 | 22.6 | 24.1 | 25.6 | 28.5 |
| 11 | 17.0 | 19.1 | 20.5 | 21.9 | 23.4 | 25.3 | 27.2 | 29.2 | 32.5 |
| 12 | 19.2 | 21.2 | 22.7 | 24.1 | 25.6 | 27.4 | 29.2 | 30.9 | 33.8 |
| 13 | 20.4 | 22.5 | 24.1 | 25.6 | 27.1 | 29.0 | 30.9 | 32.9 | 37.0 |
| 14 | 23.1 | 25.0 | 26.5 | 28.0 | 29.5 | 32.2 | 34.8 | 37.5 | 41.2 |
| 15 | 22.6 | 24.8 | 26.6 | 28.5 | 30.3 | 32.6 | 34.9 | 37.2 | 40.6 |
| 16 | 24.1 | 26.1 | 28.0 | 30.0 | 32.0 | 34.5 | 37.1 | 39.7 | 47.4 |
| 17 | 24.1 | 25.8 | 27.4 | 29.0 | 30.6 | 33.2 | 35.8 | 38.4 | 42.9 |
| 21 | 24.8 | 27.7 | 29.6 | 31.5 | 33.4 | 35.8 | 38.1 | 40.5 | 46.3 |
| 30 | 26.7 | 29.6 | 31.8 | 33.9 | 36.1 | 39.4 | 42.7 | 46.0 | 53.3 |
| 40 | 27.5 | 30.4 | 32.7 | 35.0 | 37.2 | 40.9 | 44.5 | 48.1 | 55.9 |

Modified from tables by Frisancho, A. R.: Triceps skin fold and upper arm muscle size norms for assessment of nutritional status. Am. J. Clin. Nutr., 27:1052–1058, 1974.

piratory pressures is quite useful in evaluating respiratory muscle function. This instrument consists of two gauges, one a pressure and one a vacuum gauge connected to a metal cylinder with an internal diameter of 3 cm. The cylinder is fitted with a mouthpiece proximally and closed distally, except for a 2 mm opening that prevents facial muscles from producing significant pressure variations. The patient is asked to exert maximal expiratory pressure after a deep inspiration and maximal inspiratory vacuum following complete exhalation. A similar apparatus has been used for determination of muscle strength in patients suffering from myasthenia gravis, and normal tables are available.[43a] In our preliminary data all patients who were malnourished demonstrated significant depression of maximal state inspiratory and expiratory pressures when initially evaluated and marked improvement in these values following as little as two weeks of aggressive nutritional support.

Another suggested technique for assessment of respiratory muscle function is determination of forced inspiratory volumes over $\frac{1}{2}$, 1, and 3 seconds. Normal values have not been established. Perhaps a combination of tests for maximal state inspiratory and expiratory pressures and for maximal ventilation is optimal for evaluating respiratory muscle strength and work tolerance in the malnourished patient, but further study is necessary.

Skeletal muscle strength and work tolerance tests are better standardized than tests for respiratory muscle function. Skeletal muscle assessments can be performed by all physical therapy departments, with results being relatively reproducible with patient cooperation. Impairment of muscle strength can be categorized as mild, moderate, or severe (Table 3–7). Again, serial measurements can be done to follow a patient's response to nutritional support.

At Duke University Medical Center we are currently evaluating the use of a hand dynamometer for determination of forearm and hand muscle strength and endurance. Patients are requested to compress the hand dynamometer maximally and to hold

maximal compression for a period of one minute. Work performed during that minute can be calculated from the recorded effort. In preliminary studies, both maximal strength and endurance have increased with restoration of forearm muscles during nutritional support. Patients who are not bedridden can undergo muscle group testing of the elbow and knee groups using a Cybex apparatus, which is available in many physical therapy departments. Elbow and knee muscle strength, endurance, and work output can be determined over time and compared with established normals.

*Visceral Protein Status.* Depletion of visceral protein mass is a characteristic finding in patients with kwashiorkor. The somatic protein mass is usually preserved, and patients may even be overweight, making recognition of this form of malnutrition difficult during clinical examination. Measurement of the actual mass of the viscera is obviously not possible during life. It has been proposed, however, that a fairly reliable estimate of visceral protein status can be obtained from serum concentrations of proteins synthesized by the liver. The assumption must be made that a decrease in the concentration of these proteins is primarily a direct consequence of decreased liver biosynthesis, which is due to the limited substrate supply associated with malnutrition.[44] To a great extent this is true. However, plasma protein concentrations are also dependent on rates of utilization, intravascular-extravascular transfer, catabolism, excretion, and hydration. Four serum proteins have been studied: albumin, transferrin, thyroxin-binding prealbumin, and retinol-binding protein.

Serum albumin levels are typically depressed during stress, infection and trauma, carcinoma, burns, and hypothyroidism (see Chapter 9). However, persistence of hypoalbuminemia for more than seven days suggests an actual nutritional deficiency. Albumin concentrations are not useful as an early indicator of protein malnutrition because serum levels fall and recover slowly with changes in nutrition. The sluggish response is due to the relatively long serum half-life (20 days) and also to the large pool of body albumin (4 to 5 grams per kg). Yet measurement of serum albumin is useful in documenting manifest malnutrition. The Interdepartmental Committee on Nutrition for National Defense has suggested that serum albumin concentrations of more than 3.5 grams/100 ml are normal.[45] Whitehead et al.[46] declared a serum albumin concentration of less than 3.0 grams/100 ml indicative of early kwashiorkor. In general, albumin concentrations between 2.8 and 3.5 grams/100 ml are associated with mild visceral protein depletion, between 2.1 and 2.7 grams/100 ml with moderate depletion, and less than 2.1 grams/100 ml with severe depletion (see Table 3–2).

Serum transferrin is a beta-globulin with a molecular weight of 88,000 to 90,000. It functions to transport iron in the plasma, binding 1.25 mg ferric iron per gram of protein. Normal serum concentrations of transferrin range from 250 to 300 mg/100 ml with a mean plasma pool of 5.29 grams. Serum half-life ranges from 8 to 10.4 days with an average of 8.8 days.[47] Because of the shorter serum half-life and small body pool, Blackburn et al.[40] have suggested that measurements of serum transferrin concentration more accurately reflect protein malnutrition, especially in its early stages and during recovery. Actual serum transferrin concentrations can be measured by radial immunodiffusion,[48] but a close estimate can be obtained from the more available measurement of total iron-binding capacity (TIBC), using the formula:[40]

Serum transferrin = (0.8 × TIBC) − 43

With this formula, values between 150 and 200 mg/100 ml represent mild visceral protein depletion; between 100 and 150, moderate depletion; and less than 100 mg/100 ml, severe depletion. Caution must be exercised in interpreting transferrin levels, as serum transferrin is often markedly elevated in iron deficiency,[47] reflecting the measured level of a combination of protein depletion and iron deficiency.[49]

Thyroxin-binding prealbumin, which plays a major role in the transport of thyrox-in and serves as a carrier protein for retinol-binding protein, is a third liver-dependent protein useful in visceral protein estimation.[50] Its serum half-life has been estimated as two days,[51] and therefore, it rapidly reflects changes in protein nutrition status. Ingenbleek et al.[49] reported that this blood protein was the first to fall significantly following borderline protein intake in apparently healthy children. Normal serum concentrations range from 15.7 to 29.6 mg/100 ml with a mean of 22.4 mg/100 ml. Any sudden demand for protein synthesis, such as trauma or acute infection, will rapidly depress serum prealbumin, and low levels during stress must be interpreted conservatively. Measurement of serum prealbumin is best done by radial immunodiffusion.

Retinol-binding protein is the specific protein for vitamin A alcohol transport and is linked with prealbumin in a constant molar ratio. Its serum half-life is only 10 hours, and therefore, it can reflect acute changes in protein synthesis.[52] Retinol-binding protein is filtered by the glomeruli and metabolized by the kidney. Thus, high serum levels in patients with renal disease may be misleading.[53] Its normal serum concentration ranges between 2.6 to 7.6 mg/100 ml, with a mean of 5.1 mg/100 ml.

*Immune Competence.* Moderate to severe forms of marasmus, kwashiorkor, or some combination are often associated with depression of the immune system, especially cellular immune functions.[54-57] The total lymphocyte count is depressed, especially with visceral protein depletion, to a degree related to the depletion. Total lymphocyte counts between 1200 and 2000 per cu mm are found with mild depletion, 800 and 1200 per cu mm with moderate depletion, and less than 800 per cu mm with severe depletion. Impairment of lymphocyte response to phytohemagglutinin, depressed neutrophil chemotaxis, deficiencies in IgG and $C_3$, and depression of skin test reactivity to mumps, Candida, streptokinase-streptodornase, Trichophyton, and tuberculin antigens have been observed when serum albumin concentrations fall below 3.0 grams/100 ml or when the per

**Table 3–7**   Standard muscle evaluation form (front)

| FORM M 2800 | DUKE UNIVERSITY MEDICAL CENTER<br>PHYSICAL THERAPY<br>MUSCLE EVALUATION CHART | |
|---|---|---|

### LEGEND

| N OR 100%<br>NORMAL | G OR 75%<br>GOOD | F OR 50%<br>FAIR | P OR 25%<br>POOR |
|---|---|---|---|
| FUNCTION AGAINST GRAVITY AND NORMAL RESISTANCE | FUNCTION AGAINST GRAVITY AND SOME RESISTANCE | FUNCTION AGAINST GRAVITY ONLY | FUNCTION IN HORIZONTAL PLANE |

| T OR 10%<br>TRACE | O<br>NO POWER | +. ++. +++. ++++ | |
|---|---|---|---|
| A FEW FIBERS HAVE ACTIVE FUNCTION | | SPASM ACCORDING TO SEVERITY | |

DATE OF ONSET _____

| | | | | ←——DATES——→ | | | | |
|---|---|---|---|---|---|---|---|---|
| | | | | (LEFT) TRUNK AND LEGS (RIGHT) | | | | |
| | | | | BACK | | | | |
| | | | | QUADRATUS LUMBORUM | | | | |
| | | | | ANTERIOR ABDOMINALS | | | | |
| | | | | ANTERIOR UPPER ABDOMINALS | | | | |
| | | | | ANTERIOR LOWER ABDOMINALS | | | | |
| | | | | EXTERNAL OBLIQUE | | | | |
| | | | | INTERNAL OBLIQUE | | | | |
| | | | | LATERAL ABDOMINALS | | | | |
| | | | | GLUTEUS MAXIMUS | | | | |
| | | | | ILIO PSOAS | | | | |
| | | | | SARTORIUS | | | | |
| | | | | TENSOR FASCIA LATA | | | | |
| | | | | GLUTEUS MEDIUS | | | | |
| | | | | HIP ADDUCTORS | | | | |
| | | | | INTERNAL ROTATORS | | | | |
| | | | | EXTERNAL ROTATORS | | | | |
| | | | | QUADRICEPS | | | | |
| | | | | INNER HAMSTRINGS | | | | |
| | | | | OUTER HAMSTRINGS | | | | |
| | | | | GASTROCNEMIUS | | | | |
| | | | | SOLEUS | | | | |
| | | | | ANTERIOR TIBIAL | | | | |
| | | | | POSTERIOR TIBIAL | | | | |
| | | | | PERONEUS LONGUS | | | | |
| | | | | PERONEUS BREVIS | | | | |
| | | | | EXTENSOR LONGUS DIGITORUM | | | | |
| | | | | EXTENSOR BREVIS DIGITORUM | | | | |
| | | | | EXTENSOR PROPRIUS HALLUCIS | | | | |
| | | | | FLEXOR LONGUS DIGITORUM | | | | |
| | | | | FLEXOR BREVIS DIGITORUM | | | | |
| | | | | LUMBRICALES | | | | |
| | | | | FLEXOR LONGUS HALLUCIS | | | | |
| | | | | FLEXOR BREVIS HALLUCIS | | | | |
| | | | | MEASUREMENTS | | | | |
| | | | | CALF | | | | |
| | | | | THIGH | | | | |
| | | | | LENGTH | | | | |
| | | | | CONTRACTURES AND DEFORMITIES | | | | |
| | | | | HIP | | | | |
| | | | | KNEE | | | | |
| | | | | ANKLE | | | | |
| | | | | TOES | | | | |
| | | | | SCOLIOSIS | | | | |
| | | | | ←——SIGNATURES——→ | | | | |

CHARACTERISTIC GAIT

REMARKS:

**Table 3–7** *Continued* (back)

| | | | | DATES | | | | |
|---|---|---|---|---|---|---|---|---|
| | | | | (LEFT) FACE, NECK & ARMS (RIGHT) | | | | |
| | | | | FACE | | | | |
| | | | | TONGUE | | | | |
| | | | | DEGLUTITION | | | | |
| | | | | SPEECH | | | | |
| | | | | ANTERIOR NECK | | | | |
| | | | | POSTERIOR NECK | | | | |
| | | | | ANTERIOR DELTOID | | | | |
| | | | | MIDDLE DELTOID | | | | |
| | | | | POSTERIOR DELTOID | | | | |
| | | | | UPPER TRAPEZIUS | | | | |
| | | | | MIDDLE TRAPEZIUS | | | | |
| | | | | LOWER TRAPEZIUS | | | | |
| | | | | RHOMBOIDS | | | | |
| | | | | LATISSIMUS DORSI | | | | |
| | | | | SERRATUS MAGNUS | | | | |
| | | | | CLAVICULAR PECTORALIS MAJOR | | | | |
| | | | | STERNAL PECTORALIS MAJOR | | | | |
| | | | | OUTWARD ROTATORS | | | | |
| | | | | INWARD ROTATORS | | | | |
| | | | | BICEPS | | | | |
| | | | | BRACHIORADIALIS | | | | |
| | | | | TRICEPS | | | | |
| | | | | SUPINATOR | | | | |
| | | | | PRONATORS | | | | |
| | | | | FLEXOR CARPI RADIALIS | | | | |
| | | | | FLEXOR CARPI ULNARIS | | | | |
| | | | | EXTENSOR CARPI RADIALIS | | | | |
| | | | | EXTENSOR CARPI ULNARIS | | | | |
| 1 2 3 4 | 1 2 3 4 | 1 2 3 4 | 1 2 3 4 | | 1 2 3 4 | 1 2 3 4 | 1 2 3 4 | 1 2 3 4 |
| | | | | FLEXOR PROFUNDUS DIGITORUM | | | | |
| | | | | FLEXOR SUBLIMIS DIGITORUM | | | | |
| | | | | FINGER EXTENSORS | | | | |
| | | | | LUMBRICALES | | | | |
| | | | | DORSAL INTEROSSEI | | | | |
| | | | | PALMAR INTEROSSEI | | | | |
| | | | | ABDUCTOR MINIMI DIGITI | | | | |
| | | | | OPPONENS POLLICIS | | | | |
| | | | | ABDUCTOR LONGUS POLLICIS | | | | |
| | | | | ABDUCTOR BREVIS POLLICIS | | | | |
| | | | | ADDUCTOR POLLICIS | | | | |
| | | | | FLEXOR LONGUS POLLICIS | | | | |
| | | | | FLEXOR BREVIS POLLICIS | | | | |
| | | | | EXTENSOR LONGUS POLLICIS | | | | |
| | | | | EXTENSOR BREVIS POLLICIS | | | | |
| | | | | MEASUREMENTS | | | | |
| | | | | UPPER ARM | | | | |
| | | | | LOWER ARM | | | | |
| | | | | CONTRACTURES AND DEFORMITIES | | | | |
| | | | | SHOULDER | | | | |
| | | | | ELBOW | | | | |
| | | | | WRIST | | | | |
| | | | | FINGERS | | | | |
| | | | | SIGNATURES | | | | |

REMARKS:

cent ideal body weight falls below 85.[56, 58] Depression of immune competence can often be reversed by nutritional repletion.[59-62]

Of all parameters of nutritional status, only depression of skin test reactivity has been statistically related to patient morbidity and mortality. Meakins et al.[62] studied 354 hospitalized patients and found 110 to have depressed or no skin test reactivity to mumps, tuberculin, streptokinase-streptodorinase, Candida, and Trichophyton antigens. Among 244 normal reactors there was a 3.7 per cent incidence of sepsis and 2.4 per cent incidence of death. Of the 110 immunologically depressed patients, 50 per cent had septic episodes and 23 per cent died. In serial skin testing, 135 patients remained normal or improved their reactivity with nutritional support. They had a 21 per cent sepsis rate, but only 2.1 per cent died. In contrast, among the 43 patients who had depressed reactivity and did not improve with nutritional support, there was a 65 per cent sepsis rate and 74 per cent mortality rate. Meakins et al. suggested that all nutritionally depleted patients be tested for common antigen reactivity. If the patient is shown to be anergic (fails to demonstrate at least 0.5 cm induration or erythema to any antigen after 48 to 72 hours) or relatively anergic (responds only to one antigen), vigorous nutritional support should be initiated prior to any surgical intervention, if possible, and during medical therapy. Support should continue until skin test reactivity improves or returns to normal (reactivity to two or more antigens).

## NUTRITIONAL ASSESSMENT AND THERAPY

From review of dietary adequacy, lean body mass, muscle function, visceral protein status, and immune competence, a decision can often be made about the need for nutritional support. Any patient with moderate or greater protein-calorie malnutrition, with moderate or greater hypercatabolism, or with impairment of immune competence should be considered for nutritional support. Of interest is a recent study

performed by Buzby et al.[62a] at the University of Pennsylvania. They studied 161 elective surgical patients, assessing nutritional parameters such as weight, per cent weight loss, albumin, transferrin, total protein, mid-arm muscle circumference, triceps skin-fold thickness, lymphocyte count, and delayed hypersensitivity reactivity. The patient was monitored for objective complications until death or discharge. Statistical analysis demonstrated prediction of morbidity and mortality from nutritional parameters as follows:

Predicted risk (%) = 158 − 16.6 (Albumin) − 0.78 (mm Triceps skin-fold thickness) − 0.2 (Transferrin) − 5.8 (Delayed hypersensitivity reactivity)

In Buzby's series, patients with a predicted risk of less than 30 per cent demonstrated a complication incidence of 11.7 per cent and a death rate of 2.0 per cent. Those patients with predicted risk factors of 30 to 50 per cent had a 36.8 per cent complication rate and a 7.9 per cent death rate. Patients with greater than 59 per cent predicted risk had an 81 per cent complication rate and a 59 per cent death rate.

Studies such as those of Meakins et al.[62] and Buzby et al.[62a] are beginning to demonstrate a relationship between nutritional assessment and patient prognosis. The technique of nutritional assessment, however, has only recently been considered as a factor in selection of patients for nutritional support. Tables of normal ranges for all age groups (especially 40 and older) are incomplete and of questionable accuracy. Data from nutritional assessments must, therefore, still be carefully interpreted and utilized as supportive information — not as definitive criteria — in patient selection. Clinical assessment continues to be a critical criterion of nutritional status and needs. As more studies are performed, nutritional assessment parameters will likely assume increasingly greater importance in decisions relating to nutritional support. When nutritional support is deemed advisable, such support should be an integral part of the patient's overall therapy and not just an afterthought. When there are no complicating gastrointestinal problems, oral or tube-feeding support should be attempted. When that approach fails or is inadvisable, parenteral nutritional support is required.

## SHORT BOWEL SYNDROME

Surgical resection of the gastrointestinal tract has been associated with mortality rates that vary according to the amount of bowel removed and the preoperative condition of the patient. Generally, if 40 cm or more of small bowel is preserved, oral nutrition is tolerated and most patients survive. If less than 40 cm remain, however, patients usually develop nutritional deficiency syndromes and septic complications and often expire. If they survive, these patients do not gain adequate weight and are unable to maintain employment. Factors directly influencing survival include other medical problems and prolonged preoperative illness. In addition, elderly patients do not tolerate small bowel resection as well as younger patients. Occasional exceptions to the poor clinical course that typically follows massive small bowel resection have been reported.[63, 64] Improved understanding of the metabolic effects of massive small bowel resection and aggressive nutritional support, as outlined in this section, should contribute significantly to improvement in the survival and functional capacity of these patients.

If total parenteral nutrition is given to patients with normal gastrointestinal anatomy, a marked reduction in the mass of both the large and small intestines occurs.[65, 66] The bowel becomes shortened, its wall becomes thinner, and there is a reduction in the mitotic index in the jejunal crypts. The total number of intestinal villi remains the same, but the villi are thinner and packed closer together. Electron-microscopic examination reveals no significant changes in the detailed structure, and neutral amino acid transport activity remains normal.

When, however, parenteral nutrition is administered to patients following massive small bowel resection, the remaining bowel appears to undergo adaptive hyperplasia. There is an increase in intestinal length as well as weight per centimeter.[67-69] In addition, there is an increase in mucosal cellularity, with villus enlargement resulting from an increased rate of proliferation and migration of mucosal crypt cells. These new cells are relatively immature and demonstrate decreases in both enzyme content and absorptive function.[70-72] Thus, although there is no evidence of adaptation at the cellular level, the advantage of villus hyperplasia outweighs any disadvantage of cellular immaturity. The net effect is enhanced absorption per unit of bowel length.

The mechanism for intestinal adaptation following massive resection is poorly understood (see reviews in references 72 and 72a). Adequate nutritional support may have a primary stimulatory effect on cellular mitotic activity and regeneration of new intestinal surface, or it may play only a supportive role until the adaptive process permits oral nutrition. Various humoral and neural stimuli, as well as biochemical changes in individual cells, may also contribute to adaptation.

Much information on gastrointestinal adaptation has been obtained since the development of intravenous nutrition, which allows patients with massive small bowel resection to be adequately nourished and prevents death due to starvation. According to several studies, many patients who retain the duodenum, 10 cm or more of small bowel distal to the ligament of Treitz, and part of the large bowel will eventually tolerate an oral diet and maintain body weight within 60 to 80 per cent of ideal. Distal small bowel resection is associated with a decrease in intestinal transit time, while resection of the proximal small bowel is not.[73] Loss of the ileocecal valve alone has little effect on transit time, but in combination with resection of the distal small bowel it results in a brisk diarrhea.[74] When less than 10 cm of small bowel distal to the ligament of Treitz can be salvaged, maximal intestinal adaptation may be inadequate, especially if the terminal ileum and ileocecal valve must be sacrificed. To avoid progressive metabolic wasting, continuous nutritional support should be given intravenously. With recent developments in long-term home parenteral nutrition,[75–79] even these patients can lead relatively normal lives.

Because the postoperative care of patients undergoing small bowel resection is complex and extended (perhaps requiring long-term intravenous nutrition), patient cooperation is mandatory. Young, otherwise healthy patients tolerate intestinal resection much better than elderly patients and have a greater chance of resuming an adequate oral diet. Each patient must be evaluated individually before parenteral nutrition is offered.

Some of the metabolic consequences of massive small bowel resection and their management are discussed below. Careful monitoring is essential to avoid devastating complications.

BILE SALT DEPLETION. Normally the bile salt pool measures 3 to 5 grams and cycles six to ten times a day with a loss of less than 5 per cent in the stools.[80] Bile salt resorption occurs by active transport from the terminal ileum (85 per cent) and by passive absorption from the entire gastrointestinal tract. With loss of the terminal ileum, or with rapid transit time, the enterohepatic circulation of bile salts is interrupted, and bile salts are lost in the stool. Increased bile salt concentration in the colon decreases absorption and increases excretion of water into the lumen, resulting in diarrhea. In addition, sodium, potassium, and bicarbonate ions are excreted in large amounts, and their loss may lead to severe electrolyte imbalance.[81, 82] As the bile salt pool diminishes, fat absorption is interrupted because of impaired micelle formation. Malabsorption of lipids in turn leads to steatorrhea, fat-soluble vitamin deficiencies, and deficiencies of essential fatty acids (see Chapters 10 and 11). Formation of hydroxy fatty acids in the colon by bacterial action on unsaturated fatty acids may increase diarrhea.[83] Bile salt depletion may occur within three months with the mean cholate pool decreasing by 60 per cent and

the mean chenodeoxycholate pool by 47 per cent.[84]

Treatment of complications caused by alterations in bile salt metabolism has been only partly successful. Hardison and Rosenberg[85] administered oral taurocholate in an attempt to decrease steatorrhea, but the beneficial effects were accompanied by bile salt diarrhea. Hofmann and Poley,[86] in an attempt to decrease bile salt diarrhea, administered cholestyramine orally. The results were quite satisfactory in patients with small bowel resections of less than 100 cm. Diarrhea induced by free fatty acids has been fairly well controlled with the administration of calcium carbonate, which forms non-irritating soaps.[87] Care must be taken to avoid such high doses that milk alkali syndrome occurs.

GALLSTONES. The incidence of cholelithiasis increases following small bowel resections. This may be a result of either a contracted bile salt pool with increased cholesterol concentration[88] or an altered glycine-taurine conjugation ratio.[89] No preventive therapy is available and cholecystectomy may be required. Prophylactic cholecystectomy at the time of second-look operation following small bowel resection may be indicated in selected patients.

RENAL STONES. In 1970 Hofmann et al.[90] reported two patients with recurrent calcium oxalate nephrolithiasis following ileal resection. Since then, other studies have documented that hyperoxaluria following distal small bowel resection is directly related to the amount of ileum resected and the degree of steatorrhea.[91, 92] Increases in urinary oxalate appear to be due to intraluminal and mucosal abnormalities. Steatorrhea results in increased binding of dietary calcium to free fatty acids. This leaves less calcium available to react with soluble dietary oxalate to form insoluble calcium oxalate, which is excreted in the feces. The increased soluble oxalate salts are readily absorbed through passive diffusion by the entire gastrointestinal tract. However, most oxalate is apparently absorbed in the colon because hyperoxaluria is corrected following colectomy even though severe fat malabsorption contin-

**Table 3–8**  HIGH-OXALATE  FOODS (25ng/100 grams)

| | | |
|---|---|---|
| Beans | Strawberries | Cucumbers |
| Rhubarb | Blackberries | Turnip tops |
| Parsley | Currants | Dandelion leaves |
| Spinach | Oranges | Endives |
| Cocoa | Sweet potatoes | Kale |
| Instant coffee | Plums | Peppers |
| Ovaltine | Carrots | Tea |
| Beet roots | Cola drinks | Chocolate |
| Raspberries | Celery | |

ues.[93] Another factor contributing to the intraluminal oxalate absorption is a diet high in saturated fatty acids, low in calcium, and high in oxalate. The mucosal abnormality is an increased permeability of the colonic mucosa to oxalate salts following exposure to bile salts and fatty acids.[93]

Treatment of hyperoxaluria consists of reducing dietary oxalate to less than 50 mg/day by limiting high-oxalate foods (Table 3–8); reducing saturated fats to decrease steatorrhea and replacing them with medium-chain triglycerides, which may by themselves decrease oxaluria;[94] and administering oral calcium (up to 4 grams/day) or aluminum hydroxide antacid (equivalent to 3.2 grams of elemental aluminum per day).[95] Some experimental studies support the use of cholestyramine to bind excess bile salts,[90, 91] but this may lead to more severe bile salt depletion.

GASTRIC HYPERSECRETION AND HYPERACIDITY. Intestinal resection increases gastric secretion of acidic fluid[96, 97] in direct proportion to the amount of small bowel resected.[98, 99] The hypersecretion contributes to diarrhea in at least three ways. First, the high solute load may exceed the absorptive capacity of the remaining intestine. Second, injury of the proximal intestinal mucosa by acid may impair absorption of all food and increase small bowel secretions. Third, malabsorption of fats and proteins may occur because of the acidic inactivation of the digestive enzymes lipase and trypsin. In addition to inducing diarrhea, gastric hypersecretion can also lead to peptic ulcerations and hemorrhagic gastritis, which may occasionally necessitate emergency surgery.

The mechanism that increases gastric secretion following small bowel resection remains unclear. The lack of hypersecretion following intestinal bypass procedures, along with the more marked secretion that accompanies proximal, rather than distal, small bowel resection, suggests a regulatory mechanism in the proximal small bowel. Perhaps removal of the production sites of one or more hormones normally present in the small bowel results in decreased inhibition of gastric acid secretion. Hormones that may be involved include secretin, serotonin, histaminase, cholecystokinin, pancreozymin, intestinal glucagon, vasoactive intestinal peptide, and gastric inhibitory peptide.[72] Recent studies report a significant increase in serum gastrin level following small bowel resection in man and in animals,[100, 101] gastrin being the most potent known stimulus of gastric acid secretion. Whether increased gastrin levels are due to increased gastrin production or to decreased gastrin degradation by the small bowel is unknown.[102]

Patients subjected to massive small bowel resection should be placed on vigorous antacid therapy beginning immediately after surgery and continuing for up to one year. Constipating antacids should be given orally every one to two hours either as calcium carbonate or aluminum hydroxide, and milk should be avoided. Anticholinergics may also be beneficial. Truncal vagotomy has been shown to increase gastric secretion following small bowel resection, possibly because of denervation of the small bowel. A parietal cell vagotomy at the time of small bowel resection may be useful, however, as a prophylactic procedure. The $H_2$ antagonist cimetidine has recently been shown quite effective in reducing hypersecretion, hyperacidity, and malabsorption in the short bowel syndrome.[102a,b]

*Nutritional Management.* On the second or third postoperative day, a central venous catheter should be placed and parenteral nutrition begun. Even token oral intake of clear liquids should be avoided; only antacid therapy should be administered orally. Any attempt to give fluids orally increases diarrhea and electrolyte losses, thus complicating the patient's care. If diarrhea exceeds 2 liters daily, intramuscular codeine should be given. All vitamin requirements, including those for vitamins $B_{12}$ and K, must be met. Electrolytes and minerals, including copper, magnesium, iodide, zinc, iron, and other trace elements, and essential fatty acids, must be provided.

After about 30 days, as diarrhea decreases to less than 2 to 2.5 liters per day, oral fluids may be given. Initially, only hypotonic balanced salt solutions should be used. Gradually, over a period of several weeks, a defined elemental diet that is low in fat may be added, followed by a low-fat, high-protein, solid diet. Milk products should be avoided, as an isolated lactase deficiency is likely to be present. If an intolerance of fat prevents adequate caloric intake, the medium-chain triglycerides, which are more easily absorbed, should be tried. At this point a dietician must become actively involved, as only trial and error can determine the patient's tolerance to various caloric sources. While the adaptation to an oral diet is under way, parenteral nutrition should be continued until adequate caloric intake by mouth is established. The intestine will continue to hypertrophy for two to three years following resection. Management is, therefore, a long-term process requiring close monitoring of all possible metabolic complications and perhaps repeated hospital admissions for intravenous nutrition to maintain an adequate metabolic status until adaptation of the bowel is adequate. Some patients will eventually resume a completely normal diet.

In summary, the intestinal tract does have the ability to adapt to resection if given time and proper nutritive support. Sheflan et al.[68] suggest that patients requiring small bowel resection, even if less than one foot of small intestine can be preserved, should not be denied surgical therapy. These patients should then receive intravenous nutrition early in the postoperative period and possibly repeated intravenous support over two to three years as the intestine adapts. Those patients who cannot tolerate adequate oral nutrition may be candidates for long-term home intravenous nutrition. Patients with less extensive small bowel resections will often tolerate an elemental diet with little diarrhea and good absorption in the postoperative course and can be managed without intravenous nutrition with excellent long-term results.[103]

Initially, a conservative surgical procedure designed to preserve as much intestine as possible should be undertaken. A few centimeters of the proximal jejunum can nearly always be salvaged because of overlapping blood supply. Although possible less often, an attempt to preserve the terminal ileum and ileocecal valve should be made. Similar efforts should be made to save the water- and electrolyte-absorbing surface of the right colon. Vagotomy and pyloroplasty to control gastric hypersecretion are not recommended because of their possible effects on gastric emptying.[104] The effects of parietal cell vagotomy have yet to be determined. Reversed intestinal segments or recirculating loops should not be constructed; if there is enough small bowel to form such structures, there is ample bowel for such patients to do well without them. A second-look procedure 24 hours after the initial resection is often advisable. At that time the surgeon can perform a parietal cell vagotomy, as well as an elective cholecystectomy in selected patients. Before resecting massive amounts of small bowel and offering intravenous nutritional support, the patient's general condition, age, and functional capacity must be considered.

## ACUTE PANCREATITIS

Severe acute pancreatitis is associated with an overall mortality rate of 14 to 48 per cent, owing mainly to the high incidence of renal failure (6 to 32 per cent) and respiratory failure (18 to 39 per cent) and the necessity of surgical intervention with operative mortalities of 17 to 56 per cent.[105–109] The mainstay of therapy includes passage of a nasogastric tube and continuous aspiration of gastric contents to counteract the usual ileus and to put the exocrine pancreas to rest. Although it is thought that complete bowel rest contributes to resolution of the pancreatic inflammatory process,[110] the subsequent starvation associated with the marked hypercatabolic state of acute pancreatitis is counterproductive, especially when it is extended over several weeks or more. Not only do complications of malnutrition occur, but there is also evidence that malnutrition and specific amino acid deprivation may cause or exacerbate pancreatitis.[111–113]

With renewed interest in the role of nutrition in various disease processes, researchers have studied the effects of nutritional support during treatment of severe acute pancreatitis. Experimental data have demonstrated a significant reduction of gastrointestinal, pancreatic, and biliary secretions during bowel rest and parenteral nutrition.[114, 115] For example, secretion of amylase and trypsin may decrease as much as 75 per cent. On the other hand, the secretion of insulin is strongly stimulated.[116] Clinical experience has shown nutritional support during acute pancreatitis to be relatively uncomplicated, with positive nitrogen balance easily achieved either with jejunal tube feedings or parenteral nutrition.[106, 108, 109] Electrolyte abnormalities are uncommon but respond to formula manipulations. Glucose intolerance is easily controlled by the addition of regular insulin to the infused solution. Protein intolerance is uncommon unless renal or liver failure develops. Yet it remains doubtful whether nutritional support, enteral or parenteral, plays any direct role in relief of the inflammatory process or in the reduction of morbidity or mortality except as related to malnutrition itself.[108, 109]

The current recommendation for nutritional support in patients with acute pancreatitis is limited to prevention or treatment of malnutrition. If surgical intervention is necessary, a jejunal feeding tube may be inserted. Otherwise, parenteral nutrition should be given.[117] Two statements of caution are necessary. Hypocalcemia must be vigorously treated to prevent tetany, yet hypercalcemia should be avoided, as excessive calcium infusion has been reported to induce pancreatitis.[118] Secondly, a significantly increased incidence of catheter-related sepsis has been reported in the early stages of parenteral nutrition in patients with pancreatitis,[109] and any unexplained fever demands catheter removal to avoid unnecessary morbidity. With future study, direct benefits from enteral or parenteral nutrition for patients with pancreatitis may be defined and the indications for nutritional support expanded.

## ENTEROCUTANEOUS FISTULAS

Medical and surgical management of enterocutaneous fistulas in the 1960s was associated with a mortality rate of 40 to 50 per cent.[119–123] Deaths were attributed to fluid and electrolyte imbalance (78 per cent), infection (67 per cent), and marked wasting (61 per cent).[124] The development of improved, broad-spectrum antibiotics resulted in decreased mortality and morbidity, but enterocutaneous fistulas still represented a significant risk for the patient. However, the recent addition of parenteral nutrition in management of enterocutaneous fistulas has substantially decreased the mortality rate to 4 to 20 per cent.[125–128] Several factors are responsible for this improvement. All fluids are given intravenously and oral intake is eliminated, thus decreasing intestinal secretions[114] and reducing fluid and electrolyte losses through the fistula. Electrolyte and fluid replacement becomes easier, and imbalances can be avoided. In addition, the intravenous provision of calories and protein eliminates the urgency of surgical intervention, allowing time for replacement of fluid and electrolyte losses and establishment of a normal nutritional state. Finally, some fistulas close

**Table 3-9**  PATIENTS WITH ENTEROCUTANEOUS FISTULAS (PRIMARY DIAGNOSIS, FISTULA LOCATION, AND ETIOLOGY OF FISTULAS)

| PATIENT | AGE | PRIMARY DIAGNOSIS | FISTULA LOCATION | ETIOLOGY |
|---|---|---|---|---|
| 1 | 63 | Duodenal ulcer, post vagotomy and pyloroplasty | Distal esophagus | Operative trauma |
| 2 | 43 | Aortoiliac arteriosclerosis, post-bifurcation graft | Distal ileum | Operative trauma |
| 3 | 51 | Esophageal diverticulum, post resection | Distal esophagus | Operative trauma |
| 4 | 48 | Serous cystadenoma ovary, post resection | Jejuno-colic and ileo-vaginal | Post-op. small bowel obstruction |
| 5 | 58 | Carcinoma head of pancreas, post Whipple | Gastric anastomosis | Surgical anastomosis |
| 6 | 61 | Adenocarcinoma sigmoid colon, post abdominal-perineal resection | Cecal | Post-op. peritonitis |
| 7 | 29 | Caesarian section with intestinal gangrene, post ileal-cecal resection | Ileo-colonic | Surgical anastomosis |
| 8 | 66 | Cholecystectomy | Multiple small bowel | Post-op. abscess |
| 9 | 77 | Small-bowel obstruction, post lysis adhesions | Mid-jejunum | Wound dehiscence |
| 10 | 22 | Post partum | Jejuno-vaginal | Intra-abdominal sepsis |
| 11 | 62 | Endometrial carcinoma, post exenteration, irradiation | Mid-jejunum | Irradiation enteritis |
| 12 | 58 | Crohn's disease, post cholecystectomy | Mid-jejunum | Uncertain |

| | | | |
|---|---|---|---|
| 13 | 23 | Gunshot wound left upper quadrant, post gastrostomy | Gastric | Failure of gastrostomy to close |
| 14 | 29 | Perforated gastric ulcer, post Billroth II | Cecal | Abscess |
| 15 | 55 | Duodenal ulcer, post Billroth II | Duodenal stump | Surgical anastomosis |
| 16 | 65 | Carcinoma bladder, post ileal conduit | Ileal | Abscess |
| 17 | 53 | Carcinoma colon, post anterior resection | Proximal jejunum | Abscess |
| | | Post repair jejunal fistula | Jejunal anastomosis | Surgical anastomosis |
| 18 | 38 | Abdominal abscess | Ileal | Abscess |
| 19 | 63 | Foreign body esophagus, post esophagoscopy | Distal esophagus | Esophagoscopy |
| 20 | 34 | Auto accident, blunt trauma to abdomen | Duodenal | Trauma |
| 21 | 71 | Carcinoma cervix, post irradiation | Recto-vaginal | Irradiation |
| 22 | 56 | Kicked in stomach, post-op. drainage | Duodenum | Trauma |
| 23 | 54 | Acute pancreatitis, pancreatic abscess, drainage abscess, cholecystectomy, common bile duct exploration | Mid-ileum | Pancreatic abscess |

From Grant, J. P., et al.: Parenteral nutrition in the management of enterocutaneous fistulas. N.C. Med. J., 38:327–330, 1977.

spontaneously during parenteral nutrition, thereby eliminating the need for surgery entirely. In those patients needing surgical closure of the fistula, the improved nutritional status decreases operative mortality and morbidity as well as fistula recurrence.[21, 127]

Between January, 1975, and January, 1977, 23 patients with 25 enterocutaneous fistulas were given parenteral nutrition at Duke University Medical Center.[128] The patients ranged in age from 22 to 77. Surgical procedures were the most common cause of fistula formation (Table 3–9). Of the 25 fistulas, 16 (64 per cent) closed spontaneously during parenteral nutrition (Table 3–10). Drainage from fistulas closing spontaneously was variable. In some cases drainage gradually decreased until it stopped. In other cases the decrease was sudden. Of the nine fistulas that did not close spontaneously, seven were subsequently closed surgically without complication. One patient died of sepsis not related to parenteral nutrition before fistula closure, and another was discharged with a low-output cecal fistula. No significant complication of parenteral nutrition was encountered: No electrolyte or fluid imbalance was observed, no catheter-related septicemia was identified, and no complication of catheter placement or maintenance occurred.

Our data compare favorably with data from other series, as summarized in Table 3–11. In view of the low complication rate and improvement in morbidity and mortality rates, parenteral nutrition with bowel rest should be considered for all patients with enterocutaneous fistulas. There are specific indications for early surgical intervention, as summarized by Aguirre et al.:[126] the presence of distal intestinal obstruction, bowel discontinuity as demonstrated by contrast-radiographic studies, undrained intra-abdominal abscesses, and lack of fistula closure after 30 to 90 days of parenteral nutrition.

## INFLAMMATORY BOWEL DISEASE

Surgical resection of diseased intestinal segments in patients with inflammatory bowel disease is associated with a significant incidence of recurrent disease. Consequently, surgery is often restricted to treatment of complications such as fistula formation, abscess formation, or obstruction in the case of regional enteritis, and toxic megacolon, perforation, bleeding, systemic complications, and general debility in ulcerative colitis. The effectiveness of medical therapy has been limited by the failure to identify an etiological agent. Current therapy involves intestinal antibiotics and steroids. When this non-specific therapy fails to provide symptomatic relief, patients rapidly develop nutritional deficiencies. If the disease is severe and does not respond to medical therapy, intestinal resection is often a last resort.

As early as 1939 it was recognized that surgical bypass of segments of intestine afflicted with inflammatory bowel disease often resulted in spectacular improvement of the inflamed bowel.[129] With the development of parenteral nutrition, allowing the elimination of all oral intake, several advan-

**Table 3–10**  FISTULA CLOSURE

| FISTULA LOCATION | | NUMBER | CLOSED O.R. | NOT CLOSED | CLOSED SPONT. | % SPONT. CLOSURE | DAYS TO CLOSURE |
|---|---|---|---|---|---|---|---|
| Esophageal | | 3 | 0 | 0 | 3 | 100 | 40, 26, 39 |
| Gastric | | 2 | 0 | 0 | 2 | 100 | 67, 25 |
| Duodenal | | 3 | 0 | 0 | 3 | 100 | 12. 40, 9 |
| Jejunal | | 8 | 3 | 1 | 4 | 50 | 26, 24, 15, 23 |
| Ileal | | 6 | 2 | 0 | 4 | 67 | 48, 13, 23, 21 |
| Colonic | | 3 | 2 | 1 | 0 | 0 | |
| | Total | 25 | 7 | 2 | 16 | 64 | |

**Table 3–11** INCIDENCE OF FISTULA CLOSURE WITH PARENTERAL NUTRITION

| | | CLOSURE OF FISTULAS | | | |
| AUTHOR | NUMBER OF FISTULAS | Non-op. No. (%) | Op. No. (%) | Not Closed No. (%) | Deaths No. (%) |
|---|---|---|---|---|---|
| *Sheldon[127] (1971) | 51 | 18 (35) | 28 (55) | 3 (6) | 6 (12) |
| MacFadyen[125] (1973) | 78 | 55 (70) | 17 (22) | 6 (8) | 4 (5) |
| Aguirre[126] (1974) | 38 | 11 (29) | 17 (45) | 10 (26) | 8 (21) |
| Himal[193] (1974) | 25 | 13 (52) | 10 (40) | 2 (8) | 2 (8) |
| Weisz[194] (1976) | 19 | 17 (89) | 0 (0) | 2 (10) | 2 (10) |
| Grant[128] (1977) | 25 | 16 (64) | 7 (28) | 2 (8) | 1 (4) |
| Total | 236 | 130 (55) | 79 (33) | 25 (11) | 23 (9.7) |

*Used parenteral nutrition initially and changed to oral nutrition early using nasogastric tubes or tubes inserted through the fistula.

tages over intestinal bypass were suggested. First, the entire bowel would be put to rest, thereby reducing the gastrointestinal activity in the diseased segment that results from hormonal production by the functioning, non-bypassed, normal bowel. Second, adequate nutrition could be maintained to combat marked protein depletion, possible immunological depression, and poor wound healing. Third, if nutritional support was effective in reducing intestinal inflammation, a surgical procedure in a high-risk patient would be avoided.

Since 1969 several studies have evaluated the effectiveness of parenteral nutrition in the treatment of inflammatory bowel disease.[130-134] For ease of discussion, patients can be divided into three groups based on pathological diagnosis: (1) Crohn's disease involving only the small bowel; (2) Crohn's disease involving the large bowel with or without involvement of the small bowel; and (3) ulcerative colitis. In each study, patients had been referred for palliative intestinal resection following failure of intensive medical therapy. Prior to surgical intervention all patients were placed on a course of parenteral nutrition and observed.

Patients with Crohn's disease limited to the small bowel demonstrated a 60 to 80 per cent remission in symptoms, and surgery was avoided. Patients with granulomatous colitis, with or without involvement of the small bowel, responded with clinical remission in 30 to 60 per cent of the cases. Patients with ulcerative colitis responded poorly with very few remissions, but they did demonstrate significant improvement in their nutritional status and a decrease in postoperative complications.

It should be emphasized that patients with long-standing fistulas, inadequately drained intra-abdominal abscesses, or small bowel obstruction secondary to long-standing disease should undergo surgery as soon as their nutritional status is corrected. On the other hand, patients who are not responding to medical therapy and do not require early surgical procedures should be given parenteral feeding for 30 to 40 days in hopes of spontaneous remission or at least improvement of their nutritional status prior to surgery. In some patients, use of an oral elemental diet has also been effective in inducing remissions, and this approach might be considered in selected patients.[135]

The effectiveness of parenteral nutrition in closing fistulas associated with inflammatory bowel disease is controversial. MacFadyen et al.[125] and Mullen et al.[132] reported good success. But Fischer et al.[130] found that while the fistulas may close, they often reopened later and eventually required surgical correction. At Duke University Medical Center, only two patients with fistulas due to inflammatory bowel disease have been treated with parenteral nutrition. In the first, the fistula closed after 25 days and in the second, after 35 days; fistulas in both remained closed at one-year follow-ups.

## MALIGNANT DISEASES

Malignant diseases have a devastating effect on human nutrition. Their gradual growth is often associated with poor dietary intake due to pain or partial obstruction of the gastrointestinal tract. In addition, catabolism and weight loss may result when the metabolic demands of the malignant state exceed dietary intake, which would otherwise be quite adequate. Finally, therapeutic procedures such as chemotherapy, radiotherapy, and surgery may themselves result in loss of appetite and production of nausea and diarrhea. It is not uncommon for nutritional depletion and its complications to be so severe that therapy must be withheld, discontinued, delayed, or reduced. Parenteral nutrition, by establishing and maintaining an optimal nutritional state, may significantly improve cancer therapy, in terms of both patient tolerance and long-term survival.[136-141] In addition to simply providing nutritional support to the patient, parenteral nutrition has been shown to reverse immune incompetence due to malnutrition, thus possibly improving host-tumor resistance.[142, 143] In the future, investigations may demonstrate that amino acid manipulations that deprive tumors of amino acids essential for their growth play a possible role in cancer therapy, as suggested by Demopoulas.[144] Other metabolic manipulations may also be found useful. For example, if excessive glucose is administered intravenously, some is metabolized anaerobically, resulting in lactic acidosis. The intracellular acidosis increases cellular penetrance of methotrexate[145] and may increase its antitumor effectiveness. At present, no stimulation of tumor growth by parenteral nutrition has been observed in humans.[139] In addition, detailed nitrogen utilization studies on tumor-bearing animals have demonstrated no increase in tumor protein synthesis during parenteral nutrition.[146]

The selection of patients with cancer to receive parenteral nutrition must be done carefully. Patients with terminal disease, unresponsive to all therapeutic measures, will at times demonstrate an improved sense of well-being upon institution of parenteral nutrition. When nutritional support is discontinued, however, rapid weight loss, malnutrition, and death follow. On the other hand, patients with potentially responsive tumors, especially those with low tumor burdens, are excellent candidates. In general, if the patient is severely malnourished, one to two weeks of parenteral nutrition prior to tumor therapy should be considered. If the patient is well nourished, parenteral nutrition should be initiated three to four days before tumor therapy and continued until its completion.

*Chemotherapy.* Patients to receive chemotherapy should be placed on parenteral nutrition three to four days prior to infusion of the drug or drugs and supported during and after treatment until an adequate oral diet is resumed. With this approach, a sense of well-being is often observed, and weight gain may even occur during chemotherapy.[147] Although the effect of parenteral nutrition on long-term survival has yet to be established, Copeland et al.[147] have reported a correlation between nutritional status and response to chemotherapy in patients with adenocarcinoma and squamous cell carcinoma of the lung. Others have supported Copeland's findings.[136, 139, 141] The improved

response may be due, in part, to increased tolerance to drugs[148] such as 5-fluorouracil and the resulting reduction in gastrointestinal side effects.[137] On the other hand, the severe stomatitis due to vinblastine and bleomycin in combination is unaffected,[149] and there appears to be no effect on drug-induced leukocyte depression.

*Radiotherapy.* Patients selected to receive radiotherapy often do not require nutritional support. When, however, the radiation field includes the abdomen, or large doses are given, radiation enteritis or sickness may occur. Instead of decreasing or delaying the scheduled treatment, intravenous nutrition should be begun while withholding oral intake. In general, symptoms of mucositis, nausea, vomiting, and diarrhea decrease during parenteral nutrition, allowing completion of the treatment program.[148]

*Surgery.* Patients to undergo surgery should be evaluated for their nutritional status. If they are to have a major operative procedure, and they suffer moderate to severe protein-calorie depletion, they should be given preoperative nutritional support and be maintained postoperatively with intravenous nutrition until an adequate oral diet is resumed.[138, 139] Such support will help assure wound healing and prevent complications if prolonged restriction of oral intake is necessary.[150]

Studies are in progress to determine more accurately the advantages and disadvantages of parenteral nutrition in malignant disease, and new developments are expected.

## RENAL FAILURE

Decreased or absent renal function, occurring acutely or chronically, significantly interferes with normal nutrition. The necessity of restricting water, sodium, and potassium, as well as the need to continually correct metabolic acidosis, makes adequate intake difficult and often impairs substrate utilization. To reduce the rate of nitrogenous waste accumulation in the blood, primarily as urea, moderate to severe protein restriction (20 to 40 grams per day) is often prescribed. Depending on the caloric intake and the quality of protein, catabolism and progressive debilitation may occur.

With improvement in the technique and availability of dialysis, patients with renal failure can now be managed with less severe nutritional restriction. Acute trauma, however, or severe illness may render oral intake or dialysis, or both, unsatisfactory or impossible, leading to rapid deterioration of the patient's nutritional status. Based on the finding that blood urea can function as a source of nitrogen under certain conditions in uremic patients,[151, 152] various intravenous nutritional formulas are being evaluated for their ability to reverse catabolism and establish lean tissue synthesis when oral intake or dialysis is contraindicated. The objective is to provide adequate caloric support and a minimum of high biologic value protein. The caloric source has usually been hypertonic glucose. Protein has been given as crystalline l-amino acids providing only essential or both essential and non-essential amino acids. In addition, investigation is in progress on the role of nitrogen-free alpha-keto analogs of the essential amino acids.

Infusion of only essential amino acids appears to improve the nutritional and clinical status of uremic patients in two ways: (1) Protein intake is greatly reduced, while requirements for essential amino acids are still met, and (2) the body, in the presence of adequate essential amino acids, transfers the nitrogen of urea to various carbon chains to form non-essential amino acids. Infusion of essential l-amino acids and hypertonic dextrose in patients with acute and chronic renal failure, as well as in anephric patients, has been shown to decrease blood urea nitrogen, serum potassium, magnesium, and phosphorus, thereby reducing the need for dialysis while maintaining improved or positive nitrogen balance and good nutrition.[153-157] Essential amino acids may also have a direct effect on the clinical course of acute renal failure. Abel et al.,[158] in a prospective study of patients with acute renal failure following surgical procedures, reported improved patient survival and more rapid recovery of renal function in those patients given essential amino acids and hypertonic dextrose intravenously than in patients given routine 5 per cent dextrose solutions.

Although essential amino acids are of great value in the treatment of renal failure, they are often not necessary. Routine crystalline amino acid solutions, containing both essential and non-essential amino acids, and hypertonic dextrose can be given safely to many patients with renal failure if fluid and protein tolerances are observed. Indeed, administration of routine parenteral nutrition solutions to patients with acute renal failure may enhance survival and reduce morbidity by sparing further proteolysis of renal tubular cells.[159] Solutions formulated to provide approximately 0.07 grams nitrogen per kilogram and 45 to 55 calories per kilogram per day are generally well tolerated by uremic patients.[160, 161] Dialysis should be performed if excessive fluid accumulation or excessive elevation of blood urea nitrogen is observed but is often unnecessary, depending on the degree of renal failure. If dialysis is not available or is contraindicated, and excessive fluid or urea nitrogen accumulation occurs, only hypertonic dextrose and essential amino acids should be given.

Administration of nitrogen-free alpha-keto analogs of essential amino acids, completely eliminating nitrogenous intake, remains an experimental procedure. As these compounds can be converted by transamination to their respective amino acids by uremic patients,[162, 163] they in effect provide ample essential amino acid support. Walser et al.[164, 165] developed a 20 gram protein diet supplemented with keto analogs of leucine, isoleucine, valine, methionine, and phenylalanine, along with the four remaining essential amino acids. The diet was given to patients with chronic renal failure and resulted in a significant decrease in urea accumulation, compared with the same diet supplemented with all nine essential amino acids. The keto analogs are beneficial in renal failure for several reasons: They allow complete exogenous nitrogen restriction, endogenous nitrogen may be utilized in transamination of the keto analogs to amino acids and in the synthesis of non-essential amino acids, and a direct anabolic effect, which decreases the rate of urea production by reducing turnover of endogenous protein, has been observed during analog infusion.[166] These effects act to reduce blood urea nitrogen accumulation during maintenance of adequate nutritional support. At present these compounds are unavailable commercially and are quite expensive.

## HEPATIC FAILURE

Parenteral nutrition is often necessary to maintain adequate nutrition in patients with liver failure when complications prevent or restrict oral intake. Patients suffering mild liver impairment without coma, asterixis, spontaneous ecchymosis, or jaundice, but perhaps with ascites, prolongation of the prothrombin time, and elevated sulfobromophthalein retention times, do fairly well when given standard parenteral nutrition formulas. With close supervision, salt restriction, and possibly protein restriction, they can be kept anabolic[167] (see discussion of possible hepatotoxicity of parenteral nutrition solutions in Chapter 9 on liver enzyme elevations). Gabuzda and Davidson[168] demonstrated nitrogen equilibrium, or a slight positive nitrogen balance, in patients with cirrhosis who were given adequate caloric input and 50 grams of protein orally. Intravenous administration of protein is even better tolerated, as ammonia production by enteric bacteria following oral protein intake is avoided.[169] The actual protein load infused must be adjusted to the individual patient on the basis of clinical and laboratory data.

Patients who have elevated serum ammonia and moderately severe hepatic failure, yet retain some degree of hepatic function with only mild hepatic encephalopathy, are also candidates for parenteral nutrition. Some researchers have advocated giving only essential amino acids and hypertonic dextrose because ammonia nitrogen can function as a nitrogenous source (like urea nitrogen in renal failure) for synthesis of non-essential amino acids.[170] Others have reported an improvement in hepatic encephalopathy in patients following daily infusions of hypertonic dextrose and 5.6 to 14.4 grams of nitrogen as essential and non-essential amino acids.[169] The selection of essential amino acids, or mixtures of essential and non-essential amino acids, must be based on an estimate of the liver's ability to synthesize non-essential amino acids.

Patients with severe hepatic failure and marked hepatic encephalopathy show no metabolic improvement with intravenous administration of hypertonic dextrose and either essential or routine amino acid solutions. Yet special amino acid formulas may be helpful. Plasma amino acid patterns in patients with hepatic encephalopathy due to chronic or acute liver disease are markedly abnormal.[171-173] There is an increase in the plasma concentration of straight-chain amino acids normally metabolized by the liver, including phenylalanine, tyrosine, glutamate, aspartate, and methionine. On the other hand, the branch-chain amino acids, valine, leucine, and isoleucine, which are normally metabolized by skeletal muscle, are markedly decreased because of increased portal-systemic shunting of insulin.[174] The molar ratio:

$$\frac{\text{Valine} + \text{Leucine} + \text{Isoleucine}}{\text{Phenylalanine} + \text{Tyrosine}}$$

correlates well with the grade of encephalopathy (the normal ratio of 3.0 to 3.5 may decrease to 1.0 during encephalopathy).[173] Normalization of the plasma amino acid pattern by infusion of specially formulated solutions containing increased branch-chain amino acids, decreased straight-chain amino acids, and hypertonic dextrose reduces symptoms of encephalopathy and increases survival rates in dogs[175] and man.[173] A product for oral or tube feeding use, called Hepatic-Aid, is available from McGaw Laboratories. A similar solution for intravenous infusion is being tested.

Patients with hepatic encephalopathy due to acute hepatic necrosis generally have elevated concentrations of all amino acids except the branch-chain amino acids, which are normal.[171] In these patients infusion of routine or special amino acid solutions affords little benefit.[171, 173]

## BURNS AND TRAUMA

The provision of adequate metabolic substrates to patients with burns covering 30 per cent or more of the body or with massive trauma plays a significant role in their survival. The weight loss and severe protein wasting associated with the hypermetabolic response to thermal injury or massive trauma can be reversed if an aggressive attempt is made to provide necessary carbohydrate, fat, and protein. It is often possible to provide these metabolic substrates via the gastrointestinal tract, either with an oral diet or with nasogastric feeding tubes. When enteral feedings are inadequate, supplementary caloric and nitrogenous substrates should be administered intravenously. With this approach, up to 10,000 calories a day can be given. An excellent review of the metabolic requirements and special conditions of burn patients is presented by Dr. D. W. Wilmore.[176]

## CARDIAC DISEASES

Chronic cardiac illness is often associated with progressive protein–calorie malnutrition. Patients with rheumatic heart disease, especially mitral valve disease, appear to be most severely depleted, but nearly all patients demonstrate muscular weakness and easy fatigability. The malnutrition is due to a combination of mental depression, anorexia from chronic illness, and the unpalatable nature of a low-salt diet and, at least in part, to poor cardiac output.[177] With improvements in medical and surgical technology, these patients are enjoying greater longevity but still suffer from chronic malnutrition. If subjected to major stress, such as a surgical procedure, trauma, or infection, their catabolic response far exceeds dietary intake, and rapid physical depletion occurs.

It is generally held that the heart is little altered by chronic malnutrition in that it has the capacity to utilize a wide variety of energy substrates. Yet this claim is poorly documented. It may be that malnutrition adversely alters myocardial structure and function, much as it does with the gastrointestinal tract and the liver, especially during stress, thus further compromising the already stressed heart. Recent studies suggest that adequate nutritional support may indeed significantly improve the clinical condition of patients with chronic cardiac illness,[178] improve cardiac function,[179, 180] and protect the myocardium during hypoxia.[181, 182] For these reasons it has been advocated that parenteral nutrition be given to patients with cardiac cachexia, especially those with depressed anthropometric measurements and impaired cellular immunity (anergy to skin tests and a depressed total lymphocyte count). The effects of administering parenteral nutrition *following* cardiac surgery on survival and postoperative morbidity have not been impressive, however.[183] Blackburn et al.[184, 185] have emphasized the need for two to three weeks of intensive nutritional support *preoperatively*, as well as continued postoperative support, if improved survival is to be realized. Further studies are necessary before the actual value of parenteral nutrition in cardiac malnutrition will be known.

Patients who are candidates for parenteral nutrition on criteria other than cardiac cachexia but also have heart disease should not be excluded solely on the basis of their cardiac disease. Volume restrictions may be observed by increasing the concentration of dextrose, using 50 to 70 per cent base solutions, and amino acids, using 8.5 to 10 per cent base solutions. The presence of vascular or valvular prostheses, although representing an increased risk, do not contraindicate carefully administered parenteral nutrition. Improvements in aseptic solution preparation and sterile techniques in the care of central venous lines have greatly reduced infectious complications. Such patients must, however, be carefully selected.

## OTHER USES OF PARENTERAL NUTRITION

Use of parenteral nutrition has been reported in cases of tetanus,[186] post-vagotomy gastric stasis,[187] and protein-losing enteropathy due to idiopathic intestinal lymphangiectasis.[188] There is some evidence that the mucosal erosions of the stomach associated with starvation are decreased with parenteral nutrition.[189] Parenteral nutrition has, therefore, been considered for patients at risk of developing hemorrhagic gastritis.[190] Conflicting data have been presented by Isenberg and Maxwell,[191] who found that infusion of a mixture of l-amino acids significantly stimulated gastric acid secretion in man. The role of parenteral nutrition in the aggravation or healing of gastrointestinal ulcers remains to be determined. Other uses of parenteral nutrition will likely be proposed as experience increases.

## REFERENCES

1. Holter, A.R., and Fischer, J.E.: The effects of perioperative hyperalimentation on complications in patients with carcinoma and weight loss. J. Surg. Res., 23:31–34, 1977.
2. Copeland, E.M., MacFadyen, B.V., McGown, C., and Dudrick, S.J.: The use of hyperalimentation in patients with potential sepsis. Surg. Gynecol. Obstet., 138:377–380, 1974.
3. Brunzell, J.D., Lerner, R.L., Hazzard, W.R., Porte, D., Jr., and Bierman, E.L.: Improved glucose tolerance with high carbohydrate feeding in mild diabetics. N. Engl. J. Med., 284:521–524, 1971.
4. Ernest, I., Linner, E., and Svanborg, A.: Carbohydrate-rich, fat-poor diet in diabetics. Am. J. Med., 39:594–600, 1965.
5. Cahill, G.F., Jr.: Physiology of insulin in man. Diabetes, 20:785–799, 1971.
6. Tarrant, M.E., and Ashmore, J.: Sequential changes in adipose tissue metabolism in alloxan-diabetic rats. Diabetes, 14:179–185, 1965.
7. Blackburn, G.L., Flatt, J.P., Clowes, G.H.A., and O'Donnell, T.E.: Peripheral intravenous feeding with isotonic amino acid solutions. Am. J. Surg., 125:447–454, 1973.
8. Hoover, H.C., Grant, J.P., Gorschboth, C., and Ketchum, A.S.: Nitrogen-sparing intravenous fluids in postoperative patients. N. Engl. J. Med., 293:172–175, 1975.
9. Leevy, C.M., Cardi, L., Frank, O., Gellene, R.,

and Baker, H.: Incidence and significance of hypovitaminemia in a randomly selected municipal hospital population. Am. J. Clin. Nutr., 17:259–271, 1965.
10. Bollet, A.J., and Owens, S.O.: Evaluation of nutritional status of selected hospitalized patients. Am. J. Clin. Nutr., 26:931–938, 1973.
11. Bistrian, B.R., Blackburn, G.L., Hallowell, E., and Hadelle, R.: Protein status of general surgical patients. J.A.M.A. 230:858–860, 1974.
12. Hill, G.L., Blackett, R.L., Pickford, I., Burkinshaw, L., Young, G.A., Warren, J.V., Schorah, C.J., and Morgan, D.B.: Malnutrition in surgical patients: An unrecognized problem. Lancet, 1:689–692, 1977.
13. Butterworth, C.E., Jr.: Malnutrition in the hospital. J.A.M.A., 230:879, 1974.
14. Lawson, L.J.: Parenteral nutrition in surgery. Br. J. Surg., 52:795–800, 1965.
15. Morgan, A., Filler, R.M., and Moore, F.D.: Surgical nutrition. Med. Clin. North Am., 54:1367–1381, 1970.
16. Cahill, G.F., Jr.: Starvation in man. N. Engl. J. Med., 282:668–675, 1970.
17. Gordon, J.E., and Scrimshaw, N.S.: Infectious disease in the malnourished. Med. Clin. North Am., 54:1495–1508, 1970.
18. Committee on Trauma, National Academy of Sciences–National Research Council: Postoperative wound infections: The influence of ultraviolet irradiation of the operating room and of various other factors. Ann. Surg. (Suppl.), 160:1–192, 1964.
19. Cruse, P.J.E., and Foord, R.: A five-year prospective study of 23,649 surgical wounds. Arch. Surg., 107:206–211, 1973.
20. Doekel, R. C., Jr., Zwillich, C. W., Scoggin, C. H., Kryger, M., and Weil, J.V.: Clinical semi-starvation. Depression of hypoxic ventilatory response. N. Engl. J. Med., 295:358–361, 1976.
21. Rhoads, J.E., and Alexander, C.E.: Nutritional problems of surgical patients. Ann. N.Y. Acad. Sci., 63:268–275, 1955.
22. Dudrick, S.J., and Rhoads, J.E.: Metabolism in surgical patients: Protein, carbohydrate, and fat utilization by oral and parenteral routes. In Sabiston, D.C. (ed.): Textbook of Surgery, 11th Edition. Philadelphia, W.B. Saunders Company, 1977, pp. 150–177.
23. Stein, H.D., and Keiser, H.R.: Collagen metabolism in granulating wounds. J. Surg. Res., 11:277–283, 1971.
24. Udupa, K.N., Woessner, J.F., and Dunphy, J.E.: The effect of methionine on the production of mucopolysaccharides and collagen in healing wounds of protein-depleted animals. Surg. Gynecol. Obstet., 102:639–645, 1956.
25. Irvin, T.T., and Hunt, T.K.: Effect of malnutrition on colonic healing. Ann. Surg., 180:765–772, 1974.
26. Irvin, T.T., and Goligher, J.C.: Aetiology of disruption of intestinal anastomoses. Br. J. Surg., 60:461–464, 1973.
27. Bozzetti, F., Terno, G., and Longoni, C.: Parenteral hyperalimentation and wound healing. Surg. Gynecol. Obstet., 141:712–714, 1975.

28. Rutten, P., Blackburn, G.L., Flatt, J.P., Hallowell, E., and Cochran, D.: Determination of optimal hyperalimentation infusion rate. J. Surg. Res., *18*:477–483, 1975.

29. Wilmore, D.W.: The Metabolic Management of the Critically Ill. New York, Plenum Publishing Corporation, 1977, pp. 11–14.

30. Bartlett, R.H., Allyn, P.A., Medley, T., and Wetmore, N.: Nutritional therapy based on positive caloric balance in burn patients. Arch. Surg., *112*:974–980, 1977.

31. Weir, J.B. DeV.: New methods for calculating metabolic rate with special reference to protein metabolism. J. Physiol. (London), *109*:1–12, 1949.

32. Mackenzie, T., Blackburn, G.L., and Flatt, J.P.: Clinical assessment of nutritional status using nitrogen balance. Fed. Proc., *33*:683, 1974.

33. Shizgal, H.M., Spanier, A.H., and Kurtz, R.S.: Effect of parenteral nutrition on body composition in the critically ill patient. Am. J. Surg., *131*:156–161, 1976.

34. Elwyn, D.H., Bryan-Brown, C.W., and Shoemaker, W.C.: Nutritional aspects of body water dislocations in postoperative and depleted patients. Ann. Surg., *182*:76–84, 1975.

35. Shizgal, H.M.: Total body potassium and nutritional status. Surg. Clin. North Am., *56*:1185–1194, 1977.

36. Spanier, A.H., and Shizgal, H.M.: Caloric requirements of the critically ill patient receiving intravenous hyperalimentation. Am. J. Surg., *133*:99–104, 1977.

37. Kinney, J.M., Lister, J., and Moore, F.D.: Relationship of energy expenditure to total exchangeable potassium. Ann. N.Y. Acad. Sci., *110*:711–722, 1963.

38. Moore, F.D., Olesen, K.H., McMurray, J.D., Parker, H.V., Ball, M.R., and Boyden, C.M.: The Body Cell Mass and its Supporting Environment. Body Cell Composition in Health and Disease. Philadelphia, W.B. Saunders Company, 1963.

39. Bistrian, B.R., Blackburn, G.L., Sherman, M., and Scrimshaw, N.S.: Therapeutic index of nutritional depletion in hospitalized patients. Surg. Gynecol. Obstet., *141*:512–516, 1975.

40. Blackburn, G.L., Bistrian, B.R., Maini, B.S., Schlamm, H.T., and Smith, M.F.: Nutritional and metabolic assessment of the hospitalized patient. J. Parenteral Enteral Nutr., *1*:11–22, 1977.

41. Frisancho, A.R.: Triceps skin fold and upper arm muscle size norms for assessment of nutritional status. Am. J. Clin. Nutr., *27*:1052–1058, 1974.

42. Gurney, J.M., and Jelliffe, D.B.: Arm anthropometry in nutritional assessment: Nomogram for rapid calculation of muscle circumference and cross-sectional muscle and fat areas. Am. J. Clin. Nutr., *26*:912–915, 1973.

43. Young, V.R., Havenberg, L.N., Bilmazes, C., and Munroe, H.N.: Potential use of 3-methylhistidine excretion as an index of progressive reduction in muscle protein catabolism during starvation. Metabolism, *22*:1427–1436, 1973.

43a. Black, L. F., and Hyatt, R. E.: Maximal respira-

tory pressures: Normal values and relationship to age and sex. Am. Rev. Respir. Dis., *99*:696–702, 1969.

44. Travill, A.S.: The synthesis and degradation of liver-produced proteins. Gut, *13*:225–241, 1972.

45. Interdepartmental Committee on Nutrition for Defense: Manual of Nutrition Surveys. National Institutes of Health, Bethesda, Md., 1963.

46. Whitehead, R.G., Coward, W.A., and Lunn, P.G.: Serum-albumin concentration and the onset of kwashiorkor. Lancet, *1*:63–66, 1973.

47. Awai, M., and Brown, E.B.: Studies of the metabolism of I-131-labeled human transferrin. J. Lab. Clin. Med., *61*:363–396, 1963.

48. Mancini, G., Carbonara, A.O., and Heremans, J.F.: Immunological quantitation of antigens by single radial immunodiffusion. Int. J. Immunochem., *2*:235–254, 1965.

49. Ingenbleek, Y., Van Den Schrieck, H.-G., De Nayer, P., and De Visscher, M.: Albumin, transferrin and the thyroxine-binding prealbumin/retinol-binding protein (TBPA-RBP) complex in assessment of malnutrition. Clin. Chim. Acta, *63*:61–67, 1975.

50. Ingenbleek, Y., De Visscher, M., and De Nayer, P.: Measurement of prealbumin as index of protein-calorie malnutrition. Lancet, *2*:106–108, 1972.

51. Oppenheimer, J.H., Surks, M.I., Bernstein, G., and Smith, J.C.: Metabolism of iodine-131-labeled thyroxine-binding prealbumin in man. Science, *149*:748–751, 1965.

52. Peterson, P.A.: Demonstration in serum of two physiological forms of the human retinol binding protein. Eur. J. Clin. Invest., *1*:437–444, 1971.

53. Smith, F. R., and Goodman, De W. S.: The effects of diseases of the liver, thyroid and kidneys on the transport of vitamin A in human plasma. J. Clin. Invest., *50*:2426–2435, 1971.

54. Neumann, C.G., Lawlor, G.J., Jr., Stiehm, E.R., Swendseid, M.E., Newton, C., Herbert, J., Ammann, A.J., and Jacob, M.: Immunologic responses in malnourished children. Am. J. Clin. Nutr., *28*:89–104, 1975.

55. Selvaraj, R.J., and Bhat, K.S.: Phagocytosis and leukocyte enzymes in protein–calorie malnutrition. Biochem. J., *127*:255–259, 1972.

56. Chandra, R.K.: Rosette-forming T lymphocytes and cell-mediated immunity in malnutrition. Br. Med. J., *3*:608–609, 1974.

57. Bistrian, B.R., Blackburn, G.L., Scrimshaw, N.W., and Flatt, J.P.: Cellular immunity in semistarved states in hospitalized adults. Am. J. Clin. Nutr., *28*:1148–1155, 1975.

58. Bistrian, B.R., Sherman, M., Blackburn, G.L., Marshall, R., and Shaw, C.: Cellular immunity in adult marasmus. Arch. Intern. Med., *137*:408–412, 1977.

59. Law, D.K., Dudrick, S.J., and Abdon, N.I.: Immunocompetence of patients with protein-calorie malnutrition. The effects of nutritional repletion. Ann. Intern. Med., *79*:545–550, 1973.

60. Law, D.K., Dudrick, S.J., and Abdou, N.I.: The effect of dietary protein depletion on immu-

nocompetence: The importance of nutritional repletion prior to immunologic induction. Ann. Surg., *179*:168–173, 1974.

61. Dionigi, R., Zonta, A., Dominioni, L., Gens, F., and Ballabio, A.: The effects of total parenteral nutrition on immunodepression due to malnutrition. Ann. Surg., *185*:467–474, 1977.

62. Meakins, J.L., Pietsch, J.B., Bubernick, D., Kelly, R., Rod, T., Bordon, J., and MacLean, L.D.: Delayed hypersensitivity: Indicator of acquired failure of host defenses in sepsis and trauma. Ann. Surg., *186*:241–250, 1977.

62a. Buzby, G. P., Mullen, J. L., Matthews, D. C., Hobbs, C. L., and Rosato, E. F.: Prognostic nutritional index in gastrointestinal surgery. Abst. 218, Digestive Disease Week, New Orleans, May 21–23, 1979.

63. Trafford, H.S.: The outlook after massive resection of small intestine; with a report of two cases. Br. J. Surg., *44*:10–13, 1956.

64. Chen, K.M.: Clinical survey of the patients with massive resection of small intestine during the last ten years. J. Formosan Med. Assoc., *73*:35–44, 1974.

65. Cameron, I.L., Pavlat, W.A., and Urban, E.: Adaptive responses to total intravenous feeding. J. Surg. Res., *17*:45–52, 1974.

66. Koga, Y., Ikeda, K., Inokuchi, K., Watanabe, H., and Hashimoto, N.: The digestive tract in total parenteral nutrition. Arch. Surg., *110*:742–745, 1975.

67. Weinstein, L.D., Shoemaker, C.P., and Hersh, T.: Enhanced intestinal absorption after small bowel resection in man. Arch. Surg., *99*:560–562, 1969.

68. Scheflan, M., Galli, S.J., Perrotto, J., and Fischer, J.E.: Intestinal adaptation after extensive resection of the small intestine and prolonged administration of parenteral nutrition. Surg. Gynecol. Obstet., *143*:757–762, 1976.

69. Porus, R.L.: Epithelial hyperplasia following massive small bowel resection in man. Gastroenterology, *48*:753–757, 1965.

70. Flint, J.M.: The effect of extensive resections of the small intestine. Bull. Johns Hopkins Hosp., *23*:127–144, 1912.

71. Bury, K.D.: Carbohydrate digestion and absorption after massive resection of the small intestine. Surg. Gynecol. Obstet., *135*:177–187, 1972.

72. Wright, H.K., and Tilson, M.D.: The short gut syndrome. Pathophysiology and treatment. Current Probl. Surg., June, 1971, pp. 3–51.

72a. Williamson, R.C.N., and Chir, M.D.: Intestinal adaptation. N. Engl. J. Med., *298*:1393–1402, 1444–1450, 1978.

73. Reynell, P.C., and Sprey, G.H.: Small intestinal function in the rat after massive resections. Gastroenterology, *31*:361–368, 1956.

74. Singleton, A.O., Redmond, D.C., and McMurray, J.E.: Ileocecal resection and small bowel transit and absorption. Ann. Surg., *159*:690–694, 1964.

75. Broviac, J.W., Cole, J.J., and Schribner, B.H.: A silicone rubber atrial catheter for prolonged parenteral alimentation. Surg. Gynecol. Obstet., *136*:602–606, 1973.

76. Jeejeebhoy, K.N., Zohrad, W.J., Langer, B., Phillips, M.J., Kuksis, A., and Anderson, G.H.: Total parenteral nutrition at home for 23 months without complication, and with good rehabilitation. Gastroenterology, *65*:811–820, 1973.

77. Atkins, R.C., Vizzo, J.E., Cole, J.J., Blagg, C.R., and Scribner, B.H.: The artificial gut in hospital and home. Technical improvements. Trans. Am. Soc. Artif. Intern. Organs, *16*:260–268, 1970.

78. Solassol, Cl., Joveux, H., Etco, L., Pujol, H., and Romeiu, Cl.: New techniques for long-term intravenous feeding: An artificial gut in 75 patients. Ann. Surg., *179*:519–522, 1974.

79. Riella, M.C., and Scribner, B.H.: Five years' experience with a right atrial catheter for prolonged parenteral nutrition at home. Surg. Gynecol. Obstet., *143*:205–208, 1976.

80. Borgstrom, B., Dahlqvist, A., Lundh, G., and Sjovall, J.: Studies on intestinal digestion and absorption in the human. J. Clin. Invest., *36*:1521–1536, 1957.

81. Mekhjian, H.S., Phillips, S.F., and Hofmann, A.F.: Colonic secretion of water and electrolytes induced by bile acids: Perfusion studies in man. J. Clin. Invest., *50*:1569–1577, 1971.

82. Mitchell, W.D., Findlay, J.M., Prescott, R.J., Eastwood, M.A., and Horn, D.B.: Bile acids in the diarrhea of ileal resection. Gut, *14*:348–353, 1973.

83. Soong, C.S., Thompson, J.B., Poley, J.R., and Hess, D.R.: Hydroxy fatty acids in human diarrhea. Gastroenterology, *63*:748–757, 1972.

84. Stein, T.A., and Wise, L.: Bile salt metabolism following jejunoileal bypass for morbid obesity. Ann. Surg., *185*:67–72, 1977.

85. Hardison, W.G.M., and Rosenberg, I.H.: Bile-salt deficiency in the steatorrhea following resection of the ileum and proximal colon. N. Engl. J. Med., *277*:337–342, 1967.

86. Hofmann, A.F., and Poley, J.R.: Cholestyramine treatment of diarrhea associated with ileal resection. N. Engl. J. Med., *281*:397–402, 1969.

87. LeVeen, H.H., Borek, B. Axelrod, D.R., and Johnson, A.: Cause and treatment of diarrhea following resection of the small intestine. Surg. Gynecol. Obstet., *124*:766–770, 1967.

88. Vlahcevic, Z.R., Prazich, J., and Swell, L.: Evidence that a diminished bile acid pool precedes the formation of cholesterol gallstones in man. Surg. Gynecol. Obstet., *136*:961–965, 1973.

89. Wise, L., and Stein, T.: Biliary and urinary calculi: Pathogenesis following small bowel bypass for obesity. Arch. Surg., *110*:1043–1047, 1975.

90. Hofmann, A.F., Thomas, P.J., Smith, L.H., and McCall, J.T.: Pathogenesis of secondary hyperoxaluria in patients with ileal resection and diarrhea. Gastroenterology, *58*:960, 1970.

91. Stauffer, J.Q., Humphreys, M.H., and Weir, G.J.: Acquired hyperoxaluria with regional enteritis after ileal resection. Role of dietary oxalate. Ann. Intern. Med., *79*:383–391, 1973.

92. Earnest, D.L., Johnson, G., Williams, H.E., and

Admirand, W.H.: Hyperoxaluria in patients with ileal resection: An abnormality in dietary oxalate absorption. Gastroenterology, 66:1114–1122, 1974.

93. Dobbins, J.W., and Binder, H.J.: Effect of bile salts and fatty acids on the colonic absorption of oxalate. Gastroenterology, 70:1096–1100, 1976.

94. Earnest, D.L., Williams, H.E., and Admirand, W.H.: Treatment of enteric hyperoxaluria with calcium and medium chain triglyceride. Clin. Res., 23:130, 1975.

95. Earnest, D.L., Gancher, S., and Admirand, W.H.: Treatment of enteric hyperoxaluria (EHO) with calcium and aluminum. Gastroenterology, 70:881, 1976.

96. Stassoff, B.: Experimentelle Untersuchungen über die kompensatorischen Vorgange bei Darmresektionen. Beitr. Klin. Chir., 89:527–586, 1914.

97. Osborne, M.P., Sizer, J., Frederick, P.L., and Zamcheck, N.: Massive bowel resection and gastric hypersecretion. Am. J. Surg., 114:393–397, 1967.

98. Frederick, P.L., Sizer, J.S., and Osborne, M.P.: Relation of massive bowel resection to gastric secretion. N. Engl. J. Med., 272:509–514, 1965.

99. Osborne, M.P., Frederick, P.L., Sizer, J.S., Blair, D., Cole, P., and Thum, W.: Mechanism of gastric hypersecretion following massive intestinal resection. Clinical and experimental observations. Ann. Surg., 164:622–634, 1966.

100. Straus, E., Gerson, C.D., and Yalow, R.S.: Hypersecretion of gastrin associated with the short bowel syndrome. Gastroenterology, 66:175–180, 1974.

101. Wickbom, G., Landor, J.H., Bushkin, F.L., and McGuigan, J.E.: Changes in canine gastric acid output and serum gastrin levels following massive small intestinal resection. Gastroenterology, 69:448–452, 1975.

102. Becker, H.D., Reeder, D.D., and Thompson, J.C.: Extraction of circulating endogenous gastrin by the small bowel. Gastroenterology, 65:903–906, 1973.

102a. Murphy, J.P., Jr., King, D.R., and Dubois, A.: Treatment of gastric hypersecretion with Cimetidine in the short-bowel syndrome. N. Engl. J. Med., 300:80–81, 1979.

102b. Cortot, A., Fleming, C.R., and Malagelada, J.-R.: Improved nutrient absorption after Cimetidine in short-bowel syndrome with gastric hypersecretion. N. Engl. J. Med., 300:79–80, 1979.

103. Voitk, A.J., Echave, V., Brown, R.A., and Gurd, F.N.: Use of elemental diet during the adaptive stage of short gut syndrome. Gastroenterology, 65:419–426, 1973.

104. Conn, J.H., Chavez, C.M., and Fain, W. R.: The short bowel syndrome. Ann. Surg., 175:803–814, 1972.

105. Gliedman, M.L., Bolooki, H., and Rosen, R.G.: Acute pancreatitis. Curr. Probl. Surg., Aug., 1970.

106. Lawson, D.W., Daggett, W.M., Civetta, J.M., Corry, R.J., and Bartlett, M.K.: Surgical treatment of acute necrotizing pancreatitis. Ann. Surg., 172:605–617, 1970.

107. Ranson, J.H.C., Rifkind, K.M., Roses, D.F., Fink, S.D., Eng, K., and Spencer, F.C.: Prognostic signs and the role of operative management in acute pancreatitis. Surg. Gynecol. Obstet., 139:69–81, 1974.

108. Feller, J.H., Brown, R.A., Toussaint, G.P.M., and Thompson, A.G.: Changing methods in the treatment of severe pancreatitis. Am. J. Surg., 127:196–201, 1974.

109. Goodgame, J.T., and Fischer, J.E.: Parenteral nutrition in the treatment of acute pancreatitis: Effect on complications and mortality. Ann. Surg., 186:651–658, 1977.

110. Warshaw, A.L., Imbembo, A.L., Civetta, J.M., and Daggett, W.M.: Surgical intervention in acute necrotizing pancreatitis. Am. J. Surg., 127:484–491, 1974.

111. Friedman, S.M., and Friedman, C.L.: The effect of low protein diet on the structure of the pancreas. Can. Med. Assoc. J., 55:15–16, 1940.

112. Farber, E., and Popper, H.: Production of acute pancreatitis with ethionine and its prevention by methionine. Proc. Soc. Exp. Biol. Med., 74:838–840, 1950.

113. Shaper, A.G.: Chronic pancreatic disease and protein malnutrition. Lancet, 1:1223–1224, 1960.

114. Hamilton, R.F., Davis, W.C., Stephenson, D.V., and Magee, D.F.: Effect of parenteral hyperalimentation on upper gastrointestinal tract secretions. Arch. Surg., 102:348–352, 1971.

115. Nakajima, S., and Magee, D.F.: Inhibition of exocrine pancreatic secretion by glucagon and d-glucose given intravenously. Can. J. Physiol. Pharmacol., 48:299–305, 1970.

116. Sanderson, I., and Dietel, M.: Insulin response in patients undergoing prolonged intravenous hyperalimentation. Surg. Forum, 23:64–66, 1972.

117. White, T.T., and Heimbach, D.M.: Sequestrectomy and hyperalimentation in the treatment of hemorrhagic pancreatitis. Am. J. Surg., 132:270–275, 1976.

118. Manson, R.R.: Acute pancreatitis secondary to iatrogenic hypercalcemia: Implications of hyperalimentation. Arch. Surg., 108:213–215, 1974.

119. Edmunds, L.H., Jr., Williams, G.M., and Welch, C.E.: External fistulas arising from the gastrointestinal tract. Ann. Surg., 152:445–471, 1960.

120. West, J.P., Ring, E.M., Miller, R.E., and Burks, W.P.: A study of the causes and treatment of external postoperative intestinal fistulas. Surg. Gynecol. Obstet., 113:490–496, 1961.

121. Nemhayser, G. M., and Braytom, D.: Enterocutaneous fistulas involving the jejunal-ileum. Am. Surg., 93:16–20, 1967.

122. Halversen, R.C., Hogle, H.H., and Richards, R.C.: Gastric and small bowel fistulas. Am. J. Surg., 118:968–972, 1969.

123. Lorenzo, G.A., and Beal, J.M.: Management of external small bowel fistulas. Arch. Surg., 99:394–396, 1969.

124. Chapman, R., Foran, R., and Dunphy, J.E.: Management of intestinal fistulas. Am. J. Surg., 108:157–164, 1964.

125. MacFadyen, B.V., Jr., Dudrick, S.J., and Ruberg, R.L.: Management of gastrointestinal fistulas with parenteral hyperalimentation. Surgery, 74:100–105, 1973.

126. Aguirre, A., Fischer, J.E., and Welch, C.E.: The

role of surgery and hyperalimentation in therapy of gastrointestinal–cutaneous fistulae. Ann. Surg., *180*:393–401, 1974.

127. Sheldon, G.F., Gardiner, B.N., Way, L.W., and Dunphy, J.E.: Management of gastrointestinal fistulas. Surg. Gynecol. Obstet., *133*:385–389, 1971.

128. Grant, J.P., Pittman, M.A., Maher, M.M., and Jones, R.S.: Parenteral nutrition in the management of enterocutaneous fistulas. N.C. Med. J., *38*:327–330, 1977.

129. Rhoads, J.E.: Management of regional ileitis and certain other ulcerative lesions of intestines. Pa. Med., *42*:1050–1056, 1939.

130. Fischer, J.E., Foster, G.S., Abel, R.M., Abbott, W.M., and Ryan, J.A.: Hyperalimentation as primary therapy for inflammatory bowel disease. Am. J. Surg., *125*:165–175, 1973.

131. Tamvakopoulos, S.K., Turnier, E., Barrett, M.S., and Randall, H.T.: Nutritional implications of regional enteritis. R.I. Med. J., *52*:221–223, 1969.

132. Mullen, J.L., Hargrove, W.C., Dudrick, S.J., Fitts, W.T., Jr., and Rosatto, E.F.: Ten years experience with intravenous hyperalimentation and inflammatory bowel disease. Ann. Surg., *187*:523–529, 1978.

133. Fitts, W.T., Jr.: Discussion. Am. J. Surg., *125*:173, 1973.

134. Reilly, J., Ryan, J.A., Strole, W., and Fischer, J.E.: Hyperalimentation in inflammatory bowel disease. Am. J. Surg., *131*:192–200, 1976.

135. Voitk, A.J., Echave, V., Feller, J.H., Brown, R.A., and Gurd, F.N.: Experience with elemental diet in the treatment of inflammatory bowel disease. Arch. Surg., *107*:329–333, 1973.

136. Assa, J., Schramek, A., Barzilai, A., and Weisz, G.M.: Intravenous hyperalimentation for the onco-surgical patient. J. Surg. Oncol., *6*:239–244, 1974.

137. Souchon, E.A., Copeland, E.M., Watson, P., and Dudrick. S.J.: Intravenous hyperalimentation as an adjunct to cancer chemotherapy with 5-fluorouracil. J. Surg. Res., *18*:451–454, 1975.

138. Copeland, E.M., MacFadyen, B.V., Jr., and Dudrick, S.J.: Intravenous hyperalimentation in cancer patients. J. Surg. Res., *16*:241–247, 1974.

139. DeMatteis, R., and Hermann, R.E.: Supplementary parenteral nutrition in patients with malignant disease. Cleve. Clin. Q., *40*:139–145, 1973.

140. Ford, J.H., Dudan, R.C., Bennett, J.S., and Averette, H.E.: Parenteral hyperalimentation in gynecologic oncology patients. Gynecol. Oncol., *1*:70–75, 1972.

141. Schwartz, G.F., Green, H.L., Bendon, M.L., Graham, W.P., III, and Blakemore, W.S.: Combined parenteral hyperalimentation and chemotherapy in the treatment of disseminated solid tumors. Am. J. Surg., *121*:169–173, 1971.

142. Copeland, E.M., MacFadyen, B.V., Rapp, M.A., and Dudrick, S.J.: Hyperalimentation and immune competence in cancer. Surg. Forum, *26*:138–140, 1975.

143. Copeland, E.M., MacFadyen, B.V., and Dudrick, S.J.: Effect of intravenous hyperalimentation on established delayed hypersensitivity in

the cancer patient. Ann. Surg., *184*:60–64, 1976.

144. Demopoulos, H.B.: Effects of reducing the phenylalanine–tyrosine intake of patients with advanced malignant melanoma. Cancer, *19*:657–664, 1966.

145. Meyer, J.A.: Potentiation of solid tumor chemotherapy by metabolic alterations. Ann. Surg., *179*:88–93, 1974.

146. Oram-Smith, J.C., Stein, T.P., Wallace, H.W., and Mullen, J.L.: Intravenous nutrition and tumor host protein metabolism. J. Surg. Res., *22*:499–503, 1977.

147. Copeland, E.M., MacFadyen, B.V., Lanzotti, V.J., and Dudrick, S.J.: Intravenous hyperalimentation as an adjunct to cancer chemotherapy. Am. J. Surg., *129*:167–173, 1975.

148. Copeland, E.M., and Dudrick, S.J.: Intravenous hyperalimentation as adjunctive treatment in the cancer patient. Clinical Digest, 5(1) McGaw Laboratories, Jan., 1976.

149. Copeland, E.M., MacFadyen, B.V., MacComb, W.S., Guillamondegui, O., Jesse, R.H., and Dudrick, S.J.: Intravenous hyperalimentation in patients with head and neck cancer. Cancer, *35*:606–611, 1975.

150. Heatly, H.V., and Hughes, L.E.: Preoperative intravenous nutrition in cancer patients. Proc. Int. Cancer Cong., 1975.

151. Rose, W.C., and Dekker, E.E.: Urea as a source of nitrogen for the biosynthesis of amino acids. J. Biol. Chem., *223*:107–120, 1956.

152. Giordano, C.: Use of exogenous and endogenous urea for protein synthesis in normal and uremic subjects. J. Lab. Clin. Med., *62*:231–246, 1963.

153. Dudrick, S.J., Steiger, E., and Long, J.M.: Renal failure in surgical patients. Treatment with intravenous essential amino acids and hypertonic glucose. Surgery, *68*:180–186, 1970.

154. Abel, R.M., Abbott, W.M., and Fischer, J.E.: Intravenous essential l-amino acids and hypertonic dextrose in patients with acute renal failure. Am. J. Surg., *123*:632–638, 1972.

155. Bergstrom, J., Bucht, H., Furst, P., Hultman, E., Josephson, B., Noree, L.O., and Vinnars, E.: Intravenous nutrition with amino acid solutions in patients with chronic uraemia. Acta Med. Scand., *191*:359–367, 1972.

156. Abel, R.M., Abbott, W.M., Beck, C.H., Jr., Ryan, J.A., Jr., and Fischer, J.E.: Essential l-amino acids for hyperalimentation in patients with disordered nitrogen metabolism. Am. J. Surg., *128*:317–323, 1974.

157. Kaminski, M.V., Light, J.A., and Briggs, W.A.: Parenteral nutrition with essential amino acids in pretransplantation anephrics. J. Parenteral Enteral Nutr., *2*:22–27, 1978.

158. Abel, R.M., Beck, C.H., Jr., Abbott, W.M., Ryan, J.A., Barnett, G.O., and Fischer, J.E.: Improved survival from acute renal failure after treatment with intravenous essential l-amino acids and glucose. N. Engl. J. Med., *288*:695–699, 1973.

159. Baek, S.M., Makabali, G.G., Bryan-Brown, C.W., Kusek, J., and Shoemaker, W.C.: The influence of parenteral nutrition on the course of acute renal failure. Surg. Gynecol. Obstet., *141*:405–408, 1975.

160. Doolas, A.: Planning intravenous alimentation of

surgical patients. Surg. Clin. North Am., *50*:103–112, 1970.

161. Jeejeebhoy, K.N.: Nutritional support of the azotemic patient. Urol. Clin. North Am., *1*:345–356, 1974.

162. Giordano, C., DePascale, C., Phillips, M.E., DeSanto, N.G., Furst, P., Brown, C.L., Houghton, B.J., and Richards, P.: Utilization of keto acid analogues of valine and phenylalanine in health and uremia. Lancet, *1*:178–182, 1972.

163. Gordon, R.S.: Metabolism of other D- and L-hydroxy acids. Ann. N.Y. Acad. Sci., *119*:927–941, 1965.

164. Walser, M., Coulter, A.W., Dighe, S., and Crantz, F.R.: The effects of keto-analogs of essential amino acids in severe chronic uremia. J. Clin. Invest., *52*:678–690, 1973.

165. Walser, M.: Ketoacids in the treatment of uremia. Clin. Nephrol., *3*:180–186, 1975.

166. Sapir, D.G., Owen, O.E., Pozefsky, T., and Walser, M.: Nitrogen-sparing induced by a mixture of essential amino acids given chiefly as their keto-analogues during prolonged fasting in obese subjects. J. Clin. Invest., *54*:974–980, 1974.

167. Host, W.R., Serlin, O., and Rush, B.F., Jr.: Hyperalimentation in cirrhotic patients. Am. J. Surg., *123*:57–62, 1972.

168. Gabuzda, G.J., and Davidson, C.S.: Protein metabolism in patients with cirrhosis of the liver. Ann. N.Y. Acad. Sci., *57*:776–785, 1954.

169. Silvis, S.E., and Badertscher, V.: Treatment of severe liver failure with hyperalimentation. Am. J. Gastroenterol., *59*:416–422, 1973.

170. Richards, P., Gibson, A.M., Ward, E.E., Wrong, O., and Houghton, B.J.: Utilization of ammonia nitrogen for protein synthesis in man, and the effect of protein restriction and uraemia. Lancet, *2*:845–849, 1967.

171. Rosen, H.M., Yoshimura, N., Hodgman, J.M., and Fischer, J.E.: Plasma amino acid patterns in hepatic encephalopathy of differing etiology. Gastroenterology, *72*:483–487, 1977.

172. Iob, V., Coon, W.W., and Sloan, M.: Altered clearance of free amino acids from plasma of patients with cirrhosis of the liver. J. Surg. Res., *6*:223–239, 1966.

173. Fischer, J.E., Rosen, H.M., Ebeid, A.M., James, J.H., Keane, J.M., and Soeters, P.B.: The effect of normalization of plasma amino acids on hepatic encephalopathy in man. Surgery, *80*:77–91, 1976.

174. Munro, H.N., Fernstrom, J.D., and Wurtman, J.D.: Insulin, plasma amino acid imbalance, and hepatic coma. Lancet, *1*:722, 1975.

175. Fischer, J.E., Funovics, J.M., Aguirre, A., James, J.H., Keane, J.M., Wesdorp, R.I.C., Yoshimura, N., and Westman, T.: The role of plasma amino acids in hepatic encephalopathy. Surgery, *78*:276–290, 1975.

176. Wilmore, D.W.: Parenteral nutrition in the thermally injured patient. *In* Ghadimi, H. (ed.): Total Parenteral Nutrition. New York, John Wiley & Sons, Inc., 1975, pp. 483–505.

177. Pittman, J.G., and Cohen, P.: The pathogenesis of cardiac cachexia. N. Engl. J. Med., *271*:403–409, 453–460, 1974.

178. Egdahl, R.H.: Hypertonic glucose and improved

179. critical organ performance. Surgery, *75*:145–147, 1974.

179. Abel, R.M., Fischer, J.E., Buckley, M.J., and Austen, W.G.: Hyperalimentation in cardiac surgery: A review of sixty-four patients. J. Thorac. Cardiovasc. Surg., *67*:294–300, 1974.

180. Pindyck, F., Drucker, M.R., Brown, R.S., and Shoemaker, W.C.: Cardiorespiratory effects of hypertonic glucose in the critically ill patient. Surgery., *75*:11–19, 1974.

181. Austen, W.G., Greenberg, J.J., and Piccinini, J.C.: Myocardial function and contractile force affected by glucose loading of the heart during anoxia. Surgery, *57*:839–845, 1965.

182. Hewitt, R.L., Lolley, D.M., Adrouny, G.A., and Drapanus, T.: Protective effect of glycogen and glucose on the anoxic arrested heart. Surgery, *75*:1–10, 1974.

183. Abel, R.M., Fischer, J.E., Buckley, M.J., Barnett, G.O., and Austen, W.G.: Malnutrition in cardiac surgical patients. Results of a prospective, randomized evaluation of early postoperative nutrition. Arch. Surg., *111*:45–50, 1976.

184. Blackburn, G.L., Gibbons, G.W., Bothe, A., Benotti, P.N., Harken, D.E., and McEnany, T.M.: Nutritional support in cardiac cachexia. J. Thorac. Cardiovasc. Surg., *73*:489–496, 1977.

185. Gibbons, G.W., Blackburn, G.L., Harken, D.E., Valdes, P.J., Morrehead, D., and Bistrian, B.R.: Pre and postoperative hyperalimentation in the treatment of cardiac cachexia. J. Surg. Res., *20*:439–444, 1976.

186. Parsa, M.H., Anderson, M.D., and Richter, R.W.: Central venous nutrition in severe tetanus. Arch. Surg., *105*:420–423, 1972.

187. Silverstein, M.J.: Parenteral hyperalimentation for severe postvagotomy gastric stasis: A case report. Milit. Med., *139*:212–214, 1974.

188. Wagner, A.: Treatment of protein losing enteropathy due to idiopathic intestinal lymphangiectasis by parenteral nutrition. Digestion, *2*:167–171, 1969.

189. Orane-Smith, J.C., and Rosato, E.F.: The effects of semistarvation and parenteral nutrition on the gastric mucosa of rats. Surgery, *79*:306–309, 1976.

190. Byrd, H.S., Lazarus, H.M., and Torma, M.J.: Effects of parenteral alimentation on postoperative gastric function. Am. J. Surg., *130*:688–693, 1975.

191. Isenberg, J.I., and Maxwell, V.: Intravenous infusion of amino acids stimulates gastric acid secretion in man. N. Engl. J. Med., *298*:27–29, 1978.

192. Modified from Metropolitan Life Insurance Company. Derived from data of the 1969 Build and Blood Pressure Study. Society of Actuaries.

193. Himal, H.S., Allard, J.R., Nadeau, J.E., Freeman, J.B., and MacLean, L.D.: The importance of adequate nutrition in closure of small bowel fistulas. Br. J. Surg., *61*:724–726, 1974.

194. Weisz, G.M., Barzilai, A., Assa, J., and Toledano, H.: Intravenous hyperalimentation in the management of the critically ill patient, with special reference to abdominal fistulae. Aust. N.Z. J. Surg., *46*:141–147, 1976.

# Chapter 4

# SUBCLAVIAN CATHETER INSERTION AND COMPLICATIONS

Administration of parenteral nutrition requires an easily placed, well-tolerated delivery system that is capable of remaining in place for long periods of time. The system should not restrict joint mobility or otherwise interfere with physical therapy. The high osmolality of the infused solution (up to 1500 mOsm/liter) requires administration into large veins with high blood flow to avoid severe pain, phlebitis, and hemolysis. These requirements limit the site of solution administration to the superior vena cava, right atrium, inferior vena cava, or a surgically created arteriovenous (A-V) fistula. In the superior vena cava, for example, flow is great enough to result in a dilution factor of 1:1000.

Placement of percutaneous catheters into the inferior vena cava via the femoral vein was first described by Duffy in 1949.[1] The difficulty of maintaining sterility in the groin area, however, presents a high risk of infectious complications.[2, 3] Further, an indwelling catheter may lead to inferior vena cava thrombosis and/or thromboembolic complications. However, when no other site is available, percutaneous femoral vein catherization of the inferior vena cava may be utilized for parenteral nutrition.[4, 5]

A-V fistulas or shunts of various designs have been successfully used in long-term parenteral nutrition.[6-8] Since they require an operation for insertion and, in the case of shunts, bleed profusely if the system becomes disconnected, they have not been used routinely in parenteral nutrition.

The most commonly used site for solution administration has been the superior vena cava. Long catheters inserted percutaneously into an antecubital vein may be quickly and easily advanced into the superior vena cava. Unfortunately, long plastic catheters inserted through the antecubital vein have produced a high incidence of thrombophlebitis; thus, their use is usually limited to short periods of time.[9-11] Recent experience with peripherally inserted, silicone-elastomer central venous catheters, however, has not shown a similar propensity to inflammation and thrombosis during long-term parenteral nutrition.[12, 13] These catheters, passed into the superior vena cava from the antecubital fossa, still limit flexion of the elbow and restrict physical therapy, but they can be used effectively in selected patients in whom percutaneous subclavian vein catheterization is unsuccessful or unwise.

The superior vena cava may also be cannulated via percutaneous puncture of the external jugular vein. Passage of a catheter into the superior vena cava by this route is, however, difficult and at times impossible because of the angulation between the external jugular vein and the subclavian vein. Continuous motion of the catheter with movement of the head and partial occlusion of the jugular vein by the catheter result in early phlebitis and thrombosis of the external jugular vein. Further, the presence of hair on the neck and the mobility of the neck render maintenance of a sterile dressing difficult, increasing the risk of sepsis.

Cannulation of the superior vena cava by percutaneous catheterization of the internal jugular vein is associated with a low incidence of phlebitis and thrombosis as a result of the vein's large diameter and high blood flow. However, as with cannulation of the external jugular vein, maintenance of a sterile dressing is difficult.[14] Benotti et al.[15] describe a technique for subcutaneously tunneling the catheter away from the neck and onto the anterior chest wall to facilitate dressing care. This method has reduced catheter-related sepsis.

The most commonly used site for cannulation of the superior vena cava is the subclavian vein. In 1952, Aubaniac[16] reported on 10 years of experience with percutaneous infraclavicular subclavian vein catheterization. Having worked extensively with patients in shock after military injuries, Aubaniac claimed the technique provided rapid access to the central venous system with minimal complications. Although described in 1952, it was not until 1962 that the technique was reported in the United States by Wilson et al.[17] In a footnote, these authors reported: "Since this paper was prepared, a number of pneumothoraces have occurred following subclavian cannulation by resident staff members." They suggested that the technique be performed or supervised only by experienced personnel. Over the next five years, complications of percutaneous subclavian catheterization and modifications of technique were reported in the developing literature on central venous pressure measurements in critically ill patients. In these patients, subclavian catheters were seldom left in place more than 14 days and were often used for only 3 or 4. For cases requiring prolonged central venous pressure measurements, some authorities suggested changing the catheter every 2 to 5 days to avoid subclavian vein thrombosis and infection.[18, 19] Reported complications of infraclavicular subclavian catheter placement have included pneumothorax, subclavian artery puncture, local hematomas, uncontrolled bleeding at the puncture site, improper position of the catheter tip, hemo-

mediastinum, hemothorax, injury of the brachial plexus and thoracic duct, air embolism, hydromediastinum, hydrothorax, subclavian vein thrombosis, embolism of the catheter tip, thrombophlebitis, and catheter occlusion secondary to kinks. The incidence of these complications has been greatly reduced with modifications of technique, and percutaneous puncture of the subclavian vein by the infraclavicular route is currently the procedure of choice for parenteral nutrition.

In 1965, Yoffa[20] described a supraclavicular approach to the subclavian vein. He reported only one arterial puncture and one pneumothorax in 130 catheterizations, both occurring early in his series. Parsa et al.,[21] in 1971, reported a comparative study of 225 junctional (internal jugular vein with subclavian vein), 625 infraclavicular, and 1025 supraclavicular catheterizations of the subclavian vein. He concluded that for safety, ease of puncture, and a high percentage of successful catheterizations, the supraclavicular approach was best. In his experience, maintenance of a sterile dressing posed no problem.

In this chapter the anatomy of the subclavian vein area will be reviewed. A technique for the placement of infraclavicular and supraclavicular subclavian vein catheters will be described. Other techniques, such as junctional puncture and internal jugular vein puncture, performed upon failure of the infra- and supraclavicular approaches, will not be discussed here but are described by Parsa et al.[22] Finally, recognition and management of catheterization complications will be discussed.

## ANATOMY OF THE SUBCLAVIAN VEIN AREA

The axillary vein begins at the lower border of the teres major muscle as a continuation of the basilic vein. It passes obliquely across the axilla toward the middle third of the clavicle, where it becomes the subclavian vein at the lateral border of the first rib. The subclavian vein arches behind the clavicle over the first rib anterior to the insertion of the anterior scalene muscle. At this point, just medial to the midpoint of the clavicle, the vein reaches its most cephalad position in its arch over the rib. At the medial border of the anterior scalene muscle, the subclavian vein joins the internal jugular vein to form the brachiocephalic vein. In its course behind the clavicle the subclavian vein assumes its largest diameter, 12 to 25 mm. Anteriorly, the subclavian vein is covered in its entire course by the clavicle, costoclavicular ligament, and subclavius muscle. Inferiorly, the vein rests on the first rib laterally and on the cupula of the lung medially. Hyperinflation of the lung in chronic emphysema, with protrusion of the cupula into the neck, elevates the subclavian vein above its normal position and increases the risk of puncture of the lung during catheterization of the vein. Posteriorly, as the subclavian vein crosses the first rib, it is separated from the subclavian artery by the anterior scalene muscle, which is usually more than a centimeter thick. Further medially, the internal thoracic artery, on its way into the chest, passes behind the vein. Superiorly, the suprascapular and transverse cervical branches of the thyro-cervical trunk pass in close proximity to the vein, between the scalenus anterior and sternocleidomastoid muscles. The thoracic duct enters the internal jugular vein near its junction with the left subclavian vein, passing anterior to the subclavian artery and its branches and posterior to the internal jugular vein. As the thoracic duct passes inferiorly and medially to join the internal jugular vein, it crosses in front of the anterior scalene muscle above the subclavian vein and can be damaged during subclavian vein catherization. The walls of the vein consist of a thin tunica muscularis reinforced by thick tunica fibrosa and adhere through an extension of the fascia colli media to the adjacent ligaments, fascia, and periosteum. Because of these fascial attachments the subclavian vein is not easily displaced and does not collapse, even in shock or death.

## PATIENT PREPARATION

Prior to insertion of a subclavian vein catheter, the procedure should be thoroughly explained to the patient. When the patient is properly informed, sedation will rarely be necessary. Although local anesthesia is used, the patient should be cautioned to expect some pain as the needle passes between the clavicle and first rib.

To facilitate catheter insertion, all necessary materials should be collected in advance. At Duke University Medical Center a portable cart is stocked with solutions, tubing, dressing equipment, gowns, gloves, masks, and catheters. A sterile tray, prepared by the hospital's Central Sterile Supply Department, contains all necessary hardware (Fig. 4–1). A catheter may be chosen from several that are commercially available. Optimal catheter sets include a 2 to 2¾ inch, 14-gauge needle with a 20 cm,

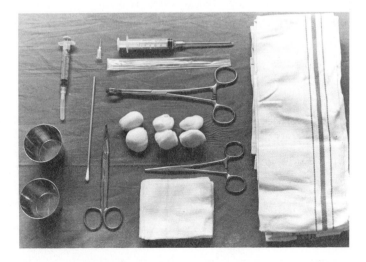

**Figure 4–1** Subclavian catheter insertion tray contains basins, clamps, syringes, and sponges required for catheter insertion.

or longer, catheter. We have found the Deseret Subclavian Set,* with a 30.5 cm radi-
opaque polyethylene catheter, removable
2¾ inch, 14-gauge needle, and blunt-tip
needle adapter, to be best suited to our
needs. The removable needle permits a
small final dressing. Catheters made of
Silastic or a similar material would be preferable, and several companies are working
on such kits. A satisfactory unit will likely
be available soon.

To provide positive pressure in the
subclavian vein, the patient should be
placed supine in the Trendelenburg position. Visible engorgement of the external
jugular vein minimizes the possibility of air
embolization, which has been reported
during the catheterization procedure (up to
100 ml air per second can pass through a
14-gauge needle).[23-25] The patient's head
should be turned slightly away from the
side of catheterization and rested flat on the
bed. A small, rolled towel placed longitu-
dinally between the scapulae from the seventh cervical vertebra to the tenth or
twelfth thoracic vertebra allows the
shoulders to fall back onto the bed. The
patient is instructed to "reach for his toes"
with both hands to bring the subclavian
vein into proper position behind the clavicle.[26] If the shoulders are drawn to a shrug-
ging position, the vein will be at a variable
distance below the lower edge of the clavicle and make catheterization difficult. Failure to achieve the exaggerated military position because of improper use of the rolled
towel, a soft bed, or a fixed shoulder girdle
(as with severe arthritis) renders insertion
of the needle at the proper horizontal angle
difficult and invites puncture of the subclavian artery or the lung (Fig. 4–2).

## INFRACLAVICULAR SUBCLAVIAN VEIN CATHETERIZATION

The physician and his assistant should
thoroughly cleanse their hands with
povidone-iodine soap. All personnel assisting in the placement of the catheter, as well
as the patient, should wear masks over

*Deseret Pharmaceutical Co., Inc., Sandy, Utah
84070, catalogue No. 755.

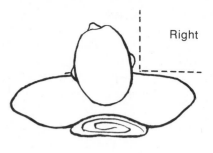

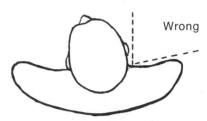

**Figure 4–2** Correct position of the patient for
insertion of subclavian catheter is the Trendelenburg position, with the arms by the side extended
toward the feet. A rolled towel is placed along the
thoracic spine to allow the shoulders to fall back
into the bed.

their noses and mouths. Sterile gowns are
preferable but not mandatory. A rectangu-
lar area from the mid-neck to below the
nipple and from the anterior axillary line to
just across the sternum is shaved. Skin
nicks should be avoided, as they provide
possible sites for infection. Some advocate
use of a depilatory instead of a razor, and
this would be acceptable.[27] The skin is
thoroughly cleansed with povidone-iodine
soap, with the scrub beginning from the
point of anticipated puncture and proceed-
ing in ever-enlarging circles to the bound-
aries of the preparation. The soap suds are
removed with a dry gauze, and a highly
volatile, fat-soluble agent (acetone or ether)
is next applied with sponges in a circular,
rubbing motion. The fat-soluble agent is
applied several times to remove fatty oils
and loose cutaneous scales both chemically
and mechanically. Cleansing is continued
until the sponges show no further debris
removal. The physician then puts on sterile
gloves and, using sterile technique, applies
several layers of povidone-iodine solution
to the skin. Sterile towels are placed so that
they expose only the medial two-thirds of
the clavicle, the sternal notch, and 1 or 2

inches of skin above and below the clavicle. Sterile gloves are then changed.

After the skin is prepared, the following anatomic landmarks are identified. The clavicular head of the sternocleidomastoid muscle as it inserts on the clavicle can be clearly defined by having the patient attempt to turn his head toward the puncture site against resistance. The anterior scalene muscle can be palpated beneath the clavicular head of the sternocleidomastoid muscle. It represents most of the muscle mass palpable in this region, as the clavicular head of the sternocleidomastoid muscle is quite thin. The anterior scalene muscle passes under the clavicle and inserts on the tubercle of the first rib. Passing the finger under the clavicle along the anterior scalene muscle, the subclavian artery can often be palpated posteriorly. The target for subclavian vein catheterization is thus identified as a postage stamp–sized area bounded inferiorly by the first rib, posteriorly by the anterior scalene muscle as it inserts upon the tubercle of the first rib, anteriorly by the clavicle, and superiorly by the tip of the finger (Fig. 4–3). The location of the subclavian vein in this area is very constant. If

displaced, it will only be more cephalad, as in the case of emphysema. It will not lie posterior to the scalene muscle. The target area contains no artery, nerve, or lung.

With a definite target area identified, the site for percutaneous needle puncture is selected. The site should provide a slightly cephalad trajectory of the needle toward the target area, usually around or slightly lateral to the midclavicular line. Occasionally a more medial puncture site with a more cephalad trajectory of the needle is necessary if the shoulders cannot be adequately drawn back onto the bed. The puncture site should permit a horizontal approach to the target area with the needle tip always anterior to the anterior scalene muscle. A small wheal of 1 per cent lidocaine without epinephrine is raised at the puncture site. No attempt should be made to anesthetize the subclavius muscle or periosteum of the clavicle. Complete anesthesia cannot be obtained, nor is it necessary, and the vein might be displaced by a large amount of fluid. A 2 to 2½ inch, 14-gauge needle is attached to a 3 ml syringe and tested to be sure no air leaks are present by occluding the tip of the needle with a gloved finger

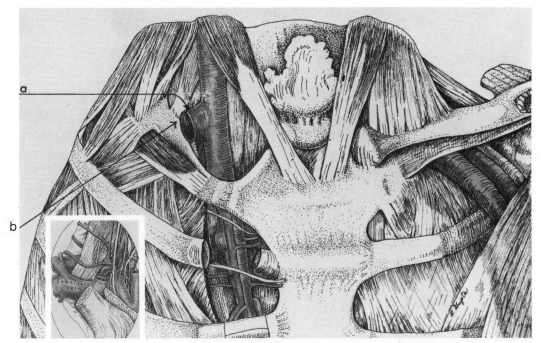

**Figure 4–3** Target area for subclavian vein puncture is defined by the first rib inferiorly, the anterior scalene muscle posteriorly, and the clavicle anteriorly. The vein will usually lie just behind the clavicle, although it may be displaced cephalad in patients with emphysema. *a,* Subclavian vein. *b,* Insertion of anterior scalene muscle on the tubercle of first rib just behind clavicle.

while applying suction to the syringe. If any leak is detected, the needle is readjusted or discarded. This procedure must be done so that no question arises during insertion of the needle as to whether the lung has been punctured if air is drawn into the syringe. The bevel of the needle should be aligned with markings on the side of the syringe. With its bevel directed anteriorly, the needle is inserted through the wheal of anesthetic agent and allowed to slip under the clavicle. With experience, "walking down the clavicle" is not necessary and should be avoided, as it can be painful both immediately and for several days. At this point, landmarks should once again be identified and the needle slowly inserted toward the target area just anterior to the anterior scalene muscle, with the syringe being held against the shoulder in a horizontal position (Fig. 4–4). Frequent small aspirations, rather than constant suctioning, should be applied to the plunger of the syringe until a free flow of blood is obtained. In our experience this usually occurs after half to three-quarters of the needle has been inserted. If the vein is not entered, the needle should be removed slowly and *completely* with gentle, intermittent aspiration. If, as occasionally occurs,

the vein has been punctured through-and-through, a return of blood into the syringe will be seen during withdrawal, and the catheter can be inserted. Upon complete removal of the needle, plugs of tissue or blood should be flushed out with air, and the target area re-evaluated. A point slightly more cephalad on the anterior scalene muscle should be selected. The temptation to direct the needle more posteriorly should absolutely be avoided, as the vein does not lie behind the anterior scalene muscle, but the subclavian artery and the cupula of the lung do. At no time should probing for the vein be done with short jabs of the needle in different directions. This markedly increases the incidence of complications. One should always withdraw the needle completely and re-evaluate the landmarks before making another pass.

Upon puncture of the subclavian vein and free return of blood into the syringe, the needle should be advanced approximately 0.5 to 1 cm to assure that its tip lies entirely within the subclavian vein; a free flow of blood should be observed as it is advanced. A clamp is applied to the hub of the needle for stabilization, and the patient instructed in the Valsalva maneuver. As the patient holds his breath, the syringe is re-

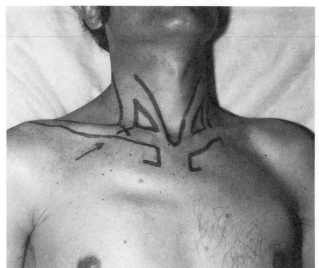

**Figure 4–4** Proper trajectory of the needle relative to the landmarks for subclavian vein catheterization.

moved from the needle hub and the end of the needle immediately occluded with the thumb to avoid aspiration of air. As the patient again holds his breath, the catheter is inserted. (Deseret catheters placed on the right side should be precut to 16 to 17 cm; those on the left to 19 to 20 cm.) To aid in passage of the catheter into the superior vena cava rather than the internal jugular or opposite subclavian vein, the catheter tip should be bent into a slight curve just prior to its insertion and the curve directed toward the heart. In addition, as the catheter will tend to flow in the direction of the needle bevel, the bevel should be directed toward the heart. Turning the patient's head toward the side of catheterization to make the angle between the subclavian and internal jugular veins more acute is of debatable value[26] but is usually done. If resistance is encountered on advancing the catheter, excessive force should not be used for fear of lacerating the vein. Rotation of the needle or catheter often will help passage and, if that fails, withdrawal of the needle approximately 2 to 5 mm may help. If, in spite of all attempts, the catheter cannot be passed, the needle and catheter should be withdrawn together and a second attempt on that side or an attempt on the opposite side made. Care must be taken to withdraw the needle and catheter simultaneously to avoid shearing of the catheter on the needle bevel and catheter embolus, which has been reported.[28] In addition, catheterization of the opposite subclavian vein should not be attempted unless the surgeon is absolutely sure that no pneumothorax was created on the first attempt. Following full insertion of the catheter, the needle is withdrawn.

In some patients whose neck or shoulders have contaminated areas, such as tracheostomies, infected wounds, or burns, it is advisable to cover the catheter dressing with a water-repellent plastic sheet and to change the dressing daily. An alternative is to tunnel the catheter subcutaneously away from the puncture site to the upper arm or lower chest between the nipple and sternum. Tunneling can be done easily with the Deseret set, in which a removable needle is used. In this instance the catheter should not be shortened. After preparing, draping, and infiltrating with lidocaine as above, a stab wound is made with a knife at the site of proposed percutaneous puncture. The subclavian vein is catheterized as above by inserting the needle through the stab wound. When the needle is removed, the catheter is positioned so its tip will lie within the superior vena cava. A subcutaneous tract is infiltrated with 1 per cent lidocaine without epinephrine, raising a small wheal at the proposed distant exit site (no further than 3½ inches away). The needle is inserted through the lidocaine wheal and advanced into the stab wound, with caution being taken to avoid puncturing the catheter (Fig. 4–5). The distal end of the catheter is inserted into the needle tip and drawn through the subcutaneous tract by slowly feeding the catheter while withdrawing the needle. The catheter is positioned so that no kinks are present and measured to assure that its tip lies in the the superior vena cava. The stab wound is irrigated with Betadine solution, closed with one or two interrupted 4-0 monofilament nylon skin sutures, and dressed with povidone-iodine ointment and a small gauze or Band-aid. Any excess catheter length is cut off so that only 4 to 5 cm protrude from the skin.

After the catheter is placed, either a needle tip guard is applied or a blunt-tip needle is inserted into the end of the catheter, depending on the type of catheter used. A sterile intravenous extension tubing is attached and an *isotonic* fluid begun at a slow rate. Placement of the catheter into a high-flow venous system is confirmed by a prompt reflux of blood into the tubing when the intravenous bottle is lowered below the level of the bed. If no blood reflux is obtained, the fluid should be stopped and the catheter repositioned or removed to avoid the risk of creating a hydrothorax or hydromediastinum.

At this point, sterile towels are removed and the area once again painted with povidone-iodine solution. A small amount of povidone-iodine ointment is applied to the catheter exit site and covered

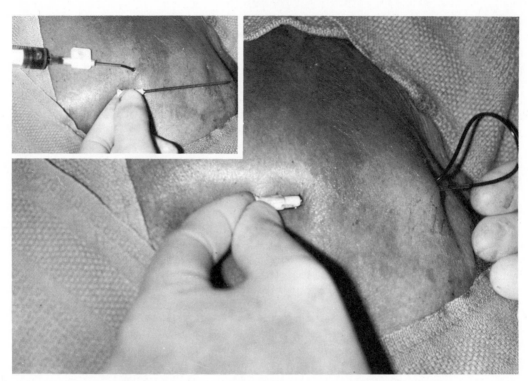

**Figure 4–5**   Subcutaneous tunneling of the catheter away from the shoulder. See text for details. The catheter is tunneled under the skin onto the chest wall using the insertion needle. Insert shows completed procedure with hub attached. A standard dressing will be applied and a single stitch placed in the small stab wound.

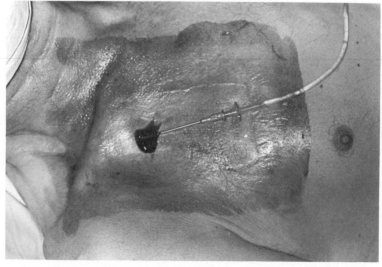

**Figure 4–6**   The catheter is draped over the anterior chest wall, slightly medial to the nipple, and covered with a 4 × 3 inch sterile gauze. The catheter is not sutured to the skin.

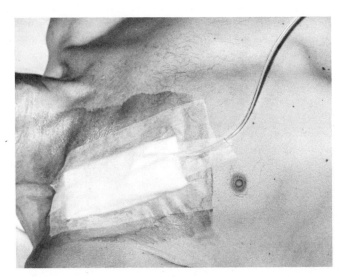

**Figure 4–7** Non-allergic paper tape is applied as an occlusive dressing, with a small opening left for exit of the catheter. Paper tape is preferred to avoid allergic reactions and to prevent buildup of adhesive residue on the skin. A third piece of tape is applied and pinched around the catheter as it exits from the dressing, to secure the catheter and to establish a tight seal.

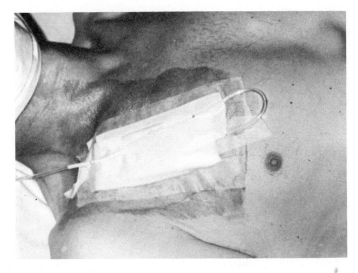

**Figure 4–8** Final position of the tubing exiting near the neck.

with a 2 × 2 inch square of Vaseline gauze to prevent absorption of the ointment into the overlying dressing. The catheter is draped over the anterior chest wall slightly medial to the nipple and the exit site covered with one 4 × 3 inch sterile gauze pad (Fig. 4–6). It is not necessary to suture the catheter to the skin if the dressing is properly applied as described below. Sutures not only serve as a nidus for skin irritation and possible infection, but they also require repeated replacement. Tincture of benzoin is sparingly applied to the skin about the 4 × 3 dressing, and paper tape is applied as an occlusive dressing (Fig. 4–7). The IV tubing is draped back over and taped to the dressing site to exit about the neck (Fig. 4–8). A chest x-ray is immediately taken to insure that no pneumothorax was created and to confirm that the catheter is properly located in the superior vena cava, no closer than 1 or 2 cm from the right atrium. Reports of perforation of the right ventricle[3, 29, 30] and right atrium,[31, 32] location of the catheter in aberrant venous channels,[33] and atrial arrhythmias due to improper positioning of the catheter[34] reinforce the need for a post-insertion chest x-ray. After x-ray confirmation of location, the hypertonic parenteral nutrition solution may be begun.

### SUPRACLAVICULAR APPROACH TO SUBCLAVIAN VEIN CATHETERIZATION

The patient is instructed about the procedure and placed in the Trendelenburg position. A right-handed physician will find a venous puncture of the left subclavian vein easiest. A wide area from the mid-neck to just above the nipple line and from the anterior axillary line to just across the sternum is shaved and cleansed with povidone-iodine soap, defatted with ether or acetone, and painted with povidone-iodine solution, as in the infraclavicular approach. The area is draped with sterile towels. Pertinent landmarks are identified, including the claviculo-sternocleidomastoid angle formed

by the lateral portion of the sternocleidomastoid muscle as it inserts upon the clavicle, the anterior scalene muscle posterior to the clavicular head of the sternocleidomastoid muscle with its insertion on the tubercle of the first rib behind the clavicle, and the subclavian artery behind the anterior scalene muscle (see Fig. 4–3). A small wheal of 1 per cent lidocaine is raised in the skin at the claviculo-sternocleidomastoid angle, just above the clavicle. A 2 to 2½ inch, 14-gauge needle is placed on a 3 ml syringe and tested to insure an airtight seal by placing a gloved finger over the tip of the needle and applying vacuum with the plunger of the syringe. The needle is then inserted through the wheal of anesthesia with its tip directed just behind the clavicle at a 45 degree angle to the sagittal plane and pointed 15 degrees forward of the coronal plane (Fig. 4–9). Thus, as the needle is advanced, it is safely moving away from the structures of the subclavian artery and cupula of the lung. The needle is very gently advanced with frequent, intermittent suction until it enters the subclavian vein, which is indicated by entry of blood into the syringe. Puncture of the vein usually occurs at a depth of 1 to 1.5 cm from the skin, but it can occur as shallow as 0.5 and as deep as 4 cm, depending on the obesity of the patient. Once within the vein, the syringe is lowered toward the shoulder to align the needle with the vein, and the bevel of the needle is directed toward the heart. As the patient performs a Valsalva maneuver, the syringe is removed, and the thumb is placed over the hub of the needle to prevent air embolization. As the patient again holds his breath, the catheter is inserted through the needle into the superior vena cava. The needle is then removed, and the catheter puncture site is dressed and attached to isotonic fluid, as described in the infraclavicular procedure. A chest x-ray is obtained to rule out an unsuspected pneumothorax and to confirm the proper position of the catheter in the superior vena cava before the administration of hypertonic fluid. When this approach is used, it is preferable to tunnel the catheter over the clavicle onto

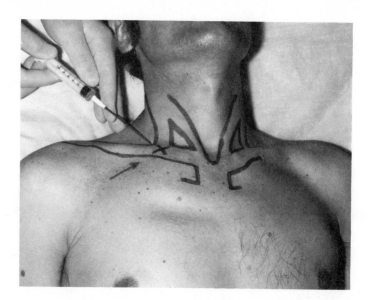

**Figure 4–9** Proper trajectory of the needle to puncture the subclavian vein from a supraclavicular approach. The needle is angled at 45 degrees to the sagittal plane and 15 degrees forward of the coronal plane.

the anterior chest wall to make dressing care easier.

In conclusion, the importance of both thorough understanding of the anatomy of the subclavian vein area and continual awareness of landmarks during catheterization cannot be overemphasized. The often quoted "blind percutaneous subclavian vein catheterization" should not be the case. Anatomical variations in this area are rare, and landmarks, in all but enormously obese patients, can be readily determined. Appreciation for the anatomical variations that do occur with chronic obstructive lung disease should help avoid pneumothoraces in these patients. Finally, there is no substitute for experience. Patients to be catheterized by inexperienced physicians should have good anatomical landmarks, and such initial catheterizations should be done as elective procedures under supervision. When emergency subclavian vein catheterization and catheterization of obese or uncooperative patients must be done, they should only be performed by experienced individuals, or else peripheral central lines should be inserted (by cutdown if necessary).

## COMPLICATION RECOGNITION AND MANAGEMENT

A summary of complications following more than 10,130 subclavian vein catheterizations reported in the English-language literature from 1956 to 1978 is given in Table 4–1. In all, 430 complications were reported (excluding failures to catheterize the vein), for a complication rate of 4.2 per cent. If only major complications are considered (242), a rate of 2.4 per cent is obtained. In another search of the literature, Burri and Krischak[35] reported a 12.5 per cent incidence of complications during placement of 17,326 catheters. When only major complications were included, an incidence of 1.4 per cent was found. Several institutions have found that experience plays a major role in complications, with very few complications occurring when catheters are inserted by physicians who have inserted 50 or more.[17, 36, 37] Recent improvements in technique, better understanding of anatomic relationships, and insistence on ideal conditions during placement have reduced complication rates to 1 per cent or less.[21, 38, 39] Nonetheless, it must be stressed

**Table 4–1**  COMPLICATIONS OF CENTRAL VEIN CATHETERIZATION

| | NO. CATHETERS | TECHNIQUE | PNEUMOTHORAX | ARTERIAL PUNCTURE | BRACHIAL PLEX. INJ. | THORACIC DUCT INJ. | SKIN BLEEDING | LOCAL HEMATOMA | HEMOMEDIASTINUM | HEMOTHORAX | HYDROMEDIASTINUM | HYDROTHORAX | SUBCUTANEOUS EMPHYSEMA | THROMBOSIS | AIR EMBOLISM | IMPROPER LOCATION | CATHETER EMBOLISM | FAILURE | REFERENCE |
|---|---|---|---|---|---|---|---|---|---|---|---|---|---|---|---|---|---|---|---|
| Keeri-Szanto (1956) | 113 | SC | 2 | 3 | | | | | | | | | | | | | | | 60 |
| Wilson (1962) | 250 | SC | | | | | | | | | | | | | | | | | 17 |
| Ashbaugh (1963) | 19 | SC | 1 | | | | | | | | | | | | | | | | 18 |
| Davidson (1963) | 100 | SC | 1 | | | | | 3 | | | | | | | | | | 6 | 61 |
| Baden (1964) | 61 | SC | | | | | | | | | 1 | 1 | | 3 | 4 | | | 10 | 43 |
| Vandeghen (1964) | 52 | SC | 1 | 10 | | | | | | | | | | | | | | 2 | 62 |
| Yarom (1964) | 200 | SC | 12 | | | | | few | 2 | | | 6 | | | | | | | 36 |
| Eastridge (1965) | 50 | ? | | | | | | | | | | | | | | | | | 19 |
| Longerbeam (1965) | 126 | SC | 5 | 3 | | | | 1 | | | | | | | | | 1 | 3 | 63 |
| Loskot (1965) | 70+ | SC | | | | | | | | | | | | | | | | 1 | 64 |
| Malinak (1965) | 113 | SC | | 1 | | | | | | | | | | | | | 1 | | 65 |
| Matz (1965) | ? | ? | 5 | | | | | | | | 1 | | | | | | | | 66 |
| Smith (1965) | 200+ | SC | 2 | | 1 | | | 1 | | 2 | 1 | | | | | | | | 52 |
| Yoffa (1965) | 130 | SPC | 1 | 1 | | | | | | | | | 1 | | | | | | 20 |
| Corwin (1966) | 98 | ? | 2 | | | | | | | | | | | | | | | 9 | 67 |
| Rams (1966) | 273 | ? | | | | | | | | | | | | | | | | | 68 |
| Atik (1967) | 300+ | SC | 3 | 3 | | | | | | | | 2 | | | | 1 | | | 69 |
| Christensen (1967) | 129 | SC | 4 | 2 | | | | 1 | | | | | | | | 8 | | 4 | 70 |
| Davis (1967) | 1 | ? | | | | | | | | | 1 | | | | | | | | 71 |
| Mogil (1967) | 219 | SC | 1 | | | 2 | | 3 | | | | | | | | | | 4 | 72 |
| Mobin-Uddin (1967) | 15 | SC | | | | | | | | | | | | | | | | | 73 |
| DeFalque (1968) | 1000 | SPC | 3 | 1 | | | | | | | | | | | | | | 1 | 74 |
| Wilson (1968) | 229 | SC | 2 | | | | | | | | | | | | | | | | 75 |
| Dudrick (1969) | 300+ | SC | | | | | | | | | | | | | | | | | 39 |
| Feiler (1969) | 704 | SC | 2 | | | | | | | | | | | 1 | | | | | 76 |
| Flanagan (1969) | 1 | SC | | | | | | | | | | | | | 1 | | | | 23 |
| Lucas (1969) | 1 | ? | | | | | | | | | | | | | 1 | | | | 77 |
| Doolas (1970) | 60 | ? | 3 | | | | | | | | | | | | | | | | 78 |
| Johnson (1970) | 2 | ? | | | | | | | | | | | | 1 | 1 | | | | 24 |
| McGovern (1970) | 25 | SC | | | | | | | | | | | | 1 | | | | | 79 |
| Bernard (1971) | 400+ | SC | 9 | 2 | | | 1 | | 1 | | | | | | | | | | 37 |
| McDonough (1971) | ? | SC | | | | | | | | | | | | 1 | | | | | 80 |
| Parsa (1971) | 1025 | SPC | | 10 | | | | | | | | | | | | | | | 21 |
| | 625 | SC | 7 | 3 | | | | | | | | | | | | | | | |
| | 225 | JC | 4 | | 7 | | | | | | | | | | | | | | |
| Baker (1972) | 30 | SC | 2 | 4 | | | | | | | | | | | | 2 | | | 81 |
| Gallitano (1972) | 600 | SC | | | | | | | | | | | | | | | | | 82 |
| Garcia (1972) | 83 | SPC | 2 | 3 | | | | | | | | | | | | | | | 83 |
| Vogel (1972) | 150 | SC | 2 | | | | | | | | | | 1 | | | | | | 38 |
| Buchsbaum (1973) | 132 | SC | 1 | | | | | | | | | | | 1 | | | | | 84 |
| Ryan (1974) | 355 | SC | | 6 | 2 | | | | | | | | | 8 | | 1 | | | 58 |
| Merk (1975) | 100 | SC | | 3 | | | | | | | | | | | | | | | 85 |
| Burri (1976) | 1098 | SC | 9 | 11 | | | | | | | | | | 15 | | 102 | | 305 | 35 |
| Armstrong (1977) | 2 | SC | | | | | | | | | | | | | | 2 | | | 86 |
| Grace (1977) | 2 | SC | | | | | | | | | | | | | | 2 | | | 87 |
| Grant | 456 | SC | 6 | 9 | 1 | | 3 | | | | | | | 8 | 1 | 50 | 1 | 3 | — |

SC = subclavian catheterization; SPC = supraclavicular catheterization; JC = junctional catheterization.

that subclavian vein catheterization is by no means a simple procedure. Prior to any attempt, a thorough review of anatomic relationship must be made. Residents learning the techniques of subclavian vein catheterization should be carefully supervised by an experienced physician. With attention to detail and proper instruction, pneumothorax, arterial puncture, hemomediastinum, hemothorax, hydromediastinum, and hydrothorax should be extremely rare, and brachial plexus or thoracic duct injury, air embolism, and catheter emboli should not occur. Some complications such as improper catheter tip locations, subclavian vein thrombosis, inadequate functioning of the catheter due to positional kinks, bleeding from puncture sites, and occasional local hematomas cannot always be avoided.

At Duke University Medical Center from June, 1973, to January, 1979, 462 catheters were placed in 414 patients with the following major complications: nine arterial punctures, treated successfully by local pressure; six pneumothoraces, one requiring a chest tube; one brachial plexus injury; and one fatal air embolus. Fifty catheters were discovered by chest x-ray to be im-

properly located, with the tips directed up into the neck, extended into the opposite subclavian vein, or coiled into the same subclavian vein. Several ended in the superior vena cava but took unusual courses (Fig. 4–10). Three patients demonstrated bleeding from small skin arterioles, which stopped with pressure in two cases and required suture ligation in the third. Our overall complication rate for catheter insertion was 15.2 per cent with a 3.7 per cent incidence of major complications. In 0.6 per cent of the patients we were unable to cannulate either the right or left subclavian vein by any percutaneous technique.

*Air Embolism.* Entry of a bolus of air into the venous system has long been recognized as a potentially dangerous event. The exact quantity of intravenous air that can lead to death is unknown but it appears to be related to the rate of entry. Tunnicliffe and Stebbing[40] administered intravenous oxygen to three patients for treatment of cyanosis in 1916 and reported a "therapeutic dose" of 10 ml/minute and a "toxic dose" of 20 ml/minute. Transient quadriplegia was noted in one patient. Yeakel[41] and Ordway[42] have reported fatal episodes follow-

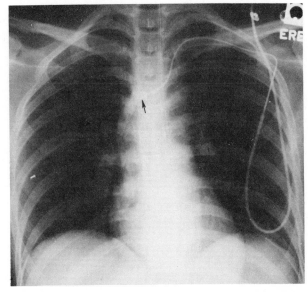

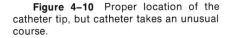
**Figure 4–10** Proper location of the catheter tip, but catheter takes an unusual course.

ing the sudden administration of 100 and 200 ml of air intravenously.

Insertion and care of central venous catheters is associated with the risk of air embolism. The first report of air embolization during catheter insertion was by Baden in 1964[43] and involved three of his patients. The first death due to air embolism during intravenous catheter insertion occurred in 1969, as reported by Levinsky.[44] Since then, 17 cases of air embolism associated with central venous catheters, including five deaths have been reported (see Table 4–1 and references 42 and 45). Air embolism may occur during catheter insertion when the syringe is removed from the needle.[24] Flanagen et al.[23] calculated that as much as 100 ml of air could pass through a 14-gauge needle in one second. Air embolization may also occur during the changing of intravenous tubing,[30] upon accidental separation of intravenous tubing from the subclavian catheter,[42] and through the subcutaneous tract, which may fail to close immediately following removal of a catheter.[46] In all instances, proper attention during care of the catheter system, as described in this chapter, can prevent embolization of air.

Clinical symptoms of air embolization depend on the quantity of air aspirated.

Aspiration of a small amount of air is usually asymptomatic. With larger air aspirations the patient may become dyspneic and possibly cyanotic and may be disoriented or even comatose. Tachycardia may be marked, and venous pressure may rise suddenly with a drop in systemic blood pressure. A loud "churning" murmur may be heard over the precordium as a result of turbulence about the pulmonary valve. The inspired air may fill both the right atrium and pulmonary artery and block blood flow (Fig. 4–11). Treatment consists of placing the patient in a left-lateral decubitus position with the head down.[47, 48] Emergency thoracotomy with needle aspiration of the right ventricle followed by direct cardiac massage has been successful in treating cardiac arrest.[49]

*Catheter Embolism.* Attempts to manipulate the catheter in and out through the insertion needle during catheter placement can result in the shearing of the catheter tip and embolization of the blood stream. This can occur surprisingly easily with little traction on the catheter and may go unrecognized until a chest x-ray is taken. The catheter will often lodge in the right atrium or ventricle but may embolize in the pulmonary artery or its tributaries. As embolized catheters can cause thrombus forma-

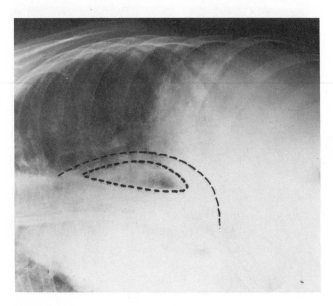

**Figure 4–11** A case of fatal air embolism during subclavian catheter insertion. Films taken at death show air-fluid level in right ventricle resulted in a complete block of the flow of blood.

tion and cardiac arrhythmias and serve as a nidus for infection, it is recommended that all be removed. Burri and Krischak[35] reviewed 208 cases of catheter embolism, 49.7 per cent of which occurred by shearing during catheter insertion as described above. Embolization of the catheter in the heart or lungs was associated with a 39.5 per cent death rate if the fragment was not removed. The preferred technique for removal is snaring of the catheter under fluoroscopy through a femoral vein approach.[50] When lodged in the pulmonary parenchyma, a thoracotomy may be necessary.

*Pneumothorax.* Most small pneumothoraces arising from subclavian vein catheterization demonstrate no progression and resolve spontaneously over several days without treatment. In a small percentage of cases, however, serial chest x-rays will demonstrate progressive enlargement of the pneumothorax, and in such cases a chest tube should be placed. If an air leak continues for several days after full lung expansion, the catheter should be removed, as it may be passing through the lung, forming a bronchopleural fistula. When the parietal pleura is penetrated during placement of a subclavian catheter, the patient often will note sharp chest pain and perhaps cough because of pleural irritation. If a patient has these symptoms during catheter insertion, the needle should be withdrawn immediately and landmarks reassessed prior to a second attempt. If the patient notes progressive pain or dyspnea, the catheterization attempt should be abandoned and a chest x-ray obtained immediately.

*Arterial Puncture.* Subclavian artery puncture with the 14-gauge needle is easily recognized both by the color of the blood aspirated and by its high pressure. Surprisingly few complications follow arterial puncture if the needle is immediately withdrawn and local pressure applied. Serial chest x-rays may demonstrate slight widening of the mediastinum, and in such cases the patient should be observed closely for possible cardiac tamponade. The possibility of creation of an A-V fistula by through-and-through puncture of the subclavian vein and puncture of the subclavian artery must be kept in mind. If the subclavian artery is punctured, the needle should be immediately withdrawn and a pressure dressing applied for five to ten minutes while the patient remains at rest. The patient should then be observed, with frequent monitoring of vital signs and serial chest x-rays.

*Improper Catheter Tip Location.* It is very important that the catheter tip be properly located in the superior vena cava for safe long-term feeding. Catheters may enter small venous tributaries, the internal jugular vein, the opposite subclavian vein, or various venous anomalies.[33] Such malpositioned catheters are associated with a higher incidence of phlebitis and may lead to thrombosis (see next section). Catheter tips located in the atrium or ventricle have been reported to perforate those chambers[29-32] and may also produce arrhythmias[34] or fibrosis of the tricuspid valve. In our experience with 50 cases in which the catheter tip was improperly located, initial attempts to reposition the tip by partially withdrawing the catheter, rotating it, and reinserting it were successful in 32 cases. In 6 cases the catheters were simply removed and new ones inserted. In 12 cases the patient was taken to the radiology department, where the catheter was manipulated under fluoroscopy. In all but 5 patients the catheters were easily positioned correctly into the superior vena cava. In the 5 cases in which the catheter was withdrawn to the point where it entered the venous system and radiographic dye injected, it was apparent that the catheter was in a tributary of the subclavian vein at right angles to the wall of the subclavian vein. Using arteriographic "J" wires these catheters can be repositioned in the superior vena cava.

Several reported instances of hydro- and hemothorax and mediastinum have been attributed to extravascular location of catheters.[36, 37, 43, 51, 52] Chest x-rays may demonstrate an aberrant catheter course, but the course may also look relatively normal. Infusion of hypertonic solutions into the pleural space or mediastinum is very irritating and can rapidly lead to severe cardiorespiratory embarrassment. Checking for free reflux of blood from the catheter by lowering the intravenous bottle below the bed, as described earlier, will aid in early diagnosis of extravascular catheter tips. A few cases in which a properly placed catheter tip eroded through the wall of the superior vena cava, resulting in hydrothorax, have also been reported.[51] Treatment consisted of catheter removal and observation.

*Subclavian Vein Thrombosis.* Subclavian vein thrombosis during parenteral nutrition has been reported to occur infrequently. In the American literature, 28 instances of thrombosis in 9674 catheterizations have been reported by 43 authors for an incidence of 0.29 per cent (see Table 4–1). A similar incidence was reported by Burri and Krischak in a review of the European literature: 0.24 per cent thrombosis in 17,326 catheterizations.[35] Yet, in their own series of 1098 catheterizations Burri and

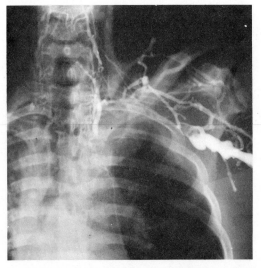

**Figure 4–12** Patient with complete occlusion of the left subclavian vein and proximal axillary vein occurring on the third day after catheter placement. Collateral flow through the internal and external jugular veins is present. The patient's left arm and neck are swollen.

Krischak encountered 15 instances of subclavian vein thrombois (1.4 per cent). We have experienced 13 instances of subclavian vein thrombosis in 462 subclavian catheters in 414 patients. In nine patients acute unilateral edema of the arm, neck, and face on the side of the catheter was observed sometime between the third and sixteenth day of therapy. Four of these patients underwent venogram studies, which demonstrated complete occlusion of the subclavian vein with moderate collateralization (Figs. 4–12 to 4–14). At an autopsy several weeks after the clinical diagnosis of subclavian vein thrombosis had been made, one patient, who did not undergo venography, was found to have a sclerosed subclavian vein on the side of the previously suspected thrombosis. One patient had bilateral facial, neck, and arm edema, symptoms of superior vena caval obstruction, and a documented pulmonary embolus (Figs. 4–15 and 4–16). The edema in all 10 patients resolved rapidly upon removal of the subclavian catheter and institution of anticoagulation with intravenous heparin. In three other patients no edema was observed, but transient episodes of acute pleuritic chest pain, shortness of breath, and mild hypoxemia occurred following removal or manipulation of the subclavian vein catheter. In each case, embolization of subclavian vein thrombi was suspected, as no pelvic thrombi or other sources were obvious. No venograms or lung scans were performed, as each episode lasted only minutes. In our series of 414 patients, therefore, five proven, four clinically apparent, and three possible episodes of subclavian vein thrombosis occurred, for a proven incidence of 1.2 per cent and a suspected incidence of 2.9 per cent.

Most patients with subclavian vein thrombosis display edema of the involved arm, neck, and face. If the catheter is malpositioned in the internal jugular vein and that vein thromboses, diplopia, generalized headache, bilateral papilledema, and sixth cranial nerve injury may occur, representing the syndrome of pseudotumor cerebri.[53] At other times recognition may be quite

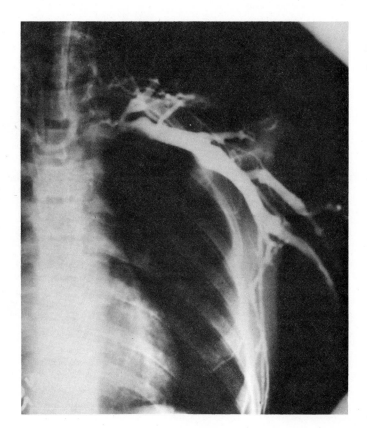

**Figure 4–13** Occlusion of proximal subclavian vein 18 days after catheter placement. Collateral flow was brisk, and minimal arm swelling was present, with no edema of the neck.

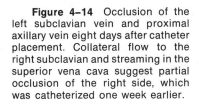

**Figure 4–14** Occlusion of the left subclavian vein and proximal axillary vein eight days after catheter placement. Collateral flow to the right subclavian and streaming in the superior vena cava suggest partial occlusion of the right side, which was catheterized one week earlier.

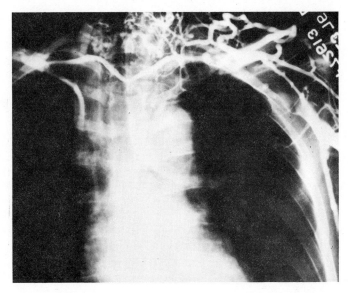

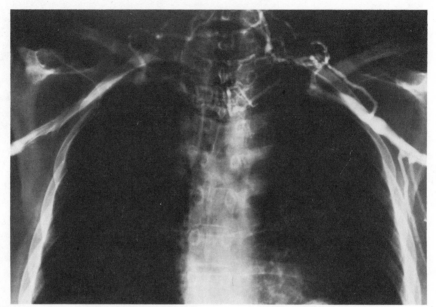

**Figure 4–15**   Patient with superior vena cava thrombosis due to subclavian catheter. Bilateral venogram demonstrates extent of occlusion and early collateral vein formation. Patient had bilateral facial, neck, and arm edema, with onset 12 days after placement of subclavian catheter.

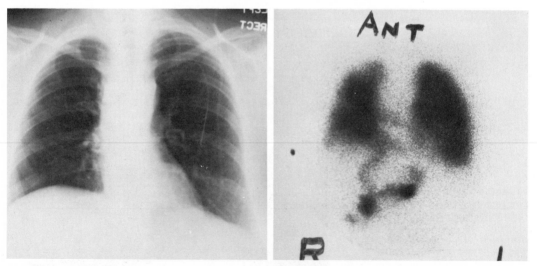

**Figure 4–16**   Chest x-ray taken just prior to bilateral venogram in patient with superior vena caval obstruction. No parenchymal defects are seen. Lung scan, however, demonstrates definite perfusion defects in the right upper and right mid-lung fields, as well as right and left bases. This case is thought to represent pulmonary emboli from superior vena caval thrombosis following placement of a subclavian catheter.

difficult. Thrombosis may first be suspected following an unsuccessful attempt to catheterize a previously cannulated vein. No other symptom may be present, and the difficulty may be falsely attributed to altered anatomy. Sepsis from an unknown source may at times be the presenting symptom of subclavian vein thrombosis following bacterial or fungal colonization. Although it was initially assumed that no significant embolic phenomena would occur from cannulation of the subclavian veins,[54] microemboli, which are often difficult to detect, and even major pulmonary emboli may well occur.[55, 56] Firor[57] attributed the death of one newborn baby to massive pulmonary emboli related to a parenteral nutrition catheter, and Ryan et al.[58] reported a similar episode in an adult. The one documented pulmonary embolus and the three transient episodes of acute pleuritic chest pain, shortness of breath, and mild hypoxemia following removal or manipulation of subclavian vein catheters in our experience add further evidence. At times, small pulmonary emboli can be documented by lung scans or pulmonary arteriograms. Whether or not emboli can be documented, if the clinical situation indicates pulmonary emboli, thrombosis of the subclavian vein must be suspected, and upper extremity venograms should be obtained.

Treatment of subclavian vein thrombosis consists of removal of the catheter and instigation of intravenous heparin. The catheter tip and blood drawn through the catheter should be cultured. Obstructive symptoms usually resolve in 24 to 48 hours, at which time a new catheter may be placed in the opposite subclavian vein and parenteral nutrition resumed, while the heparin infusion is gradually tapered over 7 to 14 days. Any troublesome bleeding from catheterization in anticoagulated patients can usually be controlled by local pressure and elevation of the head to decrease venous pressure. Alternatively, if the nutritional status of the patient permits, parenteral nutrition may be delayed until heparin therapy is discontinued, rendering placement of a new catheter safer. Eventual recannulation of the subclavian vein is thought to be possible but is not well documented. In one of our patients a catheter was placed without difficulty four months later in a previously thrombosed subclavian vein. In two others, however, a catheter could not be placed. Venograms for one of these patients demonstrated persistent subclavian vein occlusion after three years, and in the other the subclavian vein was a thin fibrotic cord at autopsy.

A possible mechanism for subclavian vein thrombosis is suggested by the appearance of well-formed, circumferential sheaths of fibrinous material around polyethylene catheters placed in the superior vena cava.[55, 56] We have confirmed the formation of fibrin sheaths in 14 patients at the time of catheter removal by injecting Renografin through the catheters after they had been withdrawn to a point where only the tip remained within the subclavian vein. In all 14 patients, well-defined tracts from the puncture site of the subclavian vein into the superior vena cava outlined the previous course of the catheter (Fig. 4–17). The earliest study, done seven days after catheter placement, demonstrated a shaggy appearing tract, suggesting an immature stage of sheath formation. Which clinical settings may lead to further deposition of thrombus and eventually complete occlusion of the subclavian vein remain to be determined. Virchow's triad of factors contributing to thrombosis includes venous stasis, hypercoagulable states, and local vessel trauma or inflammation. Preventive actions might therefore include prompt reversal of dehydration and, when possible, low-dose anticoagulation. The duration of subclavian vein catherization does not appear to play a significant role, as thrombosis occurred as early as 3 days and as late as 16 in our experience. Two reports claim avoidance of fibrin sleeve formation by use of Silastic catheters[59] or polyethylene catheters coated with graphite-benzalkonium chloride-heparin,[55] but clinical trials are needed to document any reduced incidence of subclavian vein thrombosis.

*Positional Kinking of Subclavian Catheters.* Occasionally the costoclavicular space through which subclavian catheters

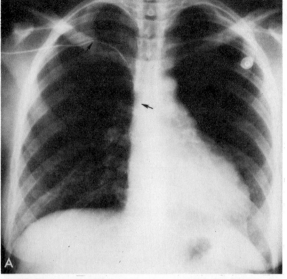

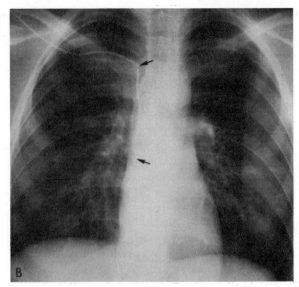

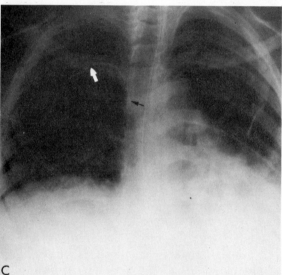

**Figure 4–17** Fibrin sheaths in the superior vena cava and subclavian veins after 8 days (a), 12 days (b), and 27 days (c) of an indwelling subclavian catheter. Arrows depict extent of sheath.

pass is so narrow that compression of the catheter occurs, and solution flow is obstructed. We have observed this in three patients, and in each case a positive pressure infusion apparatus was necessary to maintain adequate flow. Catheter kinking that obstructed solution flow has occurred in two extremely obese patients, in whom a long subcutaneous tract was present. In each case the skin had been drawn laterally prior to needle puncture in an attempt to shorten the subcutaneous tract. Apparently this stretching resulted in a right-angle kink of the catheter as it exited from the vein into the subcutaneous tissue. We now

stretch the skin toward the midline in obese patients to avoid acute catheter angulation.

## CONCLUSION

Percutaneous placement of catheters into the superior vena cava cannot be considered a routine procedure. Complication rates are related to the experience of the physician placing the catheter and increase when performed under emergency conditions. A chest x-ray must be obtained after subclavian vein catheterization, or attempted catheterization, to assure proper location of the catheter tip and to detect unsuspected complications.

We do not advocate routine changing of catheters from side to side every seven to ten days to avoid infectious complications. In our experience with 456 catheters the time a catheter is in place has had no influence on the incidence of infection. Catheters should be removed under three conditions only: at the end of therapy; upon mechanical failure, such as leaking, kinking, or obstruction; and with suspected sepsis. The exceptions to prolonged catheter life are when the catheter is placed through a burned area of skin or when exfoliative dermatitis is present, in which cases open dressings are required (see Chapter 5 on care of the catheter dressing). In these instances, catheters should be electively changed every four to seven days from one side to the other. The presence of subcutaneous emphysema about the upper chest and neck is not a contraindication to long-term subclavian vein catherization. We have treated 10 such patients, and in all, cultures of the skin puncture sites were sterile. The catheters were left in place for the duration of therapy with no catheter-related problems.

# REFERENCES

1. Duffy, B.J., Jr.: The clinical use of polyethylene tubing for intravenous therapy: A report on 72 cases. Ann. Surg., *130*:929–936, 1949.
2. Crane, C.: Venous interruption for septic thrombophlebitis. N. Engl. J. Med., *262*:947–951, 1960.
3. Henzel, J.H., and DeWeese, M.S.: Morbid and mortal complications associated with prolonged central venous cannulation. Am. J. Surg., *121*:600–605, 1971.
4. Lindenberg, J., Gjorup, S., and Aagaard, P.: Parenteral fluid administration through a catheter inserted into the inferior vena cava. Acta Chir. Scand., *117*:342–345, 1959.
5. Parsa, M.H., Ferrer, J.M., and Habif, D.V.: Long-term indwelling central venous catheters: Indications, techniques of placement, precautions and complications. A scientific exhibit, 58th Annual Clinical Congress, American College of Surgeons, Oct., 1972.
6. Scribner, B.H., Cole, J.J., Christopher, T.G., Vizzo, J.E., Atkins, R.C., and Blagg, C.R.: Long-term total parenteral nutrition. J.A.M.A., *212*:457–463, 1970.
7. Shils, M.E.: Guidelines for total parenteral nutrition, J.A.M.A., *220*:1721–1729, 1972.
8. Heizer, W.D., and Orringer, E.P.: Parenteral nutrition at home for 5 years via arteriovenous fistulae. Gastroenterology, *72*:527–532, 1977.
9. Walter, M.D., Stanger, H.A.D., and Rotem, C.E.: Complications with percutaneous central venous catheters. J.A.M.A., *220*:1455–1457, 1972.
10. Qureshi, G.D., and Lilly, E.L.: Complications of CVP catheter insertion in cubital vein. J.A.M.A., *209*:1906, 1969.
11. Hughes, E.S.R.: Collective review. Venous obstruction in upper extremity (Paget-Schroetter's syndrome): Review of 320 cases. Intern. Abstr. Surg., *88*:89–127, 1949.
12. Hoshal, V.L., Jr.: Total intravenous nutrition with peripherally inserted silicon elastomer central venous catheters. Arch. Surg., *110*:644–646, 1975.
13. MacDonald, A.S., Master, S,K.P., and Moffitt, E.A.: A comparative study of peripherally inserted silicon catheters for parenteral nutrition. Can. Anaesth. Soc. J., *24*:263–269, 1979.
14. Jernigan, W.R., Gardner, W.C., Mahr, M.M., and Milburn, J.L.: Use of the internal jugular vein for placement of central venous catheter. Surg. Gynecol. Obstet., *130*:520–524, 1970.
15. Benotti, P.N., Bothe, A., Jr., Miller, J.D.B., and Blackburn, G.L.: Safe cannulation of the internal jugular vein for long term hyperalimentation. Surg. Gynecol. Obstet., *144*:574–576, 1977.
16. Aubaniac, R.: Une nouvelle voie d'injection ou de ponction veineuse: La voie sous-claviculaire. Semin. Hop. Paris, *28*:3445–3447, 1952.
17. Wilson, J.N., Grow, J.B., Demong, C.V., Prevedel, A.E., and Owens, J.C.: Central venous pressure in optimal blood volume maintenance. Arch. Surg., *85*:55–70, 1962.
18. Ashbaugh, D., and Thomson, J.W.W.: Subclavian-vein infusion. Lancet, *2*:1138–1139, 1963.
19. Estridge, C.E., Hughes, F.A., Prather, J.R., and Clemmons, E.E.: Use of central venous pressure in the management of circulatory failure. Review of indications and technique. Am. Surg., *32*:121–125, 1966.
20. Yoffa, D.: Supraclavicular subclavian venipuncture and catheterization. Lancet, *2*:614–617, 1965.
21. Parsa, M.H., Ferrer, J.M., Habif, D.V., Forde, K.A., Sampath, A., and Lipton, R.: Experiences with central venous nutrition; problems and their prevention. Scientific exhibition presented at 57th Annual Clinical Congress, American College of Surgeons, Oct. 1971.
22. Parsa, M.H., Ferrer, J.M., and Habif, D.V.: Safe Central Venous Nutrition, Guidelines for Prevention and Management of Complications. Springfield, Ill., Charles C Thomas, Publisher, 1974.
23. Flanagan, J.P., Gradisar, I.A., Gross, R.J., and Kelly, T.R.: Air embolus — a lethal complication of subclavian venipuncture. N. Engl. J. Med., *281*:488–489, 1969.
24. Johnson, C.L., Lazarchick, J., and Lynn, H.B.: Subclavian venipuncture: Preventable complications; report of two cases. Mayo Clin. Proc., *45*:712–719, 1970.

25. Kuiper, D.H.: Cardiac tamponade and death in a patient receiving total parenteral nutrition. J.A.M.A., 230:877, 1974.
26. Land, R.E.: Anatomic relationships of the right subclavian vein. A radiologic study pertinent to percutaneous subclavian venous catheterization. Arch. Surg., 102:178–180, 1971.
27. Seropian, R., and Reynolds, B.M.: Wound infections after preoperative depilatory versus razor preparation. Am. J. Surg., 121:251–254, 1971.
28. Richardson, J.D., Grover, F.L., and Trinkle, J.K.: Intravenous catheter emboli. Experience with twenty cases and collective review. Am. J. Surg., 128:722–727, 1974.
29. Brown, C.A., and Kent, A.: Perforation of right ventricle by polyethylene catheter. South. Med. J., 49:466–467, 1956.
30. Green, H.L., and Nemir, P., Jr.: Air embolism as a complication during parenteral alimentation. Am. J. Surg., 121:614–616, 1971.
31. Johnson, C.E.: Perforation of right atrium by a polyethylene catheter. J.A.M.A., 195:584–586, 1966.
32. Friedman, B.A., and Jurgeleit, H.C.: Perforation of atrium by polyethylene CV catheter, J.A.M.A., 203:1141–1142, 1968.
33. O'Reilly, R.J.: Aberrant venous catheter position within the left chest. Contemp. Surg., 12:29–34, 1978.
34. Brady, R.E., and Weinberg, P.M.: Atrioventricular conduction disturbance during total parenteral nutrition. J. Pediatr., 88:113–114, 1976.
35. Burri, C., and Krischak, G.: Techniques and complications of administration of total parenteral nutrition. In Manni, C., Magalini, S.I., and Scrascia, E. (eds.): Total Parenteral Nutrition. New York, American Elsevier Scientific Publishing Company, 1976, pp. 306–315.
36. Yarom, R.: Subclavian venipuncture (letter to the editor). Lancet, 1:45, 1964.
37. Bernard, R.W., and Stahl, W.M.: Subclavian vein catheterizations: A prospective study. Ann. Surg., 173:184–190, 1971.
38. Vogel, C.M., Kingsbury, R.J., and Baue, A.E.: Intravenous hyperalimentation. A review of two and one-half years' experience. Arch. Surg., 105:414–419, 1972.
39. Dudrick, S.J., Wilmore, D.W., and Vars, H.M.: Long-term venous catheterization — an adjunct to surgical care and study. Curr. Top. Surg. Res., 1:325–340, 1969.
40. Tunnicliffe, F.W., and Stebbing, G.F.: Intravenous injection of oxygen gas as therapeutic measure. Lancet, 2:321, 1916.
41. Yeakel, A.E.: Lethal air embolism from plastic blood storage container. J.A.M.A., 204:267, 1969.
42. Ordway, C.B.: Air embolus via CVP catheter without positive pressure: Presentation of case and review. Ann. Surg., 179:479–481, 1974.
43. Baden, H.: Perkutan Kateterisation af v. Subclavia. Nord. Med., 71:590–593, 1964.
44. Levinsky, W.J.: Fatal air embolism during insertion of CVP monitoring apparatus. J.A.M.A., 209:966, 1969.
45. Mattox, K.L., and Bricker, D.L.: Air embolism following subclavian vein catheterization. Tex. Med., 66:74, 1970.
46. Paskin, D.L., Hoffman, W.S., and Tuddenham, W.J.: A new complication of subclavian vein catheterization. Ann. Surg., 179:266–268, 1974.
47. Durant, T.M., Long, J., and Oppenheimer, M.J.: Pulmonary (venous) air embolism. Am. Heart J., 33:269–281, 1947.
48. Oppenheimer, M.J., Durant, T.M., and Lynch, P.: Body position in relation to venous air embolism and the associated cardiovascular respiratory changes. Am. J. Med. Sci., 225:362–373, 1953.
49. Shires, T., and O'Banion, J.: Successful treatment of massive air embolism producing cardiac arrest. J.A.M.A., 167:1483–1484, 1958.
50. Block, P.C.: Transvenous retrieval of foreign bodies in the cardiac circulation, J.A.M.A., 224:241–242, 1973.
51. Rudge, C.J., Bewick, M., and McColl, I.: Hydrothorax after central venous catheterization. Br. Med. J., 3:23–25, 1973.
52. Smith, B.E., Modell, J.H., Gaub, M.L., and Moya, F.: Complications of subclavian vein catheterization. Arch. Surg., 90:228–229, 1965.
53. Saxena, V.K., Heilpern, R.J., and Murphy, S.F.: Pseudotumor cerebri. A complication of parenteral hyperalimentation. J.A.M.A. 235:2124, 1976.
54. Dudrick, S.J., Wilmore, D.W., Vars, H.M., and Rhoads, J.E.: Long-term total parenteral nutrition with growth, development and positive nitrogen balance. Surgery, 64:134–142, 1968.
55. Hoshal, V.L., Jr., Ause, R.G., and Hoskins, P.A.: Fibrin sleeve formation on indwelling subclavian central venous catheters. Arch. Surg., 102:353–358, 1971.
56. Peters, W.R., Bush, W.H., Jr., McIntyre, R.D., and Hill, L.D.: The development of fibrin sheath on indwelling venous catheters. Surg. Gynecol. Obstet., 137:43–47, 1973.
57. Firor, H.V.: Pulmonary embolization complicating total intravenous alimentation. J. Pediatr. Surg., 7:81, 1972.
58. Ryan, J.A., Jr., Abel, R.M., Abbott, W.M., Hopkins, C.C., Chesney, T. McC., Colley, R., Phillips, K., and Fischer, J.E.: Catheter complications in total parenteral nutrition. A prospective study of 200 consecutive patients. N. Engl. J. Med., 290:757–761, 1974.
59. Welch, G.W., McKeel, D.W., Silverstein, P., and Walker, H.L.: The role of catheter composition in the development of thrombophlebitis, Surg. Gynecol. Obstet., 138:421–424, 1974.
60. Keeri-Szanto, M., Fortin, G., and Rioux, A.: La voie veineuse sous-clavière en anesthesie. Can. Anaesth. Soc. J., 4:55–59, 1957.
61. Davidson, J.T., Ben-Hur, N., and Nathen, H.: Subclavian venipuncture. Lancet, 2:1139–1140, 1963.
62. Vandeghen, P., Diagneux, D., Mutsers, A., and Vanderhaeghen, N.: Le catheterisme veineux par la voie sous-clavicalaire. Rev. Franc. Gerontol., 10(Suppl):86–87, 1964.
63. Longerbeam, J.K., Vannix, R., Wagner, W., and Joergenson, E.: Central venous pressure monitoring: A useful guide to fluid therapy during shock and other forms of cardiovascular stress. Am. J. Surg., 110:220–230, 1965.

64. Loskot, F., Michaljanic, A., and Musil, J.: Right and left heart catheterization via the subclavian veins. Cardiologia, 46:114–128, 1965.
65. Malinak, L.R., Gulde, R.E., and Faris, A.M.: Percutaneous subclavian catheterization for central venous pressure monitoring: Application in obstetric and gynecologic problems. Am. J. Obstet. Gynecol., 92:477–482, 1965.
66. Matz, R.: Brief recording: Complications of determining the central venous pressure. N. Engl. J. Med., 273:703, 1965.
67. Corwin, J.H., and Moseley, T.: Subclavian venipuncture and central venous pressure: Technique and application. Am. Surg., 32:413–415, 1966.
68. Rams, J.J., Daicoff, G.R., and Moulder, P.V.: A simple method for central venous pressure measurements. Arch. Surg., 92:886, 1966.
69. Atik, M.: Application and proper interpretation of central venous pressure monitoring and the management of shock. Am. Surg., 33:118–127, 1967.
70. Christensen, K.H., Nerstrom, B., and Baden, H.: Complications of percutaneous catheterization of the subclavian vein in 129 cases. Acta Chir. Scand., 133:615–620, 1967.
71. Davis, W.S., and Akers, D.R.: Catheterization of a subclavian vein, an unusual complication. Rocky Mt. Med. J., 64:72–73, 1967.
72. Mogil, R.A., DeLaurentis, D.A., and Rosemond, G.P.: The infraclavicular venipuncture: Value in various clinical situations including central venous pressure monitoring. Arch. Surg., 95:320–324, 1967.
73. Mobin-Uddin, K., Smith, P.E., Lombardo, C., and Jude, J.: Percutaneous intracardiac pacing through the subclavian vein. J. Thorac. Cardiovasc. Surg., 54:545–548, 1967.
74. DeFalque, R.J.: Subclavian venipuncture: A review. Anesth. Analg. (Cleve.) 47:677–682, 1968.
75. Wilson, F., Nelson, J.H., and Moltz, A.: Methods and indications for central venous pressure monitoring. Am. J. Obstet. Gynecol., 101:137–151, 1968.
76. Feiler, E.M., and de Alva, W.E.: Infraclavicular percutaneous subclavian vein puncture. A safe technique. Am. J. Surg., 118:906–908, 1969.
77. Lucas, C.E., and Irani, F.: Air embolus via subclavian catheter. N. Engl. J. Med., 281:966–967, 1969.
78. Doolas, A.: Planning intravenous alimentation of surgical patients. Surg. Clin. North Am., 50:103–112, 1970.
79. McGovern, B.: Intravenous hyperalimentation. Presented at Annual Meeting, Society of Air Force Clinical Surgeons, June, 1970.
80. McDonough, J.J., and Altemeier, W.A.: Subclavian venous thrombosis secondary to indwelling catheters. Surg. Gynecol. Obstet., 133:397–400, 1971.
81. Baker, G.C., and Wilson, R.F.: Intravenous hyperalimentation. S. Afr. Med. J., 46:1493–1496, 1972.
82. Gallitano, A.L., Kondi, E.S., and Deckers, P.J.: A safe approach to the subclavian vein. Surg. Gynecol. Obstet., 135:96–98, 1972.
83. Garcia, J.M., Mispireta, L.A., and Pinho, R.V.: Percutaneous supraclavicular superior vena cava cannulation. Surg. Gynecol. Obstet., 134:839–841, 1972.
84. Buchsbaum, H.J., and White, A.J.: The use of subclavian central venous catheters in gynecology and obstetrics. Surg. Gynecol. Obstet., 136:561–563, 1973.
85. Merk, E.A., and Rush, B.F., Jr.: Emergency subclavian vein catheterization and intravenous hyperalimentation. Am. J. Surg., 129:266–267, 1975.
86. Armstrong, R., Peters, J.L., and Cohen, S.L.: Air embolism caused by fractured central venous catheter. Lancet, 1:954, 1977.
87. Grace, D.M.: Air embolism with neurological complications: A potential hazard of central venous catheters. Can. J. Surg., 20:51–53, 1977.

# Chapter 5

# CHRONIC CATHETER CARE

Patients selected for parenteral nutrition often have several factors predisposing them to infectious complications. They are usually catabolic, they often have concomitant infections, they may be receiving broad-spectrum antibiotics and perhaps steroids, and after placement of the feeding catheter, they have a foreign body within the vascular system. The placement of a central venous catheter and institution of parenteral nutrition, therefore, carry with them an obligation to maintain the system's sterility. Proper aseptic techniques for catheter insertion were discussed in Chapter 4. Aseptic preparation of the parental nutrition solution will be discussed in Chapter 8. In this chapter, catheter dressing and intravenous tubing care will be outlined. The connection tubing and the tract of the catheter to the vein are direct portals for microorganisms to enter the bloodstream and, by retrograde flow, the parenteral nutrition solution. Failure of strict asepsis at either point will significantly increase infectious complications.[1, 2]

## CARE OF INTRAVENOUS TUBING

The following list of rules is designed to assure a "closed infusion system," preventing introduction of organisms into the venous system via the tubing connecting the bottle to the patient's catheter. In most instances, changing of bottles and tubing will be done by members of the nursing staff. Frequent in-service education and close monitoring are necessary to insure observance of proper technique.

1. The intravenous administration set should be changed with each new bottle of parenteral nutrition solution. The bottle stopper should be painted with a povidone-iodine solution and allowed to stand for 60 seconds before it is pierced with the drip chamber needle. Emphasis is placed on the use of povidone-iodine instead of 70 per cent alcohol because of its broad microbial toxicity.[3-5] The old connection joint between the intravenous tubing and the patient's catheter should also be painted with povidone-iodine and allowed to stand for 60 seconds before its disconnection. After the new tubing is filled with solution, the old tubing is disconnected from the patient's catheter and the new one attached. This procedure should be done with the patient lying down to prevent air embolus.[6] Care must be taken to prevent contamination of the tubing when the new administration set is connected to either the bottle or the subclavian catheter. Connections need not be taped if they are firmly secured with a 90 degree twist as they are pushed together.

2. Proliferation of bacteria in parenteral nutrition solutions is insignificant during the first 24 hours, even at room temperature; however, in the interests of conservatism and in recognition of the possibility of atypical growth patterns, bottles of parenteral nutrition solution should be infused for no more than 12 to 18 hours. The solutions should be refrigerated until administered to inhibit bacterial and fungal growth.[2, 7] The solution should be examined against a bright

light for cloudiness or precipitants before infusion and, if abnormal, returned to the pharmacy rather than administered.

3. No stopcocks should be inserted in the administration line at any point and no piggyback injections or infusions should be given through the line.
4. No blood samples should be drawn from the catheter except to determine baseline chemistry values during its insertion or to obtain blood cultures when it is removed.
5. If the catheter becomes clotted, an attempt to free it should be made by winding the tubing tightly about the finger toward the catheter. If this procedure fails, or if a large clot is present, a member of the parenteral nutrition team should carefully irrigate the catheter at its hub under direct vision after the dressing has been removed. If irrigation fails to open the catheter, it must be removed.
6. Central venous pressure measurements can be taken through the subclavian

catheter by lowering the infusion bottle until no further solution freely drips into the patient.[8] The central venous pressure is represented by the distance between the patient's atrium and the level of fluid in the bottle exposed to atmospheric pressure (Fig. 5–1). If the closed system is broken for central venous pressure measurements, such as with insertion of a stopcock and manometer, that catheter should not be used again for infusion of parenteral nutrition solution.

## CARE OF THE CATHETER DRESSING

To assure aseptic care of the catheter puncture site, only the parenteral nutrition team should uncover or change catheter dressings. Dressings should be changed routinely every Monday, Wednesday, and Friday, as well as any time soilage occurs. The dressing should be examined at least daily to insure that it has not become soiled or wet or lost its seal. In the presence of heavy perspiration or exfoliative skin dis-

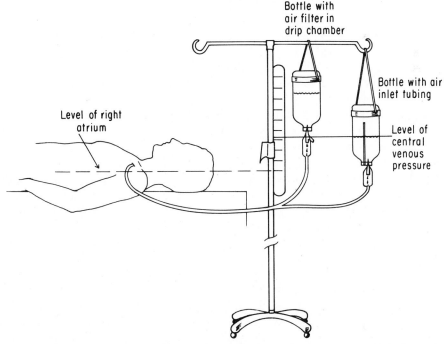

**Figure 5–1** Technique for measuring the central venous pressure with the subclavian catheter. The infusion bottle is lowered until flow stops, at which point the central venous pressure is represented by the distance between the patient's atrium and the level of fluid in the bottle exposed to atmospheric pressure. (Parsa, M. H., et al.: A new closed technique for measuring CVP. Resident Staff Phys., *17*:37–39, 1971.)

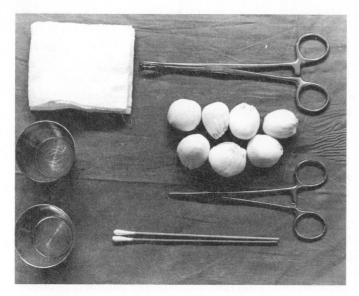

**Figure 5–2** Sterile subclavian dressing changing tray. Set includes solution cups, sponge forceps, Kelly clamp, cotton-tip applicators, and sponges.

eases, dressings may require changing daily.

To aid in dressing changes, our hospital's Central Sterile Supply Department has prepared a sterile subclavian dressing changing tray (Fig. 5–2). Minimal equipment necessary to change a dressing includes two 4 × 4 inch gauze sponges, seven gauze sponge balls, two cotton-tip applicators, two 2-ounce solution cups, one sponge forceps, and one clamp. Also available should be face masks, one bottle of acetone or ether, one bottle of 1 per cent povidone-iodine, one tube of povidone-iodine ointment, one bottle of tincture of benzoin, 2 × 2 inch sterile vaseline gauzes, sterile extension tubing, 2 inch paper tape, 2 inch adhesive tape, and 1 inch adhesive tape. If the above equipment is available, gloves need not be worn, but hands should be washed with povidone-iodine soap prior to dressing changes. If the above equipment is not available, sterile gloves should be worn. Dressings should be changed according to the following procedure:

1. Surgical masks should be worn by all personnel and by the patient. The patient is placed supine to prevent the catheter from accidentally falling out when the dressing is removed and to reduce the risk of air embolization.
2. The old dressing is carefully removed so that the underlying catheter and skin are not contaminated and the catheter remains in place.
3. A cotton-tip applicator is used to paint the connections between the extension tubing and the tubing to the bottle and between the extension tubing and catheter hub with povidone-iodine. After 60 seconds, the extension tubing is clamped. The connection between the old extension tubing and the tubing to the bottle is then separated and a new sterile extension tubing attached. After the new extension tubing is filled with fluid, the connection between the old extension tubing and the catheter hub is separated, and the new extension tubing is attached to the catheter. At this point all the old dressing can be removed.
4. The skin underlying the old bandage and extending beyond for approximately 1 inch is thoroughly defatted with acetone or ether applied with a sponge ball. Application begins at the puncture site and continues to the periphery in a circular motion. The highly volatile fat-soluble agent functions not only to defat the skin and remove old debris but also to destroy the integrity of bacterial cell walls.
5. The catheter is withdrawn 2 to 3 cm and the skin and catheter are painted with povidone-iodine.

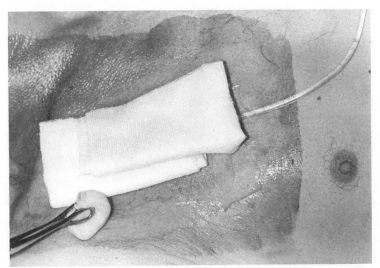

**Figure 5–3**  A sterile 3 × 4 inch gauze dressing is applied, and the skin around the dressing is painted lightly with tincture of benzoin.

6. Povidone-iodine ointment is applied around the puncture site with a cotton-tip applicator. The catheter is then reinserted to its initial position, drawing some of the ointment into the catheter tract (see Fig. 4–6). Povidone-iodine ointment is preferred to various antibiotic ointments because of its broad toxicity to both bacteria and fungi and the absence of resistant organism selection.[9] Use of antibiotic ointments has been shown to increase the incidence of fungal colonization of the catheter.[10, 11]

7. A 2 × 2 Vaseline gauze is placed over the povidone-iodine ointment to decrease absorption of the ointment into the overlying dressing and to add another barrier to contamination of the catheter in case the dressing becomes soiled.

8. The catheter hub and extension tubing are placed over the anterior chest wall medial to the nipple, and a sterile 4 × 3 gauze is placed over the Vaseline gauze and catheter hub. A 3 to 4 cm area around the dressing is painted with tincture of benzoin and allowed to dry (Fig. 5–3).

9. As the arm is slightly abducted and the neck rotated away from the dressing, 2 inch paper tape is applied in two strips on either side of the 4 × 3 dressing, angled at the top to form an inverted V, with the tubing exiting from the lower border of the dressing (Fig. 5–4). The paper tape must be applied carefully to avoid wrinkles around the edges or breaks in the seal. Next a 2 inch piece of paper tape is placed from the top down over the middle of the dressing, overlapping the paper tape strips and extending down the tubing, which exits from the inferior border of the dressing. The tape is pinched under the tubing as it exits from the inferior border of the dressing and then secured to the anterior chest wall in a butterfly fashion (see Fig. 4–7). This technique assures a good seal around the entire dressing and secures the catheter in position, preventing its accidental removal. The intravenous tubing is draped back over the dressing and taped so that it exits by the neck over the shoulder (see Fig. 4–8).

In rare instances, such as with burns or extensive exfoliative dermatitis, the catheter must be inserted through eschar or denuded skin or close to these areas, and application of an occlusive dressing is impossible. Although such situations should be avoided if possible, these catheters can be maintained with "open dressings." The catheter is secured to the shoulder with a nylon suture. Initially and every four hours, the puncture site must be

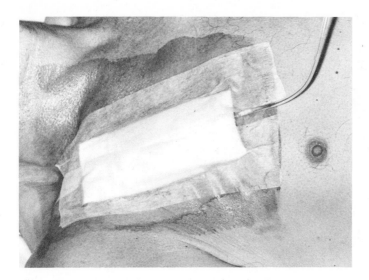

**Figure 5–4** Strips of 2 inch paper tape are applied, with a small slit left for exit of the catheter from the lower end.

cleansed with hydrogen peroxide or saline and painted widely with povidone-iodine solution, followed by application of povidone-iodine ointment and a povidone-iodine gauze. Care must be taken to minimize touch contamination. These catheters should be routinely changed every seven to ten days.

## CONCLUSION

With proper care, infectious complications related to subclavian vein catheters should be infrequent. Continual emphasis on aseptic techniques through in-service education and monitoring of patient care is essential.

## REFERENCES

1. Miller, R. C., and Grogan, J. B.: Incidence and source of contamination of intravenous nutritional systems. J. Pediatr. Surg., 8:185–190, 1973.
2. Deeb, E. N., and Natsios, G. A.: Contamination of intravenous fluids by bacteria and fungi during preparation and administration. Am. J. Hosp. Pharm., 28:764–767, 1971.
3. Connell, J. F., Jr., and Rousselot, L. M.: Povidone-iodine. Extensive surgical evaluation of a new antiseptic agent. Am. J. Surg., 108:849–855, 1964.
4. Polk, H. C., Jr., and Ehrenkranz, N. J. (eds.): Therapeutic Advances and New Clinical Implications: Medical and Surgical Antisepsis with Betadine Microbicides. The Purdue Frederick Company, U.S.A., Yonkers, N.Y., 1972.
5. Shelanski, H. A., and Shelanski, M. V.: PVP-iodine: History, toxicity and therapeutic uses. J. Int. Coll. Surg., 25:727–734, 1956.
6. Green, H. L., and Nemir, P., Jr.: Air embolism as a complication during parenteral alimentation. Am. J. Surg., 121:614–616, 1971.
7. Brennan, M. F., O'Connell, R. C., Rosol, J. A., and Kundsin, R.: The growth of *Candida albicans* in nutritive solutions given parenterally. Arch. Surg., 103:705–708, 1971.
8. Parsa, M. H., Ferrer, J. M., and Habif, D. V.: A new, closed technique for measuring CVP. Resident Staff Phys., 17:37–39, 1971.
9. Vanderwyk, R. W.: Microbicidal Effectiveness of Betadine Surgical Scrub (povidone-iodine) versus Hexachlorophene. The Purdue Frederick Company, U.S.A., Yonkers, N.Y., 1971.
10. Norden, C. W.: Application of antibiotic ointment to the site of venous catheterization — a controlled trial. J. Infect. Dis., 120:611–615, 1969.
11. Zinner, S. H., Denny-Brown, B. C., Braun, P., Burke, J. P., and Kass, E. H.: Risk of infection with intravenous indwelling catheters: Effect of application of antibiotic ointment. J. Infect. Dis., 120:616–619, 1969.

# Chapter 6

# BASIC HUMAN METABOLISM RELATING TO PARENTERAL NUTRITION

To estimate daily metabolic requirements during intravenous nutrition, it is necessary to understand normal metabolic requirements and the effects of short- and long-term starvation and acute trauma on those requirements. This chapter will review principles of human metabolism related to intravenous nutrition. Owing to the complex nature of the subject, the discussion will at times be cursory, and the reader is encouraged to refer to the cited literature and recent books[1-4] for further review.

## NORMAL BODY COMPOSITION

A 70 kg human is composed of approximately 55 per cent water, 40 per cent organic materials, and 5 per cent minerals.[5] The actual water content is inversely related to the amount of body fat and diminishes progressively with age.[6] Itemization of the body's organic materials and caloric equivalents indicates approximately 166,000 total calories to be present (Table 6–1).[7] Of the 6 kg of body protein, muscle protein accounts for 4 kg and hemoglobin for 1 kg. The remaining 1 kg is located in various body organs, with serum protein representing a very small fraction.[8] During starvation the body's organic materials are utilized to provide energy for essential metabolic processes. There is a limit, however, to this self-cannibalism, as loss of more than a third of the total body weight during stress or prolonged starvation is often fatal.[7, 9-11]

**Table 6–1** CALORIC EQUIVALENTS OF ORGANIC COMPONENTS IN A 70 kg HUMAN

| KG | SUBSTANCE | CALORIC EQUIVALENT |
|---|---|---|
| 15.0 | Fat (intracellular triglyceride) | 141,000 |
| 6.0 | Protein | 24,000 |
| 0.225 | Glycogen | 900 |
| 0.02 | Extracellular glucose | 80 |
| 0.0003 | Plasma free fatty acids | 3 |
| 0.003 | Plasma triglycerides | 30 |
| | | Total    166,013 |

Modified from Cahill, G. F., Jr.: Starvation in man. N. Engl. J. Med., *282*:668–675, 1970. Reprinted by permission from the New England Journal of Medicine.

## NORMAL NUTRITIONAL REQUIREMENTS

*Calories.* The traditional unit of energy used in clinical nutrition in the United States is the kilocalorie (kcal). This unit represents the amount of heat required to raise the temperature of 1 kg of water from 14.5° to 15.5° C at standard atmospheric pressure. The average daily caloric intake for a 70 kg man is 2,700 kcal. Approximately 324 kcal are provided by dietary protein (81 grams), 1126 kcal by fat (125 grams), and 1250 kcal by carbohydrate (312 grams). Basal caloric requirements in kcal/hour, or minimal caloric requirements to maintain body weight in healthy, trained subjects at rest, may be determined by finding the rel-

evant value on a basal metabolic rate chart (Fig. 6–1)[12] and multiplying by the patient's body surface area (Fig. 6–2).[13]

*Protein.* Recommended oral protein intake for adults is 0.8 gram/kg/day. Most oral diets contain more than this recommended amount. The minimal amount of protein required to maintain positive nitrogen balance in healthy adults has been estimated by two methods. In the first, called the factorial method, nitrogen requirements were estimated by measuring nitrogen losses during complete protein restriction. Healthy young adults placed on protein-free diets demonstrate a progressive decrease in urinary nitrogen loss, which plateaus after seven to ten days at about 37 mg/kg/day.[14-17] About 12 mg ni-

| AGE IN YEARS | kcal/sq m/hr | |
|---|---|---|
| | *Men* | *Women* |
| 1 | 53.0 | 53.0 |
| 2 | 52.4 | 52.4 |
| 3 | 51.3 | 51.2 |
| 4 | 50.3 | 49.8 |
| 5 | 49.3 | 48.4 |
| 6 | 48.3 | 47.0 |
| 7 | 47.3 | 45.4 |
| 8 | 46.3 | 43.8 |
| 9 | 45.2 | 42.8 |
| 10 | 44.0 | 42.5 |
| 11 | 43.0 | 42.0 |
| 12 | 42.5 | 41.3 |
| 13 | 42.3 | 40.3 |
| 14 | 42.1 | 39.2 |
| 15 | 41.8 | 37.9 |
| 16 | 41.4 | 36.9 |
| 17 | 40.8 | 36.3 |
| 18 | 40.0 | 35.9 |
| 19 | 39.2 | 35.5 |
| 20 | 38.6 | 35.3 |
| 25 | 37.5 | 35.2 |
| 30 | 36.8 | 35.1 |
| 35 | 36.5 | 35.0 |
| 40 | 36.3 | 34.9 |
| 45 | 36.2 | 34.5 |
| 50 | 35.8 | 33.9 |
| 55 | 35.4 | 33.3 |
| 60 | 34.9 | 32.7 |
| 65 | 34.4 | 32.2 |
| 70 | 33.8 | 31.7 |
| 75 and over | 33.2 | 31.3 |

**Figure 6–1** Normal basal metabolic rates at different ages for each sex. (Reprinted by permission from Plenum Medical Book Company, New York, as published in Wilmore, D. W.: The Metabolic Management of the Critically Ill, 1977.)

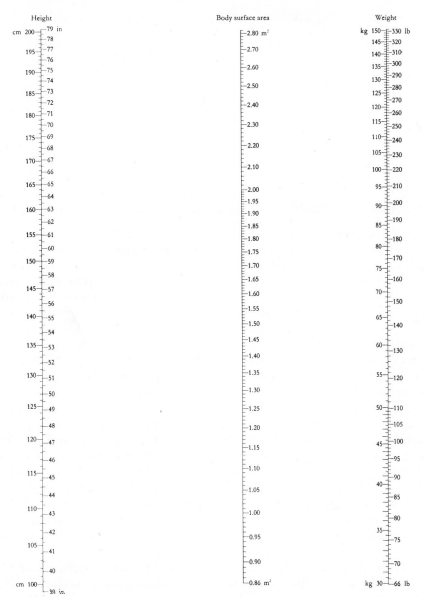

**Figure 6-2**   Nomogram for determination of body surface area from height and weight. (From Diem, K., and Lentner, C., eds.: Scientific Tables, 7th Edition. Basle, Switzerland, Ciba-Geigy Limited, 1970.)

trogen per kilogram per day are excreted in the feces. This represents unabsorbed gastrointestinal secretions and desquamated cells.[15, 17] Nitrogen lost through the skin amounts to about 3 mg/kg/day.[18] Small amounts of nitrogen are also excreted in the breath as ammonia, in menstruation and seminal ejaculation, and in the saliva, sputum, and nasal secretions. These average about 2 mg/kg/day.[19] Summation indicates an average nitrogen loss of 54 mg/kg/day. Converted to dry protein (conversion factor N × 6.25), this represents an average of 0.34 gram/kg/day. To maintain nitrogen balance, an equivalent amount of protein must be replaced daily.

The second method bases nitrogen requirements on the minimum protein intake necessary to maintain nitrogen equilibrium. Various studies utilizing different protein sources, such as whole egg, cow's milk, soy flour, and rice, indicate that the minimum protein intake ranges from 0.38 to 0.52 gram/kg/day.[17, 20, 21]

**Table 6–2**  ESSENTIAL AMINO ACIDS IN ADULT HUMAN DIET

| AMINO ACID | MINIMAL DAILY REQUIREMENT (grams) | RECOMMENDED SAFE INTAKE (grams) |
|---|---|---|
| Lysine | 0.80 | 1.60 |
| Tryptophan | 0.25 | 0.50 |
| Phenylalanine | 1.10 | 2.20 |
| Methionine | 1.10 | 2.20 |
| Threonine | 0.50 | 1.00 |
| Leucine | 1.10 | 2.20 |
| Isoleucine | 0.70 | 1.40 |
| Valine | 0.80 | 1.60 |

From Rose, W. C., et al.: Amino acid requirements of man; valine requirement; summary and final observations. J. Biol. Chem. *217*:987–995, 1955.

Ideally, the two methods should provide similar values. The higher protein requirement found with the second method suggests that dietary proteins are used somewhat inefficiently. To compensate for this inefficiency, an intake of 0.43 gram protein per kilogram is accepted as the minimum daily requirement. A study of elderly patients suggested that their minimum protein requirement was 0.6 gram/kg/day, which is 40 per cent greater than for younger adults.[22] The above estimates for protein requirements apply only to the trained healthy adult in a basal state. As will be discussed later, the protein requirements of traumatized and stressed patients are significantly greater than the minimum daily requirements (see Chapter 7).

In addition to protein needs, essential amino acid requirements must also be met. In the healthy adult, there are eight essential amino acids (Table 6–2). In spite of many difficulties in determining dietary requirements for essential amino acids,[23] there is fairly close agreement between reports.[24, 25] The most thorough and widely accepted study of essential amino acid requirements for the adult human is that of Rose et al. in 1954 and 1955 (Table 6–2).[26–31] Several studies on the essential amino acid requirements of elderly patients have given contradictory results.[32–35]

The studies by Rose were performed with orally administered protein, of which more than 99 per cent is absorbed in the small bowel. During digestion and absorption, protein is hydrolyzed to free amino acids and small peptides.[36] The peptides are hydrolyzed to free amino acids within the mucosal cell for absorption as such into the portal vein. Aspartic and glutamic acids are transaminated to oxaloacetate and α-ketoglutarate in the intestinal mucosa, with only a fraction entering the systemic blood. In addition, absorbed amino acids pass directly to the liver, where many are metabolized. Elwin[37] estimated that 57 per cent of absorbed amino acid nitrogen in dogs passed out of the liver into the blood as urea, 6 per cent was secreted from the liver as plasma protein, 14 per cent was retained in the liver as protein, and only 23 per cent passed into the systemic circulation as free amino acids. Analysis of these free amino acids indicated that hepatic metabolism was primarily of straight-chain amino acids, while branch-chain amino acids (isoleucine, leucine, and valine) passed into the systemic circulation.[38, 39]

When commercially available amino acid solutions are administered intravenously, bypassing the liver, the amino acid composition of the blood is markedly altered, reflecting the composition of the infused amino acid solution.[40–43] In particular, isoleucine, leucine, and valine concentrations are much lower, while other amino acid concentrations are considerably higher than normal. In addition, there is some indication that nitrogen given intravenously, rather than orally, is more readily taken up by peripheral tissues than by the liver and is not as available for the synthesis of plasma proteins.[44, 45] It thus becomes important to determine both total protein and essential amino acid requirements during intravenous feeding. These studies have yet to be done. Furst et al.[46] measured nitrogen balance in healthy women given 5 grams amino acid nitrogen intravenously per day with varying proportions as essential amino acids. Although they did not attempt to determine the minimum requirements for non-essential or essential amino acids, their study did show that not more than 700 mg/kg/day total amino acids with 140 mg/kg/day as essential amino acids were required to maintain nitrogen balance. Nitrogen balance studies similar to those performed by Rose et al. are needed to determine requirements of intravenously administered non-essential and essential amino acids. From such studies, more nearly ideal amino acid solutions could be formulated.

The amount of intravenously administered nitrogen necessary to establish positive nitrogen balance can be determined clinically in individual patients by using the factorial method. The estimated insensible loss of 5 mg/kg/day nitrogen is added to nitrogen losses measured in 24-hour urine collections. An additional 12 mg/kg/day are added to replace nitrogen losses from the gastrointestinal tract. The daily nitrogen input is simply increased until calculations show a positive nitrogen balance.

*Fats.* The average fat intake ranges from 100 to 180 grams/day for adults. Saturated fatty acids account for approximately 37 per cent, oleic acid 40 per cent and linoleic acid about 12 per cent of the total. Under normal conditions, 95 per cent or more of ingested fat is absorbed in the proximal small bowel. Since 1929, with the work of Burr and Burr,[47] it has been recognized that three polyunsaturated fatty acids cannot be synthesized by man: linoleic, arachidonic, and linolenic. These fatty acids, which are made by plants from oleic acid, have been considered essential to the diet. Yet, the importance of linolenic acid remains to be established, as it appears to compensate for only part of deficiencies of the other two fatty acids. Arachidonic acid can be synthesized in man in the presence of adequate linoleic acid. It appears, therefore, that only linoleic acid is actually essential in the diet of man.

Linoleic acid composes 8 to 10 per cent of the adipose tissue depot. This can amount to as much as 700 grams linoleic acid in the normal individual — enough to meet the body's requirements for months, or even years. Initially, essential fatty acid deficiency was observed only in thin patients after prolonged fasting or in newborn infants. More recently, however, deficiencies in adults have been observed within the first month of fat-free parenteral nutrition (see Chapter 9). The infusion of hypertonic dextrose with parenteral nutrition greatly reduces lipolysis and limits release of endogenous linoleic acid. The daily requirements for linoleic acid must, therefore, be provided during parenteral nutrition. The minimal requirement for linoleic acid is estimated to be between 25 and 100 mg/kg/day.[48–51] Studies of infused fat (Intralipid) suggest that more linoleic acid may be necessary when given intravenously.[51, 52] Cutaneous manifestations of essential fatty acid deficiency, as well as some systemic effects, can be corrected with application of 2 to 3 mg/kg/day linoleic acid to the skin.[53]

*Carbohydrates.* The average diet contains about 312 grams carbohydrate, representing about 1250 kcal. Cellulose and pentosans cannot be digested by man and are excreted in the feces. Polysaccharides are degraded to monosaccharides in the gut by pancreatic enzymes. It is as monosaccharides (glucose, fructose, and galactose) that carbohydrate is absorbed, mainly in the proximal small bowel by an active transport process.[54] Both fructose and galactose are rapidly converted by the liver to glucose, the major carbohydrate of human metabolism. When glucose intolerance prevents adequate caloric support, as may occur in patients with pancreatic dysfunction, stress, shock, or marked malnutrition, or in the elderly or very young, exogenous insulin can be added to enhance glucose utilization without apparently interfering with the endogenous insulin response.[55, 56]

## METABOLIC EFFECTS OF SHORT-TERM STARVATION

When dietary intake is abruptly interrupted, the body rapidly turns to endogenous, "stored" calories to provide energy for essential functions. Initially, the central nervous system is dependent on glucose as an energy substrate, requiring 100 to 150 grams/day and metabolizing it completely to carbon dioxide and water.[57] If this requirement is not met, a rapid alteration of neuronal activity, accompanied by personality changes, confusion, lethargy, and coma, follows. Irreversible damage occurs if carbohydrate deprivation is prolonged. The renal medulla, bone marrow, red blood cells, and peripheral nerves require a total of 30 to 40 grams glucose a day and metabolize it to lactate and pyruvate.[58-60] The lactate can be recycled back to glucose through the Cori cycle in the liver and kidney, a process that utilizes energy derived from oxidation of fatty acids.[61] The pyruvate can serve as a metabolic substrate in the formation of ATP or for gluconeogenesis in the liver (Fig. 6-3). Fibroblasts and phagocytes derive most of their energy from the anaerobic metabolism of glucose to lactate.[60] The liver derives much of its energy from the oxidation of free fatty acids to acetoacetate, acetone, and β-hydroxy-

butyrate (the ketone bodies). The heart, skeletal muscle, and renal cortex, although utilizing glucose for a major share of their energy during normal nutrition, can and do utilize free fatty acids and ketone bodies during starvation.[60]

Since glycogen and extracellular glucose reserves are small (see Table 6-1), and since muscle glycogen cannot be converted to blood glucose because of a lack of glucose-6-phosphatase in muscle, man depends mainly on gluconeogenesis to meet obligatory glucose requirements. The normal glycolysis pathway is shown in Figure 6-3. Although most steps are reversible, three enzymes are necessary for gluconeogenesis to occur. The first is a specific phosphatase ① capable of converting fructose diphosphate to fructose-6-phosphate. This enzyme is highly active during conditions of fasting, diabetes, and glucocorticoid excess. This increased activity aids in conversion of glycerol, derived from hydrolysis of triglycerides, into glucose.[58] Phosphoenolpyruvate carboxykinase ② catalyzes the conversion of oxalacetate to phosphoenolpyruvate. This step permits oxalacetate, and any substance that can be transformed into oxalacetate, such as aspartate, to serve as substrates for gluconeogenesis. Finally, pyruvate carboxylase ③ catalyzes conversion of pyruvate to oxalacetate, thereby al-

**Figure 6-3** Glycolysis

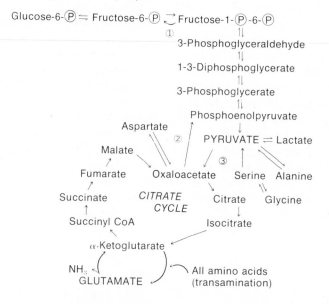

lowing lactate, alanine, serine, and similar substances to enter gluconeogenesis upon their conversion into pyruvate. It is apparent from Figure 6–3 that such substrates as lactate, pyruvate, glycerol, dicarboxylic acids, and amino acids can all be utilized for gluconeogenesis.

Gluconeogenesis occurs mainly in the liver and kidney, with up to half of the total glucose produced derived from the kidney as starvation continues.[62] The main substrate for gluconeogenesis in the kidney is glutamine,[63] with other amino acids being converted into it by transamination (see Fig. 6–3). The main nitrogenous by-product is ammonia, which is partly excreted in the urine and partly reutilized in protein synthesis. The main amino acid substrate for gluconeogenesis in the liver is alanine.[64] Felig[65] and Mallette et al.[66] proposed a glucose-alanine cycle between skeletal muscle and the liver (Fig. 6–4). The branch-chain amino acids (valine, leucine, and isoleucine) are preferentially transaminated in muscle and provide the major source of nitrogen for the synthesis of alanine from pyruvate.[67-69] The nitrogenous by-product of liver gluconeogenesis is urea, which is partly excreted in the urine and partly reutilized in protein synthesis.

During starvation approximately 75 grams of body protein and 160 grams of adipose tissue are metabolized each day for every 1800 kcal utilized.[59, 60] All endogenous proteins are utilized, including those that play important metabolic roles, such as plasma and liver proteins and digestive enzymes.[8, 70, 71] Serum albumin is used in the ratio of 1 gram albumin to 30 grams tissue protein lost.[72] The most clini-cally evident protein loss, however, is from skeletal muscles.

Lipolysis, which is quite sensitive to serum insulin levels,[73] releases free fatty acids and glycerol. The free fatty acids cannot participate directly in gluconeogenesis[8, 56] but serve as an energy source in the liver for the Cori cycle[61] and generate acetyl coenzyme A, which enhances the conversion of pyruvate to oxalacetate.[74] The glycerol is readily converted to glucose but is of minor consequence, providing only about 18 grams glucose per 24 hours.[59] Metabolism of triglycerides is associated with a slight elevation of free fatty acids to greater than 1.0 mEq per liter[75] and an elevation of serum ketone bodies (starvation ketosis) to 1 to 1.5 mmoles per liter.[76] Starvation ketosis may provide the signal for reduction in alanine synthesis by muscle and facilitate the conversion of the central nervous system to ketone body metabolism, as discussed below.[77]

## METABOLIC EFFECTS OF PROLONGED STARVATION

With prolonged fasting there is a gradual decrease in metabolic rate and total body energy expenditure. This decreased metabolic activity is manifested by diminished muscle activity, increased sleep, and decreased core temperature. There is a gradual shift to the use of fats for energy and decreased requirements for glucose. Protein catabolism falls from 75 grams to 20 grams/day, and the efficiency of amino acid reutilization increases, resulting in a marked decrease in excretion

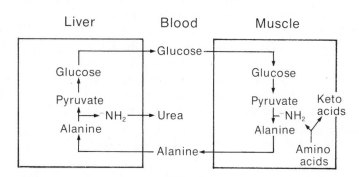

**Figure 6–4** Glucose-alanine cycle. (From Felig, P.: The glucose-alanine cycle. Metabolism, 22:179–207, 1973; Mallette, L. E., et al.: Effects of glucagon on amino acid transport and utilization in the perfused rat liver. J. Biol. Chem., 244: 5724–5728, 1969.)

of blood urea nitrogen to 3 to 5 grams/day.[14, 60, 78] As starvation continues, the central nervous system gradually converts to metabolism of ketone bodies for energy, and after three weeks, only a small glucose requirement remains.[79, 80] Consequently, gluconeogenesis decreases, and protein catabolism provides as little as 5 per cent of the total daily calories. Adipose tissue becomes an important energy substrate, with 60 per cent of the total caloric expenditure derived from metabolism of fat to carbon dioxide, 10 per cent from conversion of free fatty acids to ketone bodies, and 25 per cent from metabolism of ketone bodies by peripheral tissues.[16] Ketosis increases with ketone body production and represents a physiologic response to starvation. The provision of fluid requirements as 5 per cent dextrose solutions, long advocated to decrease proteolysis and starvation ketosis,[7, 23, 81, 82] has recently come under question. The actual effect of administration of 100 to 150 grams dextrose a day is a combination of (1) reduced requirements for gluconeogenesis from amino acids and glycerol and (2) an increased endogenous insulin release, which reduces lipolysis, increases protein synthesis, and increases requirements for gluconeogenesis. Indeed, improved nitrogen sparing has been demonstrated with the addition of 3 per cent amino acid solutions to isotonic carbohydrate solutions or to sterile water in both non-stressed and stressed patients.[76, 83, 84]

## ACUTE STRESS

*Catabolic Response.* When starvation is complicated by acute trauma or severe stress, marked alterations in metabolism occur, as first described by Cuthbertson in 1930.[85] These dramatic changes, termed "the catabolic response," are typified by increased oxygen consumption and also increased urinary losses of nitrogen in great excess of the amount of tissue injured. Cuthbertson suggested that this response was beneficial, supplying calories and amino acids needed following injury

or during acute stress.[86] Indeed, it does appear that there are synthetic needs for carbohydrate intermediates not provided by fatty acid metabolism but met by increased protein degradation.[87] In addition, protein catabolism may provide the amino acids acutely needed for synthesis of blood and structural proteins and various enzymes.[88] For whatever purpose, protein catabolism commonly results in the loss of 40 grams nitrogen or more a day, approximating 1 kg wet muscle tissue.[60] Most of the nitrogen is excreted in the urine as urea. Additional losses include hemorrhage (1 liter whole blood is equivalent to 30.4 grams nitrogen), transudates and exudates, wound drainage, and intestinal losses. The level of previous nutrition strongly influences nitrogen excretion during the catabolic response.[89-91] Patients who are severely protein-depleted have the smallest increases in losses of urinary urea nitrogen and, in general, have a poorer clinical prognosis.[92]

Cuthbertson stated that the net nitrogen loss associated with catabolic responses could not be avoided during the first eight days, even with maximal nutritional support.[86, 93] The development of parenteral nutrition has demonstrated that this is not true.[94-97] Administration of parenteral nutrition does not prevent the catabolic response, but rather apparently overwhelms the associated negative nitrogen balance. In our experience, achievement of early positive nitrogen balance has not been difficult. In the following cases (Fig. 6–5), nitrogen balance was determined from measured inputs and calculated outputs according to the factorial method. Urinary nitrogen levels were determined by the micro-Kjeldahl technique.

Patient E.N. underwent partial gastrectomy for retroperitoneal lymphoma invading and obstructing the stomach. Parenteral nutrition was begun on the second postoperative day. Positive nitrogen balance was obtained by the next day.

Patient R.N. had squamous cell carcinoma on the floor of the mouth and

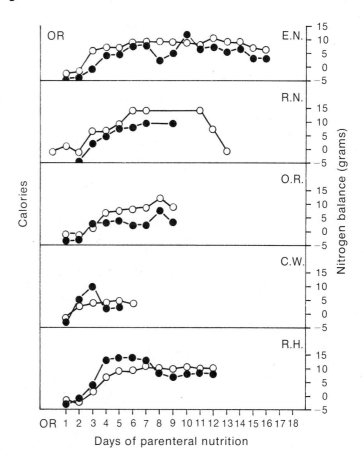

**Figure 6–5** Nitrogen balance studies in postoperative patients demonstrating rapid establishment of positive nitrogen balance (see text). ○–○, Calories infused; •–•, nitrogen balance.

underwent a wide local resection. He was given parenteral nutrition the second day after surgery and was in positive nitrogen balance within 24 hours.

Patient O.R. underwent a radical hysterectomy for stage II carcinoma of the cervix and received parenteral nutrition three days later. Again, within 24 hours she was in positive nitrogen balance.

Patient C.W. underwent bypass of a small bowel obstruction due to metastatic carcinoma of the ovary. She was started on parenteral nutrition during the first postoperative day and was in positive nitrogen balance within 24 hours.

Patient R.H. had a total pelvic exenteration for recurrent carcinoma of the cervix. She was placed on parenteral nutrition the third day following surgery and was in positive nitrogen balance 24 hours later.

*Electrolyte and Acid-Base Changes.* Electrolyte losses after trauma or during stress reflect cellular destruction arising from either the trauma itself or subsequent proteolysis. In the urine, excretion of potassium, phosphate, sulfate, and magnesium, as well as creatinine, creatine, and uric acid, are all elevated.[68] Retention of bicarbonate and sodium due to aldosterone activity results in a persistently acidic urine and the development of mild metabolic alkalosis. The alkalosis may be aggravated by blood transfusions because of the oxidation of citrate to bicarbonate. Further, loss of hydrogen ions through nasogastric suction and hyperventilation from excitement and central nervous system stimulation can add to the alkalosis. It is not uncommon for blood pH to increase to 7.5 or 7.6.

**Table 6–3** HORMONAL CHANGES IN VARIOUS STATES OF NUTRITION

| HORMONE | EFFECT | STARVATION | | D5W | STRESS |
|---|---|---|---|---|---|
| | | *Marasmus* | *Kwashiorkor* | | |
| Catecholamines | Catabolic | sl ↑ | sl ↑ | ± | ⤊ |
| Glucocorticoids | Catabolic | ⇈ | ↑ | nl | ⤊ |
| Growth hormone | Anabolic | ↑ | ⇈ | nl | ↑ |
| Androgens | Anabolic | nl | nl | nl | ↓ |
| Insulin:glucagon ratio | Anabolic: catabolic | ↓ | ↓ | nl to sl ↑ | ⇊ |
| Aldosterone | Sodium retention | sl ↑ | ↑ | nl to sl ↑ | ⇈ |
| Antidiuretic hormone | Water retention | sl ↑ | sl ↑ | nl | ⇈ |

nl = normal; sl = slight; ↑ ( ↓ ) = increase (decrease); ⇈ (⇊) = moderate increase (decrease); ⤊ (⤋) = marked increase (decrease).

## ENDOCRINE RESPONSE TO STARVATION AND STRESS

Endocrine responses to starvation and stress are often complex (Table 6–3). To simplify this discussion, the endocrine response will be divided into substances enhancing catabolism, those stimulating anabolism, and those influencing fluid and electrolyte balance. The degree of stimulation and the relative potency of each hormone determines the overall host response.

## CATABOLIC HORMONES

*Catecholamines.* The adrenalin response to stress and injury was first described by Cannon in 1939.[98] The two catecholamines, epinephrine and norepinephrine, are secreted following a large variety of stimuli, including excitement, fear, anger, tissue injury, and fractures.[99] Epinephrine, which is secreted only by the adrenal medulla, stimulates hepatic glycogenolysis and gluconeogenesis, inhibits secretion of insulin,[100] inhibits uptake of glucose by peripheral tissues,[101] favors release of amino acids from muscle, and directly stimulates hydrolysis of fat.[99, 102–104] Norepinephrine, produced throughout the body at nerve synapses and also by the adrenal medulla, has less marked metabolic activity but does stimulate fat hydrolysis.[104, 105] Because of their

extremely short biologic half-lives, the metabolic effects of catecholamines are transient, lasting only 24 to 48 hours.[106, 107] During severe stress or trauma, however, their effects may be prolonged by continued secretion and can contribute to tissue ischemia. Both epinephrine and norepinephrine greatly increase metabolic activity and account for the posttraumatic hypermetabolic response and increased heat production. In addition to their direct metabolic effects, catecholamines stimulate release of glucagon from the pancreas[108] and adrenocorticotrophic hormone (ACTH) from the pituitary, resulting in glucocorticoid and aldosterone secretion.

*Glucocorticoids.* Elevations of both free and conjugated 17-hydroxycorticosteroids to two to five times normal are characteristic of trauma.[109–112] With minimal injury, elevations are transient, lasting only 7 to 10 days.[106] With prolonged stress or injury, the free and conjugated steroids can remain elevated for weeks or months, leading to hypertrophy of the adrenal cortex. Corticoids, in addition to their steroid effects, increase total body fat and augment lipolysis,[58] inhibit protein synthesis, facilitate amino acid mobilization from skeletal muscle,[113] and decrease renal tubular reabsorption of amino acids, increasing amino aciduria.[114] In addition, corticosteroids induce transaminating enzymes for gluconeogenesis,[115, 116] suppress insulin secretion,[117] and liberate glucagon.[118] They further enhance the conversion of lactic acid to glycogen[119, 120] and protect the lysosomal membrane against pH changes.[121]

## ANABOLIC HORMONES

*Growth Hormone.* Human growth hormone is produced by the acidophilic cells of the anterior pituitary gland. It stimulates nitrogen, phosphorus, and potassium retention, and also lypolysis, fatty acid oxidation, and ketogenesis.[122] In addition, it inhibits insulin,[123] thereby depressing glucose uptake by muscle and subsequently elevating blood glucose levels, and stimulates synthesis of chondroitin sulfate and collagen. During starvation or hyperglycemia, blood levels of human growth hormone may be elevated two to three times above normal. Stress, such as in hypoglycemia, exercise, hemorrhage, surgery, burns, and sepsis, is also a strong growth hormone stimulant.[72, 112, 124–126] Ingestion of high-protein meals and infusion of amino acids (especially arginine) are both potent stimulators of growth hormone secretion in the absence of fasting or stress.

*Androgens.* Testosterone is considered the major androgen.[127] The normal female produces 0.34 mg/day and the male 7 mg/day. This hormone has potent anabolic activity, stimulating retention of nitrogen, potassium, phosphorus, and calcium and increasing lean body and visceral protein masses. It may also function to decrease amino acid catabolism. Little change is seen in androgen production during fasting and only a slight decrease follows stress.

*Insulin and Glucagon.* Secretions of the pancreatic islet cells play a major role in the regulation of body fuels. Insulin, secreted by the beta cell, functions as a potent anabolic hormone. It promotes storage of exogenous glucose, inhibits gluconeogenesis and glycogenolysis,[76] strongly inhibits lypolysis,[73] and favors protein synthesis. Glucagon, on the other hand, secreted by the pancreatic alpha cell, is a potent catabolic hormone. It acts

to prevent hypoglycemia by stimulating gluconeogenesis, glycogenolysis, proteolysis, and lypolysis.[128, 129] The pancreatic delta islet cells are interposed between the alpha and beta cells and may regulate both by secretion of the inhibitory hormone somatostatin.[129, 130] The interreactions between the pancreatic islet cells result in very precise glucose homeostasis. The absolute concentrations of insulin and glucagon appear not to be as important in glucose homeostasis as the insulin:glucagon molar ratio.[131, 132] Following an overnight fast, or elective surgery, the insulin:glucagon molar ratio is only slightly depressed from its normal level of about 4.0, favoring moderate gluconeogenesis.[133–135] Further starvation, up to six to eight days, and any condition of stress are associated with a marked depression of the ratio to as low as 0.4,[133–137] strongly favoring catabolism. The increased glucagon secretion is felt to play a prominent role in stimulating the glucose-alanine cycle of catabolism, as discussed above.[138] With prolonged starvation there is an increased production of ketone bodies, which in turn stimulate the release of insulin.[76] As discussed earlier, insulin inhibits lipolysis, thereby reducing ketosis. Further, the increased insulin:glucagon molar ratio reduces the rate of catabolism. Metabolic processes during starvation and stress are thus finely regulated by various feedback mechanisms.

In non-diabetic subjects, infusion of carbohydrate results in an increased insulin:glucagon ratio as high as 70,[133] while infusion of amino acids decreases it. The simultaneous infusion of hypertonic dextrose and amino acids, as in total parenteral nutrition, has a synergistic effect on insulin release and results in a marked increase in the insulin:glucagon ratio favoring anabolism.[128, 139, 140]

Certain diseases may be associated with hyperglucagonemia, which makes the establishment of anabolism during parenteral nutrition more difficult. Glucagon is cleared from the plasma by the liver[141, 142] and by the kidney.[143] In either hepatic or renal failure, decreased glucagon clearance can become significant. Further, diabetic patients often demonstrate baseline hyperglucagonemia, an exaggerated release of glucagon with protein meals, and a paradoxical increase in glucagon with carbohydrate infusion.[133]

## FLUID AND ELECTROLYTE BALANCE

*Aldosterone.* Aldosterone secretion decreases renal excretion of sodium and bicarbonate while increasing potassium losses. By increasing sodium ion concentrations in the serum and thus serum osmolarity, the extracellular fluid volume is increased. Aldosterone secretion is increased by catecholamines and hyponatremia. In addition, isotonic hypovolemia stimulates renin release by the renal juxtaglomerular apparatus; this promotes angiotensin formation, which in turn stimulates aldosterone release.[144, 145] Uncomplicated starvation is associated with only small increases in aldosterone secretion, while the major fluid shifts of trauma may result in marked increases.

*Antidiuretic Hormone.* Antidiuretic hormone (ADH) inhibits free-water clearance by the kidneys.[109, 146–148] Clinical situations associated with hypovolemia or hyperosmolality stimulate the release of antidiuretic hormone, which results in an increase in intravascular volume and a decrease in osmolality.

As discussed above, the two hormones of fluid and electrolyte balance respond primarily to decreased intravascular volume and decreased serum osmolality. After surgery, trauma, or prolonged malnutrition, patients will often be markedly dehydrated, with depleted intravascular volumes. Initiation of parenteral nutrition in these patients may be associated with marked initial fluid retention until the intravascular volume is replenished. Solution formulas reflecting normal serum electrolyte content are most effective in replacing the intravascular volume, while hypotonic electrolyte solutions are contraindicated and can lead to the syndrome of "inappropriate ADH secretion" with excessive shifting of fluid into extravascular spaces.[149, 150]

## RECOVERY FROM STARVATION AND STRESS

If the hospital course remains uncomplicated, the metabolic and endocrine changes of acute stress or injury usually run their course in the first two to seven days. With aggressive nutritional support, patients can usually be converted to an anabolic state soon after trauma or stress, decreasing their metabolic losses and possibly shortening their recovery period. Normal nitrogen anabolism occurs at a rate of approximately 3 to 5 grams nitrogen per 70 kg per day.[151] It is, therefore, possible to predict the approximate duration of metabolic recovery by dividing the estimated total nitrogen loss by the average daily gain. The actual time required to replace all nitrogen losses is somewhat longer than calculated, since maximum anabolism is not immediately obtained nor always maintained. During recovery, essential amino acid, total protein, and caloric requirements are all greater than normal.[106, 152] After nitrogen losses have been restored, fat is gained almost exclusively for several weeks or months until the normal body fat stores are regained.[68] In this phase, nitrogen balance is zero, although carbon balance is positive.

## CONCLUSION

This chapter has dealt with normal metabolic requirements as well as the metabolic effects of starvation and acute stress. An understanding of these metabolic requirements, as well as those for vitamins, electrolytes, and minerals, which will be discussed in later chapters, is mandatory for the proper administration of parenteral nutrition. Every effort should be made to recognize and assess catabolic losses and to avoid significant nutritional depletion by providing adequate nutritive support early. If nutritional support is provided before marked wasting occurs, an anabolic state is more easily obtained and maintained. Freeman and MacLean[153] reported that the protein requirement for nitrogen balance in normal subjects maintained on a protein-deficient diet and subsequently fed intravenously was 33 per cent higher than that of subjects on normal diets prior to intravenous alimentation. The difficulty of achieving anabolism is increased when acute stress or injury is superimposed on malnutrition. With vigorous nutritional support the morbidity and mortality associated with prolonged starvation and acute stress should be appreciably reduced.

## REFERENCES

1. American College of Surgeons, Committee on Pre- and Postoperative Care: Manual of Surgical Nutrition. Philadelphia, W. B. Saunders Company, 1975.
2. Lee, H. A.: Parenteral Nutrition in Acute Metabolic Illness. New York, Academic Press, Inc., 1974.
3. Wilkinson, A.: Parenteral Nutrition. Edinburgh, Churchill Livingstone, 1972.
4. Ghadimi, H.: Total Parenteral Nutrition. New York, John Wiley & Sons, Inc., 1975.
5. Kinney, J. M., and Moore, F. D.: Surgical metabolism and metabolism of body fluids. In Zimmerman, L., and Levine, R. (eds.): Physiological Principles of Surgery. Philadelphia, W. B. Saunders Company, 1964.
6. Edelman, I. S., and Leibman, J.: Anatomy of body water and electrolytes. Am. J. Med., 27:256–277, 1959.
7. Cahill, G. F., Jr.: Starvation in man. N. Engl. J. Med., 282:668–675, 1970.
8. Dudrick, S. J., and Rhoads, J. E.: Metabolism in surgical patients: Protein, carbohydrate and fat utilization by oral and parenteral routes. In Sabiston, D. C. (ed.): Davis-Christopher Textbook of Surgery, 11th Edition. Philadelphia, W. B. Saunders Company, 1977, p. 152.
9. Studley, H. O.: Percentage of weight loss: basic indicator of surgical risk in patients with chronic peptic ulcer. J.A.M.A. 106:458–460, 1936.
10. Lawson, L. J.: Parenteral nutrition in surgery. Br. J. Surg., 52:795–800, 1965.
11. Morgan, A., Filler, R. M., and Moore, F. D.: Surgical nutrition. Med. Clin. North Am., 54:1367–1381, 1970.
12. Fleisch, A.: Le metabolism basal standard et sa determination au moyen du "Metabolicalculator." Helv. Med. Acta, 18:23, 1951.
13. Diem, K., and Lentner, C. (eds.): Scientific Tables, 7th Edition. Basle, Switzerland, Ciba-Geigy Limited, 1970.
14. Munro, H. N.: General aspects of the regulation of protein metabolism by diet and hormones. In Munro, H. N., and Allison, J. B. (eds.): Mammalian Protein Metabolism, Vol. I. New York, Academic Press, Inc., 1964, pp. 382–413.
15. Young, V. R., and Scrimshaw, N. S.: Endogenous nitrogen metabolism and plasma free amino acids in young adults given a "protein-free" diet. Br. J. Nutr., 22:9–20, 1968.
16. Owen, O. E., Felig, P., Morgan, A. P., Wahrem, J., and Cahill, G. F., Jr.: Liver and kidney metabolism during prolonged starvation. J. Clin. Invest., 48:574–583, 1969.
17. Calloway, D. H., and Margen, S.: Variation in endogenous nitrogen excretion and dietary nitrogen utilization as determinants of human protein requirement. J. Nutr., 101:205–216, 1971.
18. Sirbu, E. R., Margen, S., and Calloway, D. H.: Effect of reduced protein intake on nitrogen loss from the human integument. Am. J. Clin. Nutr., 20:1158–1165, 1967.
19. Calloway, D. H., Odell, A. C. F., and Margen, S.: Sweat and miscellaneous nitrogen losses in human balance studies. J. Nutr., 101:775–786, 1971.
20. Bricker, M., Mitchell, H. H., and Kinsman, G. M.: The protein requirements of adult human subjects in terms of the protein contained in individual foods and food combinations. J. Nutr., 30:269–283, 1945.
21. Inone, G., Fujita, Y., and Nujama, Y.: Personal communication as reported by Munro, H. N.: Basic concepts in the use of amino acids and protein hydrolysates for parenteral nutrition. Drug Intel. Clin. Pharm., 6:216–224, 1972.
22. Kountz, W. B., Hofstatter, L., and Ackermann, P. G.: Nitrogen balance studies in four elderly men. J. Gerontol., 6:20–33, 1951.
23. Calloway, D. H., and Spector, H.: Nitrogen balance as related to caloric and protein intake in active young men. Am. J. Clin. Nutr., 2:405–411, 1954.
24. Irwin, M. I., and Hegsted, D. M.: A conspectus of research on amino acid requirements of man. J. Nutr. 101:539–566, 1971.
25. Fisher, H., Brush, M. K., and Griminger, P.: Reassessment of amino acid requirements of young women on low nitrogen diets. II. Leucine, methionine, and valine. Am. J. Clin. Nutr., 24:1216–1223, 1971.
26. Rose, W. C., Lambert, G. F., and Coon, M. J.: Amino acid requirements of man; general procedures; tryptophan requirement. J. Biol. Chem., 211:815–827, 1954.
27. Rose, W. C., Leach, B. E., Coon, M. J., and Lambert, G. F.: Amino acid requirements of man; phenylalanine requirements. J. Biol. Chem., 213:913–922, 1955.
28. Rose, W. C., Borman, A., Coon, M. J., and Lambert, G. F.: Amino acid requirements of man; lysine requirements. J. Biol. Chem., 214:579–587, 1955.
29. Rose, W. C., Coon, M. J., Lockhart, H. B., and Lambert, G.: Amino acid requirements of

man; threonine and methionine requirements. J. Biol. Chem., 215:101–110, 1955.

30. Rose, W. C., Eades, C. H., Jr., and Coon, M. J.:
Amino acid requirements of man; leucine
and isoleucine requirements. J. Biol.
Chem., 216:225–234, 1955.

31. Rose, W. C., Wixom, R. L., Lockhart, H. B.,
and Lambert, G. F.: Amino acid requirements of man; valine requirement; summary and final observations. J. Biol. Chem.,
217:987–995, 1955.

32. Tuttle, S. G., Swendseid, M. E., Mulcare, D.,
Griffith, W. H., and Bassett, S. H.: Study
of the essential amino acid requirements of
men over fifty. Metabolism, 6:564–573,
1957.

33. Tuttle S. G., Swendseid, M. E., Mulcare, D.,
Griffith, W. H., and Bassett, S. H.:Essential
amino acid requirements of older men in
relation to total nitrogen intake. Metabolism, 8:61–72, 1959.

34. Tuttle, S. G., Bassett, S. H., Griffith, W. H.,
Mulcare, D. B., and Swendseid, M. E.: Further observations on the amino acid requirements of older men. II. Methionine
and lysine. Am. J. Clin. Nutr., 16:229–231,
1965.

35. Watts, J. H., Mann, A. N., Bradley, L., and
Thompson, D. J.: Nitrogen balances of men
over 65 fed the FAO and milk patterns of
essential amino acids. J. Gerontol., 19:370–
374, 1965.

36. Fauconneau, G., and Michel, M. C.: The role of
the gastrointestinal tract in the regulation of
protein metabolism. In Monro, H. H. (ed.):
Mammalian Protein Metabolism, Vol. 4.
New York, Academic Press, Inc., 1970, pp.
481–522.

37. Elwyn, D. H.: The role of the liver in regulation
of amino acid and protein metabolism. In
Munro, H. H. (ed.): Mammalian Protein
Metabolism, Vol. 4. New York, Academic
Press, Inc., 1970, pp. 523–558.

38. Miller, L. L.: The role of the liver and the non-
hepatic tissues in the regulation of free amino
acid levels in the blood. In Holden, J. T. (ed.):
Amino Acid Pools. Amsterdam, Elsevier/
North Holland Biomedical Press, 1962, pp.
708–721.

39. Mimura, T., Yamada, C., and Swendseid, M.
E.: Influence of dietary protein levels and
hydrocortisone administration on the
branched-chain amino acid transaminase
activity in rat tissues. J. Nutr., 95:493–497,
1968.

40. Elman, R.: Amino-acid content of blood following intravenous injection of hydrolyzed casein. Proc. Soc. Exp. Biol. Med. 37:437–440,
1937.

41. Ghadimi, H., Abaci, F., Kumar, S., and Rathi,
M.: Biochemical aspects of intravenous alimentation. Pediatrics, 48:955–965, 1971.

42. Stegink, L. D., and Baker, G. L.: Infusion of
protein hydrolysates in the newborn infant: Plasma amino acid concentrations. J.
Pediatr., 78:595–602, 1971.

43. Dudrick, S. J., MacFadyen, B. V., Jr., Van
Buren, C. T., Ruberg, R. L., and Maynard,
A. T.: Parenteral hyperalimentation. Meta-

bolic problems and solutions. Ann. Surg.,
176:259–264, 1972.

44. Christensen, H. N., Lynch, E. L., Decker, D.
G., and Powers, J. H.: The conjugated,
non-protein, amino-acids of plasma. IV. A
difference in the utilization of the peptides
of hydrolysates of fibrin and casein. J. Clin.
Invest., 26:849–852, 1947.

45. Furst, P., Jonsson, A., Josephson, B., and Vinnars, E.: Distribution on muscle and liver
vein protein of $^{15}N$ administered as ammonium acetate to man. J. Appl. Physiol.,
29:307–312, 1970.

46. Furst, P., Josephson, B., and Vinnars, E.: The
effect on the nitrogen balance of the ratio
essential–nonessential acids in intravenously
infused solutions. Scand. J. Clin. Lab. Invest., 26:319–326, 1970.

47. Burr, G. O., and Burr, M. M.: A new deficiency
disease produced by the rigid exclusion of
fat from the diet. J. Biol. Chem., 82:345–
367, 1929.

48. Holman, R. T.: Essential fatty acid deficiency.
In Holman, R. T. (ed.): Progress in the
Chemistry of Fats and Other Lipids, Vol. 9,
Part 2. Oxford, Pergamon Press Ltd., 1968,
p. 285.

49. Hansen, A. E., Haggard, M. E., Boelsche, A.
N., Adam, D. J. D., and Wiese, H. F.: Es-
sential fatty acids in infant nutrition. J.
Nutr., 66:565–576, 1958.

50. Caldwell, M. D., Jonsson, H. T., and Othersen,
H. B., Jr.: Essential fatty acid deficiency in
an infant receiving prolonged parenteral alimentation. J.Pediatr., 81:894–898, 1972.

51. Collins, F. D., Sinclair, A. J., Royle, J. P.,
Coats, D. A., Maynard, A. T., and Leonard, R. F.: Plasma lipids in human linoleic
acid deficiency. Nutr. Metab., 13:150–167,
1971.

52. Jeejeebhoy, K. N., Zohrab, W. J., Langer, B.,
Phillips, M. J., Kuksis, A., and Anderson,
G. H.: Total parenteral nutrition at home
for 23 months without complication and
with good rehabilitation. A study of technical and metabolic features. Gastroenterology, 65:811–820, 1973.

53. Press, M., Hartop, P. J., and Prottey, C.: Correction of essential fatty-acid deficiency in
man by the cutaneous application of sun-
flower-seed oil. Lancet, 1:597–598, 1974.

54. McCoy, S., and Drucker, W. R.: Carbohydrate
metabolism. In American College of Surgeons, Committee on Pre- and Postoperative Care: Manual of Surgical Nutrition.
Philadelphia, W. B. Saunders Company,
1975, pp. 13–15.

55. Dudrick, S. J., Long, J. M., Steiger, E., and
Rhoads, J. E.: Intravenous hyperalimentation. Med. Clin. North Am., 54:577–589,
1970.

56. Dennis, C., and Grosz, C. R.: A quarter century
of intracaval feeding. Surg. Gynecol. Obstet., 135:883–889, 1972.

57. Ferrendelli, J. A.: Cerebral utilization of non-
glucose substrates and their effect in hypoglycemia. In Plum, F. (ed.): Brain Dysfunction in Metabolic Disorders. New York,
Raven Press, 1974, p. 113.

58. Levine, R., and Haft, D. E., Carbohydrate homeostasis. N. Engl. J. Med., 283:175–183, 1970.
59. Cahill, G. F., Jr., Herrera, M. G., Morgan, A. P., Soeldner, J. S., Steinke, J., Levy, P. L., Reichard, G. A., Jr., and Kipnis, D. M.: Hormone-fuel interrelationships during fasting. J. Clin. Invest., 45:1751–1769, 1966.
60. Cahill, G. F., Jr., Felig, P., and Marliss, E. P.: Some physiological principles of parenteral nutrition. In Nahas, G., and Fox, C. (eds.): Body Fluid Replacement in the Surgical Patient, Part IV. New York, Grune & Stratton, Inc., 1969, pp. 286–295.
61. Exton, J. H.: Progress in endocrinology and metabolism, gluconeogenesis. Metabolism, 21:945–990, 1972.
62. Owen, O. E., Felig, P., Morgan, A. P., Wahren, J., and Cahill, G. F., Jr.: Liver and kidney metabolism during prolonged starvation. J. Clin. Invest., 48:574–583, 1969.
63. Pitts, R. F.: Renal production and excretion of ammonia. Am. J. Med., 36:720–742, 1964.
64. Saudek, C. D., and Felig, P.: The metabolic events of starvation. Am. J. Med., 60:117–126, 1976.
65. Felig, P.: The glucose-alanine cycle. Metabolism, 22:179–207, 1973.
66. Mallette, L. E., Exton, J. H., and Park, C. R.: Effects of glucagon on amino acid transport and utilization in the perfused rat liver. J. Biol. Chem., 244:5724–5728, 1969.
67. Felig, P., Owen, O. E., Wahren, J., and Cahill, G. F., Jr.: Amino acid metabolism during prolonged starvation. J. Clin. Invest., 48:584–594, 1969.
68. Moore, F. D.: Homeostasis: Bodily changes in trauma and surgery. In Sabiston, D. C. (ed.): Davis-Christopher Textbook of Surgery, 11th Edition. Philadelphia, W. B. Saunders Co., 1977, pp. 27–64.
69. Felig, P., and Wahren, J.: Muscle nitrogen repletion after protein ingestion: Key role of branched chain amino acids and evidence of a new defect in diabetes. Clin. Res., in press.
70. Whipple, G. H.: The Dynamic Equilibrium of Body Proteins. Springfield, Ill., Charles C Thomas, Publisher, 1956.
71. Filkins, J. P.: Lysosomes and hepatic regression during fasting. Am. J. Physiol., 219:923–927, 1970.
72. Elman, R.: Parenteral Alimentation in Surgery. New York, Hoeber Medical Books (Harper & Row, Publishers, Inc.) 1947.
73. Tarrant, M. E., and Ashmore, J.: Sequential changes in adipose tissue metabolism in alloxan-diabetic rats. Diabetes, 14:179–185, 1965.
74. Scrutton, M. C., and Utter, M. F.: The regulation of glycolysis and gluconeogenesis in animal tissues. Annu. Rev. Biochem., 37:249–302, 1968.
75. Issekutz, B. Jr., Boatz, W. M., Miller, H. I., and Paul, P.: Turnover rate of plasma FFA in humans and in dogs. Metabolism, 16:1001–1009, 1967.
76. Blackburn, G. L., Flatt, J. P., Clowes, G. H. A., Jr., O'Donnell, T. F., and Hensle, T. E.: Protein sparing therapy during periods of starvation with sepsis or trauma. Ann. Surg., 177:588–594, 1973.
77. Sherwin, R. S., Hendler, R. G., and Felig, P.: Effect of ketone infusion on amino acid and nitrogen metabolism in man. J. Clin. Invest., 55:1382–1390, 1975.
78. Rand, W. M., Young, V. R., and Scrimshaw, N. S.: Change of urinary nitrogen excretion in response to low-protein diets in adults. Am.J. Clin. Nutr., 29:639–644, 1976.
79. Owen, O. E., Morgan, A. P., Kemp, H. G., Sullivan, J. M., Herrera, M. G., and Cahill, G. F., Jr.: Brain metabolism during fasting. J. Clin. Invest., 46:1589–1595, 1967.
80. Skoloff L.: Metabolism of ketone bodies by the brain. In Creger, W. P.: Annual Review of Medicine, Vol. 24. Palo Alto, Calif., Annual Reviews, Inc., 1973.
81. Gamble, J. L.: Physiological information gained from studies on the life raft ration. Harvey Lect., 42:247–273, 1947.
82. Randall, H. T.: Fluid and electrolyte therapy. In American College of Surgeons, Committee on Pre- and Postoperative Care: Manual of Preoperative and Postoperative Care. Philadelphia, W. B. Saunders Company, 1967, p. 24.
83. Blackburn, G. L., Flatt, J. P., Clowes, G. H. A., and O'Donnell, T. E.: Peripheral intravenous feeding with isotonic amino acid solutions. Am. J. Surg., 125:447–454, 1973.
84. Hoover, H. C., Grant, J. P., Gorschboth, C. and Ketcham, A. S.: Nitrogen-sparing intravenous fluids in postoperative patients. N. Engl. J. Med., 293:172–175, 1975.
85. Cuthbertson, D. P.: The disturbance of metabolism produced by bony and non-bony injury, with notes on certain abnormal conditions of bone. Biochem. J., 24:1224–1263, 1930.
86. Cuthbertson, D. P.: Further observations on the disturbance of metabolism caused by injury, with particular reference to the dietary requirements of fracture cases. Br. J. Surg., 23:505–520, 1936.
87. Coleman, S. E.: Metabolic interrelationships between carbohydrates, lipids, and proteins. In Bondy, P. K.: Diseases of Metabolism. Philadelphia, W. B. Saunders Company, 1969, p. 89.
88. Blackburn, G. L., and Flatt, J. P.: Metabolic response to illness: Role of protein-sparing therapy. Compr. Ther., 1:23–29, 1975.
89. Munro, H. N., and Cuthbertson, D. P.: The response of protein metabolism to injury. Biochem J., 37:XII, 1943.
90. Abbott, W. E., and Albertsen, K.: The effect of starvation, infection and injury on the metabolic processes and body composition. Ann. N.Y. Acad. Sci., 110:941–964, 1963.
91. Johnston, I. D. A.: The endocrine response to trauma. In Scientific Basis of Medicine: Annual Review. London, Oxford University Press, 1968, pp. 224–241.
92. Kinney, J. M.: Calories-nitrogen–disease and injury relationships. In Symposium on Total Parenteral Nutrition. Chicago, American Medical Association, 1972, pp. 35–45.

93. Cuthbertson, D. P., Fell, G. S., and Tilstone, W. J.: Nutrition in the post-traumatic period. Nutr. Metab., 14:92–109, 1972.

94. Rush, B. F., Jr., Richardson, J. D., and Griffen, W. O.: Positive nitrogen balance immediately after abdominal operations. Am. J. Surg., 119:70–76, 1970.

95. VanWay, C. W., III, Meng, H. C., and Sandstead, H. H.: Nitrogen balance in postoperative patients receiving parenteral nutrition. Arch. Surg., 110:272–276, 1975.

96. Loirat, Ph., Rohan, J. E., Chapman, A., Beaufils, F., David, R., and Nedey, R.: Positive nitrogen balance in hypercatabolic states: Results obtained with parenteral feeding after major surgical procedures. Europ. J. Intensive Care Med., 1:11–17, 1975.

97. Byrd, H. S., Lazarus, H. M., and Torma, M. J.: Effects of parenteral alimentation on postoperative gastric function. Am. J. Surg., 130:688–693, 1975.

98. Cannon, W. B.: The Wisdom of the Body. New York, W. W. Norton & Co., Inc., 1939, pp. 263–285.

99. Walker, W. F., Zileli, M. S., Reutter, F. W., Shoemaker, W. C., Friend, D., and Moore, F. D.: Adrenal medullary secretion in hemorrhagic shock. Am. J. Physiol., 197:773–780, 1959.

100. Porte, D., Jr., and Robertson, R. P.: Control of insulin secretion by catecholamines, stress, and the sympathetic nervous system. Fed. Proc., 32:1792–1796, 1973.

101. Kinney, J. M., Long, C. L., and Duke, J. H.: Carbohydrate and nitrogen metabolism after injury. In Porter, R., and Knight, J. (eds.): Energy Metabolism in Trauma. London, J. & A. Churchill, 1970, p. 103.

102. Hammond, W. G., Aronow, L., and Moore, F. D.: Studies in surgical endocrinology. III. Plasma concentrations of epinephrine and norepinephrine in anesthesia, trauma and surgery, as measured by a modification of the method of Weil-Malherbe and Bone. Ann. Surg., 144:715–732, 1956.

103. De Bodo, R. C., and Altszuler, N.: Insulin hypersensitivity and physiological insulin antagonists. Physiol. Rev., 38:389–445, 1958.

104. Havel, R. J., and Goldfien, A.: The role of the sympathetic nervous system in the metabolism of free fatty acids. J. Lipid Res., 1:102–108, 1959.

105. Walker, W. F., Reutter, F. W., Zileli, M. S., Friend, D., and Moore, F. D.: Effects of infusion of norepinephrine on blood hormone levels, electrolytes and water excretion in man. J. Surg. Res., 1:272–277, 1961.

106. Moore, F. D.: Metabolic Care of the Surgical Patient. Philadelphia, W. B. Saunders Company, 1959, p. 460.

107. Groves, A. C., Griffiths, J., Leung, F., and Meek, R. N.: Plasma catecholamines in patients with serious postoperative infection. Ann. Surg., 178:102–107, 1973.

108. Gerich, J. E., Karam, J. H., and Forsham, P. H.: Stimulation of glucagon secretion by epinephrine in man. J. Clin. Endocrinol. Metab., 37:479–481, 1973.

109. Hume, D. M.: The neuro-endocrine response to injury: Present status of the problem. Ann. Surg., 138:548–557, 1953.

110. Moore, F. D., Steenburg, R. W., Ball, M. R., Wilson, G. W. and Myrden, J. A.: Studies in surgical endocrinology. I. The urinary excretion of 17-hydroxycorticoids, and associated metabolic changes, in cases of soft tissue trauma of varying severity and in bone trauma. Ann. Surg., 141:145–174, 1955.

111. Gold, N. I., Smith, L. L., and Moore, F. D.: Cortisol metabolism in man: Observations of pathways, pool sizes of metabolites, and rates of formation of metabolites. J. Clin. Invest., 38:2238–2252, 1959.

112. Ross, H., Johnston, I. D. A., Welborn, T. A., and Wright, A. D.: Effect of abdominal operation on glucose tolerance and serum levels of insulin, growth hormone, and hydrocortisone. Lancet, 2:563–566, 1966.

113. Clark, I.: Effect of cortisone upon protein synthesis. J. Biol. Chem., 200:69–76, 1953.

114. Albanese, A. A., Lorenze, E. J., and Orto, L. A.: Nutritional and metabolic effects of some newer corticosteroids. New York J. Med., 61:3998–4002, 1961.

115. Welt, I. D., Stetten, D., Jr., Ingle, D. J., and Morley, E. H.: Effect of cortisone upon rates of glucose production and oxidation in the rat. J. Biol. Chem., 197:57–66, 1952.

116. Schumner, W.: The metabolic effects of trauma. Contemporary Surg., 1:39–45, 1972.

117. Perley, M., and Kipnis, D. M.: Effects of glucocorticoids on plasma insulin. New Engl. J. Med., 274:1237–1241, 1966.

118. Marco, J., Calle, C., Roman, D., Diaz-Fierros, M., Villanueva, M. L., and Valverde, I.: Hyperglucagonism induced by glucocorticoid treatment in man. New Engl. J. Med., 288:128–131, 1973.

119. Oji, N., and Shreeve, W. W.: Gluconeogenesis from 14-C and 3H-labeled substrates in normal and cortisone-treated rats. Endocrinology, 78:765–772, 1966.

120. Friedmann, N., Exton, J. H., and Park, C. R.: Interaction of adrenal steroids and glucagon on gluconeogenesis in perfused rat liver. Biochem. Biophys. Res. Commun., 29:113–119, 1967.

121. Janoff, A., Weissmann, G., Zweifach, B. W., and Thomas, L.: Pathogenesis of experimental shock. IV. Studies on lysosomes in normal and tolerant animals subjected to lethal trauma and endotoxemia. J. Exp. Med., 16:451–466, 1962.

122. Drenick, E. J., Gold, E. M., and Elrick, H.: Acute symptomatic ketoacidosis following growth hormone administration in prolonged fasting. Metabolism, 19:608–613, 1970.

123. Levine, R.: Analysis of the actions of the hormonal antagonists of insulin. Diabetes, 13:362–365, 1964.

124. Glick, S. M., Roth, J., Yalow, R. S., and Berson, S. A.: The regulation of growth hormone secretions. Recent Prog. Horm. Res., 21:241–283, 1965.

125. Dillon, R. S.: Handbook of Endocrinology. Philadelphia, Lea & Febiger, 1973, pp. 167–173.

126. Wright, P. D., and Johnston, I. D. A.: The effect of surgical operation on growth hormone levels in plasma. Surgery, *77*:479–486, 1975.

127. Paulsen, C. A.: The testes. *In* Williams, R. H. (ed.): Textbook of Endocrinology, 5th Edition. Philadelphia, W.B. Saunders Company, 1974.

128. Unger, R. H., and Orci, L.: Physiology and pathophysiology of glucagon. Physiological Rev., *56*:778–826, 1976.

129. Liljenquist, J. E., Mueller, G. L., Cherrington, A. D., Keller, V., Chiasson, J. L., Perry, J. M., Lacy, W. W., and Rabinowitz, D.: Evidence for an important role of glucagon in the regulation of hepatic glucose production in normal man. J. Clin. Invest., *59*:369–374, 1977.

130. Orci, L., and Unger, R. H.: Hypothesis: functional subdivision of islets of Langerhans and possible role of D-cells. Lancet, *2*:1243–1244, 1975.

131. Parrilla, R., Goodman, M. N., and Toews, C. J.: Effect of glucagon:insulin ratios on hepatic metabolism. Diabetes, *23*:725–731, 1974.

132. Unger, R. H.: Alpha- and beta-cell interrelationships in health and disease. Metabolism, *23*:581–593, 1974.

133. Unger, R. H.: Glucagon physiology and pathophysiology. New Engl. J. Med., *285*:443–448, 1971.

134. Lindsey, A., Santeusanio, F., Braaten, J., Faloona, G. R., and Unger, R. H.: Pancreatic alpha-cell function in trauma. J.A.M.A., *227*:757–761, 1974.

135. Pozefskyy, T., Tancredi, R. G., Moxley, R. T., Dupre, J., and Tobin, J. D.: Effects of brief starvation on muscle amino acid metabolism in nonobese man. J. Clin. Invest., *57*:444–449, 1976.

136. Unger, R. H.: Glucagon physiology and pathophysiology: Abnormal alpha cell function as a characteristic of human diabetes mellitus. New Engl. J. Med., *285*:443–449, 1971.

137. Meguid, M. M., Brennan, M. F., Aoki, T. T., Muller, W. A., Ball, M. R., and Moore, F. D.: Hormone-substrate interrelationships following trauma. Arch. Surg., *109*:776–783, 1974.

138. Muller, W. A., Rocha, D., Faloona, G. R., and Unger, R. H.: Alanine-glucagon relationships in the control of gluconeogenesis. Clin. Res., *19*:480, 1971. (abstract)

139. Dudrick, S. J., Long, J. M., and Steiger, E.: Intravenous hyperalimentation. Med. Clin. North Am., *84*:577–589, 1970.

140. Floyd, J. C., Jr., Fajans, S. S., Pek, S., Thiffault, C. A., Knopf, R. T., and Conn, J. W.: Synergistic effect of essential amino acids and glucose upon insulin secretion in man. Diabetes, *19*:109–115, 1970.

141. Assan, R.: *In vivo* metabolism of glucagon, *In* Lefebvre, P. J., and Unger, R. H. (eds.): Glucagon, Molecular Physiology, Clinical and Therapeutic Implications. Oxford, Pergamon Press Ltd., 1972, pp. 47–59.

142. Kakiuchi, S., and Tomizawa, H. H.: Properties of glucagon-degrading enzyme of beef liver. J. Biol. Chem., *239*:2160–2164, 1964.

143. Lefebvre, P. J., and Luyckx, A. S.: Effect of acute kidney exclusion by ligation of renal arteries on peripheral plasma glucagon levels and pancreatic glucagon production in the anesthetized dog. Metabolism, *24*:1169–1176, 1975.

144. Skillman, J. J., Lauler, D. P., Hickler, R. B., Lyons, J. H., Olson, J. E., Ball, M. R., and Moore, F. D.: Hemorrhage in normal man: Effect on renin, cortisol, aldosterone, and urine composition. Ann. Surg., *166*:865–885, 1967.

145. Hayes, M. A., Williamson, R. J., and Heidenreich, W. F.: Endocrine mechanisms involved in water and sodium metabolism during operation and convalescence. Surgery, *41*:353–386, 1957.

146. Ganong, W. F.: Review of Medical Physiology. Los Altos, Calif., Lange Medical Publications, 1963, pp. 162–163.

147. Shu'ayb, W. A., Moran, W. H., Jr., and Zimmermann, B.: Studies of the mechanism of antidiuretic hormone secretion and the post-commissurotomy dilutional syndrome. Ann. Surg., *162*:690–701, 1965.

148. Kerrigan, G. A., Talbot, N. B., and Crawford, J. D.: Role of neurohypophyseal–antidiuretic-hormone–renal system in everyday clinical medicine. J. Clin. Endocrinol., *15*:265–275, 1955.

149. Drucker, W. R., and Wright, H. K.: Physiology and pathophysiology of gastrointestinal fluids. Current Problems in Surgery. Chicago, Year Book Medical Publishers, Inc., 1964, p. 63.

150. Hoye, R. C., Bennett, S. H., Geelhoed, G. W., and Gorschboth, C.: Fluid volume and albumin kinetics occurring with major surgery. J.A.M.A., *222*:1255–1261, 1972.

151. Shils, M. E.: Guidelines for total parenteral nutrition. J.A.M.A., *220*:1721–1729, 1972.

152. Lawson, L. J.: Parenteral nutrition in surgery. Br. J. Surg., *52*:795–800, 1965.

153. Freeman, J. P., and MacLean, L. D.: Intravenous hyperalimentation: A review. Can. J. Surg., *14*:180–194, 1971.

# Chapter 7

# ADMINISTRATION OF PARENTERAL NUTRITION SOLUTIONS

The provision of sufficient calories and nitrogen to convert a metabolic state from catabolism to anabolism entails significant alterations in fluid, electrolyte, and mineral requirements. Methods for determining these requirements and suggestions for administering parenteral nutrition will be discussed in this chapter. In addition, standard orders for monitoring patients and providing nursing care will be outlined.

## FLUID REQUIREMENT

Requirements for fluid can be estimated from body weight (Fig. 7–1) or from body surface area (Fig. 7–2). Determinations made from body weight slightly overestimate fluid requirements of obese patients and underestimate requirements of thin patients. Use of body surface area, in which both height and weight are considered, is more accurate. Either method indicates adequate fluid levels for normal urinary excretion (1200 to 1500 ml/day) and replacement of normal insensible losses (500 to 1000 ml/day). Adjustments must be made for other measured losses (those from diuresis, diarrhea, and various drainage tubes), unmeasurable losses (third-space fluid following surgery or trauma and losses from burns or wounds), and losses associated with elevated temperature (360 ml per degree C per day). Patients breathing humidified air, either by mask or by endotracheal tube, lose less fluid a day from their lungs than patients breathing room air, and in some instances they may gain water.

Both the body weight and the body surface formulas assume that 350 to 500 ml/day of endogenous water will be produced from oxidation of body fat (1 gram fat = 9 calories = 1 ml water) and proteolysis (1 kg body cell mass loss = 800 to 850 ml water). When patients are given parenteral nutrition and converted to an anabolic state, endogenous water production is greatly reduced, increasing daily fluid requirements. To determine fluid requirements during parenteral nutrition, therefore, basic fluid requirements should first be estimated. To this value, 800 to 1000 ml water should be added to substitute for endogenous water production (350 to 500 ml) and to provide new intracellular water (400 to 500 ml). Other unusual losses, measurable and unmeasurable, must also be replaced with appropriate electrolyte solutions (Table 7–1)

Significant fluid shifts accompany the onset of anabolism and account for early changes seen in body weight. With starvation there is a mild loss of total body water (TBW) with a shift of intracellular water (ICW) to extracellular water (ECW) spaces. Even with adequate fluid administration, ICW may be 18 to 20 per cent below normal and ECW 10 to 15 per cent above normal. If dehydration is also present, ICW losses are about the same, but ECW and TBW losses increase.[1, 2] When adequate nutrition is

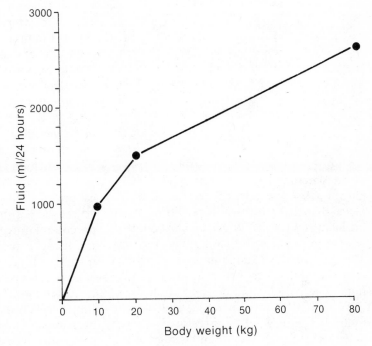

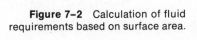

**Figure 7–1** Calculation of fluid requirements based on body weight.

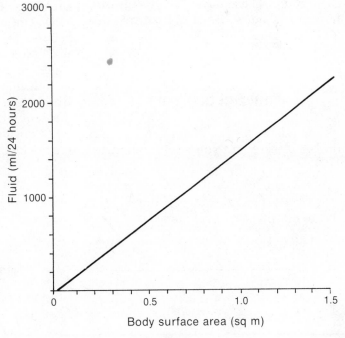

**Figure 7–2** Calculation of fluid requirements based on surface area.

**Table 7-1** APPROXIMATE ELECTROLYTE CONCENTRATIONS OF VARIOUS BODY FLUIDS (mEq/liter)

| SOURCE | VOLUME/DAY | Na | K | Cl | HCO₃ |
|---|---|---|---|---|---|
| Gastric | 2000 to    pH < 4 | 60 | 10 | 90 | — |
|  | 2500       pH > 4 | 100 | 10 | 100 | — |
| Pancreas | 1000 | 140 | 5 | 75 | 90 |
| Bile | 1500 | 140 | 5 | 100 | 35 |
| Small bowel | 3500 | 100 | 15 | 100 | 25 |
| Diarrhea | 1000 to 4000 | 60 | 30 | 45 | 45 |
| Urine | 1500 | 40 | 40 | 20 | — |
| Sweat |  | 50 | 5 | 55 | — |

given parenterally, the normal ECW:ICW ratio is first established by losing ECW faster than ICW increases, resulting in an initial weight loss. Vogel et al.[3] reported weight losses of up to 3.6 kg over the first four to five days of parenteral nutrition, with the largest losses seen in severely malnourished patients. After one to four days, TBW and ICW both increase, and normal hydration and weight are restored. Thereafter, weight increases at an average of 0.2 to 0.5 kg/day, representing gains in lean body mass. It is not unusual, however, for body weight to fluctuate by as much as 1 kg daily despite steady fluid and caloric infusion. In addition, weight may remain unchanged for several days. The average gain observed in our series of 414 patients was 0.4 kg/day (Fig. 7–3).

## CALORIC REQUIREMENTS

Requirements for protein and calories during disease and stress are interrelated and roughly proportional to the degree of injury, stress, or infection. Studies of nitrogen balance during constant infusion of adequate nitrogen have demonstrated a proportional relationship between nitrogen retention and level of caloric support.[2, 4, 5] Similarly, with fixed, adequate caloric intake, patients show improved nitrogen retention with increasing nitrogen infusion (Fig. 7–4).[6] Studies undertaken to determine the ideal calorie:nitrogen ratio for tissue synthesis at varying levels of stress have concluded that intake of 120 to 180 kcal per gram of nitrogen is optimal.[7, 8] In clinical practice, one can generally meet estimated caloric requirements by administering a parenteral nutrition solution with that calorie:nitrogen ratio and then making adjustments until an appropriate nitrogen balance is achieved.

In Chapter 3 a method for estimating basal caloric expenditure from the basal metabolic rate (BMR) and oxygen consumption was presented. Kinney et al.[9] measured actual caloric expenditures in surgical patients with varying degrees of stress and trauma. They used prolonged measurements of gas exchange and nitrogen excretion and compared those measurements to calculated basal metabolic rates. Uncomplicated, elective surgical procedures elevated caloric expenditure by a maximum of 10 per cent over the BMR. Caloric expenditure increased 10 to 25 per cent during major trauma, 20 to 50 per cent during extensive infections and 50 to 125 per cent with burns.

Consideration must also be given to energy losses due to fever. DuBois,[10] study-

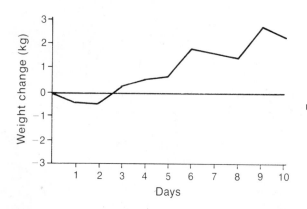

**Figure 7-3** Weight gain during parenteral nutrition.

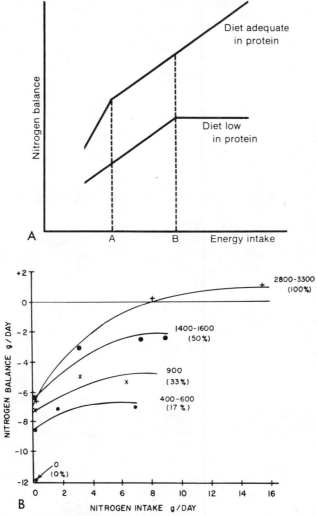

**Figure 7–4** Diagram showing relationship between nitrogen and energy intake and nitrogen balance. Under normal conditions, nitrogen balance is improved by an increase in either nitrogen or energy intake as long as an adequate intake of each is present. A. Nitrogen balance related to energy intake on diets of differing protein level. At energy intakes below point A, efficiency of dietary nitrogen utilization is impaired. At intakes of energy above point B, a lack of adequate dietary nitrogen prevents improved nitrogen balance. B. Nitrogen balance related to nitrogen intake on diets of differing caloric intake. Upon intake of adequate calories, nitrogen balance is directly related to nitrogen intake. (Part A from Munro, H.N.: General aspects of the regulation of protein metabolism by diet and by hormones. *In* Munro, H.N., and Allison, J.B. (eds.): Mammalian Protein Metabolism, Vol. 1. New York, Academic Press, Inc., 1964, pp. 267–319. Part B from Wilmore, D.W.: The Metabolic Management of the Critically Ill. New York, Plenum Press, 1977, p. 197.)

ing various types of infectious diseases, found an average increase in caloric expenditure of 10 to 13 per cent over BMR per day per degree C. It should be emphasized that the metabolic rate of hospitalized, disease-stressed patients rarely exceeds twice basal level, and this should be considered the upper limit of caloric expenditure in critically ill, bed-ridden patients. It is our experience, as well as that of others,[7, 10] that provision of adequate nitrogen and measured or calculated caloric requirements based on caloric expenditure often does not result in weight gain or positive nitrogen balance. Empirically, 40 to 60 per cent more calories appear to be necessary. Based on the above considerations, caloric requirements for a 32-year-old male with a body surface area of 1.7 sq m can be calculated as in Table 7–2.

Spanier and Shizgal[2] correlated changes in body cell mass with caloric sup-

**Table 7-2**  CALCULATION OF CALORIC REQUIREMENTS OF STRESSED PATIENTS*

| CONDITION | BMR | STRESS COMPONENT BMR | STRESS COMPONENT Cal. | CALORIC REQUIREMENT (BMR + STRESS + 50%) |
|---|---|---|---|---|
| Normal | 1500 | — | — | 2250 |
| Mild stress | 1500 | 0% | 0 | 2250 |
| Moderate stress | 1500 | +20% | 300 | 2700 |
| Major sepsis | 1500 | +40% | 600 | 3150 |
| Major burn | 1500 | +80% | 1200 | 4050 |

*Add 13 per cent of basal metabolic rate (BMR) for each degree C of fever per day. Figures are based on 32-year-old male with a 1.7 sq m surface area.

port (nitrogen infusion was constant). They found that an average of 46 kcal/kg/day was required to maintain body cell mass, with more necessary for growth. Other studies by Hartley and Lee[4] and Long et al.[5] likewise found 43 to 46 kcal/kg/day to be minimal caloric support for maintenance of nitrogen equilibrium. For a 70 kg man this represents 3,220 kcal/day and compares favorably with the data in Table 7-2. Caldwell et al.[11] found 35 kcal/kg/day necessary for nitrogen equilibrium, which is also in fair agreement.

Many caloric sources have been tried, including fructose, galactose, xylitol, sorbitol, alcohol, and fat emulsions. In general, none has been found superior to glucose, and several have undesirable side effects.[12] A healthy adult can normally metabolize 0.3 to 0.4 gram/kg/hour intravenous glucose.[13-15] In some instances, up to 1.2 grams/kg/hour have been given without adverse effects.[16] Provision of 600 to 800 grams glucose, however, without administering high volumes of fluid, requires a hypertonic solution (20 to 25 per cent), which can only be given through a catheter in a central vein. An isotonic fat solution, on the other hand, is relatively well tolerated when given through peripheral veins. Up to two thirds of the daily caloric requirements can be given safely as fat.[17] The two solutions available in the United States are Intralipid (Cutter Labs) and Lyposyn (Abbott Labs). Intralipid is a 10 per cent soybean oil emulsion with 1.2 per cent egg yolk phospholipids, 2.25 per cent glycerin, and water. The major fatty acids of this emulsion are linoleic (54 per cent), oleic (26 per cent), palmitic (9 per cent), and linolenic (8 per cent). Lyposyn is a 10 per cent safflower oil emulsion with 1.2 per cent egg phospholipids, 2.5 per cent glycerin, and water. Major fatty acids are linoleic (77 per cent), oleic (13 per cent), palmitic (7 per cent), and stearic (2.5 per cent). The osmolarity of these solutions is between· 280 and 300 mOsm/liter, with a pH between 5.5 and 9.0 and fat particle sizes of 0.4 to 0.5 microns. They provide 1.1 kcal per milliliter.

Although in many ways these are ideal solutions, preliminary data have shown fat to have less nitrogen-sparing effect than glucose. Long et al.[18] related nitrogen excretion to: $17.44 - 1.997 \times \log_e$ (glucose intake kcal/sq m/day) $+ 0.0752$ (resting metabolic rate kcal/sq m/hour). Fat was thought to play an insignificant role. Indeed, in severely traumatized patients Long found a progressive decrease in nitrogen retention during isocaloric support as the percentage of total calories provided by glucose decreased and Intralipid increased.[19] Paradis et al.[20] found that a solution containing 68 per cent of non-protein calories as lipid and having 5 per cent fructose and 3.5 per cent amino acids was able to maintain normal body mass but could not replenish a depleted body mass over a period of 15 days. The tendency of fat to induce less nitrogen retention than glucose may be explained, in part, by studies with dogs in which marked decreases in utilization of long-chain free fatty acid occur during shock induced by cardiac tamponade or endotoxin. It is thought that the carnitine-dependent transport mechanism is interrupted, and long-chain fatty acids cannot enter the mitochondria to undergo oxidation.[21] On the other hand, Jeejeebhoy has reported positive nitrogen balanced in stressed patients who derived 83 per cent of the non-protein calories from lipid; however, their nitrogen retention was less than that of patients receiving isocaloric and isonitrogenous infusions of hypertonic dextrose.[22]

A few complications following Intralipid infusion have been reported. They include a fat-overload syndrome[23] and increased lithogenesis of the bile.[24]

Until further studies demonstrate definite metabolic advantages to fat infusion, all patients should receive calculated caloric requirements as glucose, and fat emulsions should be used mainly to meet essential fatty acid requirements. When glucose intolerance occurs due to pancreatic dysfunction, stress, shock, infection, or marked malnutrition, insulin should be added to the solution to enhance glucose utilization. In addition to its effects on glucose utilization, insulin is a potent anabolic hormone and can contribute to tissue synthesis and weight gain. (See further discussion in Chapter 6 — Endocrine Response to Stress; Chapter 7 — Other Additives: Insulin; and Chapter 9 — Failure to Establish Anabolism).

The value of calories in excess of calculated requirements is debatable. Nitrogen appears to be replaced at a finite rate, with excess nitrogen catabolized or excreted in the urine.[25] Further, the administration of calories in excess of metabolic requirements increases lipogenesis and the deposition of fat in the liver, occasionally leading to acute, painful hepatomegaly.[26, 27] Long et al.[28] associated infusion of greater than 3000 kcal/day parenteral nutrition with respiratory quotients above 1.0, which implied fat synthesis. They suggested that the extra calories were not required. Excessive generation of carbon dioxide associated with respiratory quotients greater than 1.0 during aggressive carbohydrate infusion has been implicated by some as a contributing factor in patients who cannot be weaned from respirators because of hypercarbia. Yet Spanier and Shizgal[2] claimed infusion of excessive calories assisted in correction of preexisting deficits of body cell mass. The value of "hyper" alimenta-

tion, that above calculated requirements, remains to be determined. There are data suggesting that man cannot exceed two times his basal energy expenditure during any stressful event other than exercise and severe burns, and that nutritional support at that level is unnecessary except in those conditions.[29]

## NITROGEN REQUIREMENTS

Standard parenteral nutrition solutions contain 4 to 5 per cent protein with 6 to 6.6 grams nitrogen per liter in a calorie:nitrogen ratio of 120 to 180:1. Administration of 2.5 to 3.5 liters a day, therefore, provides 15 to 23 grams nitrogen per day, which is usually sufficient to establish positive nitrogen balance in the presence of adequate caloric support. In patients with protein intolerance due to renal or hepatic dysfunction, or patients with unusual nitrogen needs, an estimate of the actual nitrogen requirement can be made by using the factoral method. A 24-hour urine collection is assayed for total nitrogen excretion (by the micro-Kjeldahl method). The resulting figure is then increased by 5 mg/kg/day nitrogen for insensible losses and about 12 mg/kg/day for gastrointestinal losses. If the calculation of total urinary nitrogen by the micro-Kjeldahl method is not available from the laboratory, it can be estimated by measuring 24-hour urinary excretion of urea nitrogen and adding a constant factor of 2.0 grams nitrogen.[30] If proteinuria is present, an additional nitrogen loss of N = grams protein loss ÷ 6.25 occurs. The amount of infused nitrogen is increased or decreased until a positive nitrogen balance of 2.0 to 5.0 grams/day is obtained. Unlike orally ingested nitrogen, which has a delayed effect on nitrogen balance,[31, 32] there is no delay in utilization or excretion of intravenously administered amino acids; this allows nitrogen balances to be calculated on a day-to-day-basis.[32] Studies of minimum intravenous nitrogen requirements for persons receiving adequate non-protein calories (150 or more kcal per gram nitrogen) have suggested that a minimum of 64 mg/kg/day nitrogen as crystalline amino acids and 128 mg/kg/day nitrogen as a protein hydrolysate are necessary to maintain positive nitrogen balance during minimal stress.[33] Greater amounts of nitrogen are required to maintain balance in malnourished patients with moderate to severe stress. Hartley and Lee[4] found 240 mg/kg/day minimal for routine postoperative patients, and Bozzetti[34] reported requirements of 240 to 416 mg/kg/day. Loirat et al.,[35] studying stressed patients, reported 9 to 18 grams nitrogen/sq m/day necessary to establish and maintain positive nitrogen balance. Burn patients required up to 20.7 to 25.5 grams nitrogen/sq m/day during the acute catabolic phase.[31]

## ELECTROLYTE AND MINERAL REQUIREMENTS

Table 7–3 and Figure 7–5 summarize the electrolyte and mineral requirements of 314 adult patients given parenteral nutrition at Duke University between January, 1975, and January, 1978. The requirements of anabolic patients are quite different from those of patients receiving insufficient calories and nitrogen. Proteolysis during administration of 5 per cent dextrose solutions and uncomplicated starvation is association with metabolism of 300 to 400 grams/day lean body mass, which releases about 250 to 300 ml intracellular fluid. With more marked catabolism, 500 to 800 ml intracellular water may be released from proteolysis. This intracellular fluid provides a large part of the daily requirements of potassium, magnesium, sulfate, and phosphate (Table 7–4)[30]. With parenteral nutrition, not only is release of intracellular fluid from proteolysis reduced, but new cell synthesis requires additional electrolytes and minerals.

Wide ranges of electrolyte and mineral requirements are seen. The amounts given to an individual patient must be based on serum concentrations, known losses, and estimated renal function. Patients often pass through three phases of electrolyte and mineral requirements during the first three to five days of support, necessitating fre-

**Table 7–3** ELECTROLYTE AND MINERAL REQUIREMENTS DURING PARENTERAL NUTRITION (normal range of daily requirements)

| | |
|---|---|
| Sodium | 60 to 150 mEq as sodium chloride and sodium lactate. |
| Potassium | 70 to 150 mEq as potassium chloride and potassium phosphate. |
| Chloride | Equal to Na to prevent acid-base disturbances. |
| Calcium | 0.2 to 0.3 mEq/kg/day added as calcium gluconate. |
| Magnesium | 0.35 to 0.45 mEq/kg/day added as magnesium sulfate. Give more if increased losses are present. |
| Phosphorus | 7 to 10 mmoles per 1000 kcal, extremely variable—adjust to keep serum concentrations normal. |
| Vitamins | 0.5 amp MVI daily, folic acid 0.1 to 0.25 mg/day, vitamin C 1 mg/day, all added to the feeding solution. 100 $\mu$g vitamin $B_{12}$ is given intramuscularly each month, and 5 mg vitamin K is given intramuscularly each week. |
| Albumin | Up to 25 grams salt-poor albumin may be added per bottle until a normal serum albumin is obtained. |
| Insulin | 0 to 350 units regular insulin are added to each bag, based on blood sugars (see Table 7–5). As glucosuria can occur during hypokalemia in spite of adequate insulin secretion, serum potassium must be checked before insulin is given. Urinary potassium excretion should be equal to or greater than 40 mEq/liter. |

quent changes in solution composition. During the first 24 to 48 hours, total body deficits of electrolytes and minerals must be replaced. The second phase begins sometime during the first 24 hours and lasts for two to three days. It follows conversion to an anabolic state and is associated with increased requirements for potassium, magnesium, and phosphorus. After deficit replacement and establishment of anabolism, a relatively stable period of electrolyte and mineral requirements follows.

With the introduction of parenteral nutrition as a tool to study human metabolism, it has been possible to define interrelationships between various metabolic substrates. One study of interest was pub-

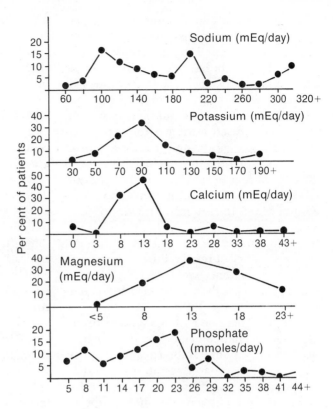

**Figure 7–5** Electrolyte requirements during parenteral nutrition.

**Table 7–4** COMPOSITION OF BODY FLUIDS (mEq/liter)

| | EXTRACELLULAR FLUID | | INTRACELLULAR FLUID |
|---|---|---|---|
| | Plasma | Interstitial | |
| Cations | | | |
| Sodium | 142 | 146 | 10 |
| Potassium | 5 | 4 | 150 |
| Calcium | 5 | 3 | 0 |
| Magnesium | 3 | 2 | 40 |
| Total | 155 | 155 | 200 |
| | | | |
| Anions | | | |
| Chloride | 103 | 115 | 0 |
| Bicarbonate | 27 | 30 | 10 |
| Protein | 16 | 1 | 40 |
| Sulfate | 1 | 1 | 10 |
| Phosphate | 2 | 2 | 140 |
| Organic Acid | 6 | 6 | 0 |
| Total | 155 | 155 | 200 |

After Bland, J. H.: Clinical Metabolism of Body Water and Electrolytes. Philadelphia, W. B. Saunders Company, 1963.

lished by Rudman et al.[37] They concluded:

Data show that repletion of protoplasm and extracellular fluid of wasted adults by intravenous hyperalimentation is retarded or abolished if N, P, Na, or K is lacking. Repletion of bone minerals does not occur in absence of Na or P but proceeds in absence of N or K. Repletion of adipose tissue proceeds in the absence of N, P, K, or Na. Thus, quality of weight gained by underfed adult patients during hyperalimentation depends on elemental composition of the infusion.

Withdrawal of N, P, Na, or K impaired or abolished retention of other elements. Removal of N halted retention of P, K, Na, and Cl; withdrawal of K stopped retention of N and P; and removal of Na or P interrupted retention of all other elements. Weight gain continued . . . despite zero or negative elemental balances of N, K, P, and sometimes Na and Cl. Calculations showed that weight gained during infusion of fluids lacking N, P, K, or Na consisted largely of adipose tissue, with little or no contribution by protoplasm or extracellular fluid.

To provide maximum benefits with parenteral nutrition, all serum electrolyte and mineral concentrations should be maintained within normal limits.

*Sodium.* Approximately 80 per cent of the body's sodium is metabolically available, the rest being firmly bound in bone.

Sodium exists predominately as an extracellular ion, and consequently, requirements are unaltered by parenteral nutrition. If the patient has been on intravenous solutions of 5 per cent dextrose and salt, and the serum sodium concentration has been normal, the same amount of sodium should be infused during parenteral nutrition. If the patient has not previously been on intravenous therapy, infusion of 1.4 to 2.0 mEq/kg/day (60 to 150 mEq/day) sodium is satisfactory. Greater amounts should be administered to patients known to have large sodium losses or to be sodium-depleted, and lesser amounts administered in the presence of renal failure or heart disease. Adjustments in sodium infusion should be based thereafter on blood chemistries.

Sodium may be added as the chloride, lactate, or acetate salt and should be distributed evenly in the solution administered each day. Lactate and acetate salts should be avoided in patients with severe liver disease. Sodium bicarbonate should not be added because of the reactions of bicarbonate with other added ions.

*Potassium.* 35 to 45 mEq/kg of potassium are present in the body. Most potassium is located within cells (75 per cent of the body potassium is within the muscle mass), where it is the major cation (see Table 7–4). Only 50 to 60 mEq are present in extracellular fluid. Serum concentrations are greatly influenced by shifts in the acid-base balance and, therefore, only indirectly reflect total body potassium stores (Fig. 7–6).[38] A more reliable indication of potassium deficiency, in the presence of normal renal function, is urinary potassium concentration, which should be greater than or equal to 40mEq/liter. This measurement can be done on random urine samples but becomes more accurate with 24-hour collections.

Potassium ion is important in glucose uptake and glycogen synthesis by cells.[39-41] Hypokalemia can result in glucosuria in spite of adequate insulin release (see Chapter 9). In addition, an intracellular ratio of

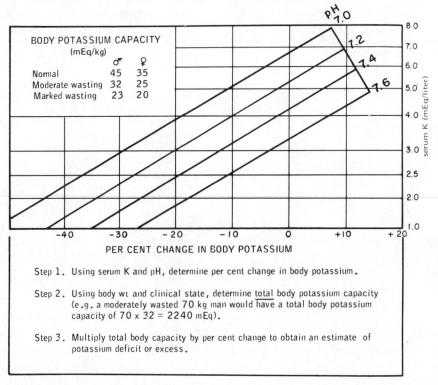

**Figure 7–6** Calculation of body potassium stores with corrections for acid-base abnormalities. (From Condon, R. E., and Nyhus, L. M.: Manual of Surgical Therapeutics, 2nd Edition. Boston, Little, Brown & Company, 1972, p. 200.)

potassium:nitrogen of 3.5:1 must be maintained for optimal protein synthesis.[42] To assure optimal metabolic conditions, serum potassium concentration should be maintained in the high normal range. If the patient has been receiving 5 per cent dextrose intravenously and has a stable serum potassium, an additional 30 to 40 mEq/day are required when parenteral nutrition is started. If the patient has not been on intravenous therapy, 1.2 to 1.5 mEq/kg/day potassium should be given initially unless marked potassium deficiency or significant renal failure is present. It is not unusual for potassium requirements to approach, or exceed, 2.5 mEq/kg/day, and potassium supplementation must be reviewed daily with monitoring of serum concentrations and estimated losses. Bernard and Stahl[43] have suggested that potassium balance during parenteral nutrition (measured either by changes in total body potassium using $^{40}K$, or by studies of 24-hour potassium input and output) can be used to measure the effects of nutritional support. The more potassium retained by the body, the greater the increase in lean body mass.

Potassium may be given as either the chloride, the phosphate, or the acetate salt and should be added evenly to the solution administered each day.

*Chloride.* Chloride is present in the human mostly as an extracellular ion, although gastric mucosal cells producing hydrochloric acid contain significant amounts also. Approximately 27 to 30 mEq/kg chloride ion is metabolically active. The main effect of chloride ion excess or deficiency is on acid-base balance (see Chapter 9). Chloride ion concentration in parenteral nutrition solutions should be adjusted to equal sodium ion by adding non-chloride salts of sodium and potassium.

*Calcium.* Between 1000 and 1500 grams calcium are present in the body, with virtually all located in bone apatite. The normal daily oral requirement is 30 to 40 mEq, of which only 5 to 40 per cent is absorbed.[44] There are few studies of calcium requirements during parenteral nutrition, and the amount to be infused daily is not well established. Wittine et al.[45] reported

that infusion of 0.25 mEq/kg/day calcium maintained a neutral to positive calcium balance during parenteral nutrition. Their study agrees with our findings that 0.2 to 0.3 mEq/kg/day calcium is adequate. One would expect little difference in requirements whether a patient was anabolic or catabolic, as calcium is not an important soft-tissue intracellular ion. Daily calcium supplementation should not be based solely on serum concentrations, however. Many patients receiving parenteral nutrition have low serum protein concentrations, and because approximately 60 per cent of serum calcium is bound to protein, primarily albumin, they also have low serum calcium concentrations. The clinically important ionized calcium concentration may, however, be normal. Reference to charts relating serum calcium to serum protein concentration may be helpful (Fig. 7–7),[46] and many hospital laboratories can now measure ionized calcium concentrations.

Plasma calcium plays a major role in the regulation of parathormone (PTH) secretion. If serum calcium falls below 10 mg/100 ml, PTH secretion increases. If serum calcium is elevated above 10 mg/100

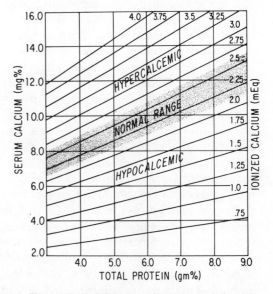

**Figure 7–7** Influence of serum protein concentration on ionized calcium. (From McLean, F. C., and Hastings, A. B.: Clinical estimation and significance of calcium-ion concentrations in the blood. Am. J. Med. Sci., *189*:601–613, 1935.)

ml, PTH secretion is suppressed. PTH, in addition to its regulatory role on serum calcium concentration, decreases tubular reabsorption of phosphate and bicarbonate by the kidney through its action on the proximal renal tubule. This in turn leads to increased reabsorption of chloride and mild hyperchloremic renal tubular acidosis.[47] Excessive calcium infusion may be associated with hyperphosphatemia and hypochloremic metabolic alkalosis. Inadequate calcium supplementation may result in hypophosphatemia and hyperchloremic acidosis. In addition, excessive infusion of calcium or vitamin D with parenteral nutrition has been reported to induce pancreatitis.[48]

If patients are immobilized, urinary excretion of calcium may exceed 10 to 15 mEq/day, with gradual depletion of bone calcium, hypercalcemia, and nephrolithiasis.[49] Such patients should undergo vigorous physical therapy.

Calcium may be given as the gluconate, glucoheptonate, or glucoceptate salt. The chloride salt is somewhat less soluble and should not be used.

*Magnesium.* Of the approximately 2000 mEq of magnesium in the body, 60 per cent is firmly bound to bone and unavailable for metabolism. The remaining magnesium is largely intracellular. Because of low serum concentrations and a slow rate of magnesium exchange, serum magnesium concentrations do not accurately reflect total body content. Nonetheless, since total body magnesium is difficult to measure clinically, intravenous magnesium supplementation is directed toward establishing and maintaining normal serum concentrations. In most patients, intravenous magnesium requirements range from 0.35 to 0.45 mEq/kg/day and are somewhat greater than the recommended oral intake (0.25 to 0.35 mEq/kg/day).[50] Some patients, especially those with gastrointestinal losses, require as much as 30 to 40 mEq/day magnesium to maintain normal serum values. The actual amount of magnesium administered should be based on serum concentrations, but if these are not available at the start of therapy, the patient should be given 0.35

mEq/kg/day until serum concentrations are known. Low serum magnesium concentrations should be corrected gradually over several days, not through large amounts over a short period of time.

Magnesium should be added to each bag or bottle as magnesium sulfate, thus providing needed sulfate ions as well.

*Phosphate.* Phosphate ion plays a significant role in human metabolism. It is involved in energy transfer and oxygen transport and release,[51] and it influences leukocyte phagocytosis and microbial resistance.[52] Failure to provide adequate phosphorus can result in rapid development of clinically significant hypophosphatemia (see Chapter 9). Sheldon and Grzyb[53] recommend infusion of 7 to 9 mmoles potassium dihydrogenphosphate per 1000 kcal in parenteral nutrition solutions. Some patients, however, require only 3 mmoles phosphate per 1000 kcal, while others need more than 17 mmoles per 1000 kcal. Actual phosphate supplementation must be based on serum phosphate concentration until a more accurate method for determination of body pools is available. When beginning parenteral nutrition, if serum phosphate concentration is normal, the patient should receive 7 to 9 mmoles phosphate per 1000 kcal. If serum phosphate is low, an additional 3 to 5 mmoles of phosphate as a potassium salt should be given per 1000 kcal. The level should be increased as necessary to establish and maintain normal serum concentrations. Even though many protein hydrolysate solutions contain phosphate ion, some in appreciable amounts (Table 7–5), phosphate supplementation is often necessary. Apparently the phosphate in protein hydrolysate solutions is bound in a way that renders it metabolically unavailable.

## VITAMINS

Both fat- and water-soluble vitamins must be given during parenteral nutrition. Stress, high carbohydrate and protein loads, and positive nitrogen balance all greatly increase normal vitamin require-

**Table 7–5** ELECTROLYTE COMPOSITION OF AMINO ACID SOLUTIONS (mEq/liter)

| PRODUCT | Na | K | Cl | Mg | Ca | $HPO_4^=$ | ACETATE | PROTEIN NITROGEN (grams/liter) |
|---|---|---|---|---|---|---|---|---|
| Hydrolysate Solutions | | | | | | | | |
| Amigen 5% | 35 | 19 | 20 | 2 | 5 | 30 | – | 50/6.5 |
| Amigen 10% | 60 | 31 | 44 | 4 | 10 | 60 | – | 100/13 |
| Aminosol 5% | 10 | 17 | 7 | 0 | 0 | 0 | – | |
| CPH 5% | 39 | 18 | 14 | 2 | 6 | 14 | | |
| Hyprotogen 5% | 25 | 18 | 18 | 2 | 5 | 25 | | |
| Amino Acid Solutions | | | | | | | | |
| Aminosyn 3.5% | 40 | 18.4 | 40 | 3 | 0 | 0 | 27 | |
| Aminosyn 7% | 0 | 5.4 | 0 | 0 | 0 | 0 | | 75/12 |
| FreAmine II 8.5% | 10 | 0 | 0 | 0 | 0 | 20 | 0 | 78/12.5 |
| Travasol 5.5% | 70 | 60 | 70 | 10 | 0 | 60 | 100 | 55/9.24 |
| Travasol 8.5% | 70 | 60 | 70 | 10 | 0 | 60 | 130 | 85/14.2 |
| Travasol 5.5% (no lytes) | 3 | 0 | 22 | 0 | 0 | 0 | 35 | 55/9.24 |
| Travasol 8.5% (no lytes) | 3 | 0 | 34 | 0 | 0 | 0 | 52 | 85/14.2 |
| Veinamine 8.0% | 40 | 30 | 50 | 6 | 0 | 0 | 50 | 80/13.3 |

ments, and many patients have vitamin deficiencies prior to instigation of parenteral nutrition. A thorough discussion of vitamins in parenteral nutrition, their function and estimated requirements, as well as available solutions, is given in Chapter 11. Vitamins may be administered daily in one bottle or, preferably, divided equally in the administered solution.

## OTHER ADDITIVES

*Albumin.* Although administered amino acids are utilized in the synthesis of serum albumin, usually several weeks pass before parenteral nutrition has any significant effect on serum albumin concentration. If serum albumin is less than 2.5 mg per 100 ml, therefore, 12.5 grams of salt-poor albumin may be added per liter of parenteral nutrition solution for four to seven days or until serum albumin concentration returns to 4.0 mg per 100 ml. If at this point albumin infusion is stopped, serum albumin concentrations will fall rapidly because of equilibration with the albumin pool. Albumin infusion should thus be continued at 12.5 to 25 grams per day until the albumin pool is replenished and endogenous albumin production becomes adequate to maintain normal serum concentrations — usually three to five additional

days unless there are ongoing losses. Albumin is compatible with parenteral nutrition solutions at all concentrations.

*Heparin.* Administration of parenteral nutrition solution through subclavian catheters is occasionally complicated by occlusion of the catheter by clotted blood, even when infusion pumps with empty bottle alarms are used. As little as five to ten minutes interruption in solution flow can result in blood backing up into the catheter and clotting. If not immediately cleared, the clot may become firmly attached to the catheter and necessitate separating the infusion line at the catheter hub and flushing with saline — a dangerous procedure at best. The addition of 1000 units heparin per liter of solution completely eliminates catheter clotting (500 units heparin per liter is inadequate). Blood may still back up into the subclavian catheter occasionally, but neither clotting nor adherence of the clots is a problem, and solution flow can be reestablished without flushing. Measurement of prothrombin time and clotting time in more than 100 patients has demonstrated no anticoagulant effect from the administered heparin.

*Insulin.* Serum glucose concentrations should remain within normal limits during parenteral nutrition, although concentrations of 130 to 140 mg per 100 ml are often seen and accepted. The pancreatic beta cell produces increasing quantities of insulin in response to increasing glucose loads. There is, however, a time lag and a limit. Further, very young and very old patients and those with stress or severe malnutrition may exhibit insulin resistance.[54] At the beginning of therapy and beyond a maximal endogenous insulin response, exogenous insulin is often necessary. Fifty-two per cent of 414 patients at Duke University Medical Center between January, 1975, and January, 1979, required insulin supplementation ranging initially from 12 to 300 units per day. A third required insulin throughout infusion of the hypertonic dextrose solution. Infusion of exogenous insulin is thought not to interfere with the pancreatic response and endogenous insulin secretion.[55, 56] Insulin supplementation needs to be reduced or discontinued, therefore, after three to six days in about 40 per cent of those patients initially requiring insulin. Although a precipitous fall in blood sugar concentration may occur during insulin infusion as endogenous insulin secretion becomes adequate or insulin resistance decreases, it does not make removal of exogenous insulin from the parenteral nutrition solution urgent. Blood sugar concentrations as low as 30 and 40 mg per 100 ml have been observed by the author without a single clinical finding of hypoglycemia. It is thought that infusion of carbohydrate plus insulin meets the demands of the tissues effectively with a high carbohydrate turnover in spite of low serum concentrations. This is *not* the case with sudden discontinuation of the parenteral nutrition solution (especially if exogenous subcuticular insulin has been given) when severe hypoglycemic damage can occur (see Chapter 9 concerning hypoglycemia).

Maintenance of normal serum glucose is important for two reasons. First, elevated glucose concentrations suggest poor utilization of infused carbohydrate. Second, there is some suggestion that hyperglycemia contributes to infectious complications, fungal infections in particular. To avoid large fluctuations in blood sugar concentrations, insulin should not be given intermittently as subcutaneous or intramuscular injections. Instead, it should be added directly to the parenteral nutrition solution in amounts necessary to lower the serum glucose concentration to less than 150 mg/100 ml. Insulin is fully compatible with parenteral nutrition solutions at all concentrations.[57] Some controversy remains as to the adherence of insulin to glass bottles or plastic bags. Studies on insulin added to parenteral nutrition solutions have demonstrated from 53 to nearly 100 per cent recoverability.[58-60] The decreased adherence of insulin to solutions of parenteral nutrition, compared to solutions containing no amino acids or albumin, is attributed to preferential binding of insulin to amino acids and albumin.[61]

If the patient has been on intravenous therapy with 5 per cent dextrose, and the blood glucose has been consistently within normal limits, insulin will often not be required during parenteral nutrition (Table 7–6). If, however, glucose has ranged between 130 and 150 mg per 100 ml, 6 to 10 units regular insulin should be added to the nutrition solution per 250 grams of glucose given. If blood glucose has ranged from 150 to 200 mg per 100 ml, 12 to 18 units regular insulin should be added. If blood glucose has been over 200 mg per 100 ml on 5 per cent dextrose, 25 units or more of regular insulin per 250 grams glucose should be added. In some patients it may be helpful to leave additional orders for regular insulin administration based on urinary glucose spillage. Doses of 5 to 8 units for 3+ glucosuria, and 10 to 12 units for 4+ glucosuria, should be given every four to six hours. The insulin should

**Table 7–6** ADDITION OF REGULAR INSULIN TO INITIAL PARENTERAL NUTRITION SOLUTION

| BLOOD SUGAR CONCENTRATION DURING 5% DEXTROSE INFUSION | AMOUNT OF REGULAR INSULIN TO BE ADDED PER 250 GRAM DEXTROSE |
|---|---|
| ≤ 120 mg per 100 ml | 0 units |
| 130 to 150 mg per 100 ml | 6 to 10 units |
| 150 to 200 mg per 100 ml | 12 to 18 units |
| ≥ 200 mg per ml | 25 units or more |

be given intramuscularly to avoid the sporadic absorption that may occur with subcutaneous injections and to give more rapid effect (the half-life of intramuscular insulin is about two hours, compared to four hours for subcutaneous insulin).[62, 63] When new orders are written, the amount of intramuscular insulin given during the previous 24 hours may be added to the parenteral nutrition solution for the next 24 hours. If no glucosuria occurs, regular insulin should be added based on daily blood glucose concentrations. In this manner the amount of regular insulin added is increased until the desired result is obtained. Up to 350 units of regular insulin per 250 grams glucose have been necessary to maintain blood sugar levels below 150 mg per 100 ml in stressed patients with severe hepatic and renal disease, even when there was no prior pancreatic disease. A word of caution: At no time should insulin be given unless potassium supplementation is adequate and the serum potassium concentration is normal.

## WRITING PARENTERAL NUTRITION SOLUTION ORDERS

Many amino acid solutions are available commercially. Crystalline amino acid solutions (composed entirely of levorotatory amino acids) provide the most metabolically useful amino acids and are the preferred solutions (see Chapter 8). However, each amino acid solution has a different electrolyte and mineral composition, which must be taken into consideration when writing solution orders (see Table 7–5).

It is best to distribute electrolyte, mineral, and vitamin additions evenly among the bottles given each day unless well-documented incompatibilities exist (see Chapter 8). In some instances, such as with water-soluble vitamins, the additive may be lost rapidly in the urine if all is given in one bottle. In other instances, absence of a component for 8 to 16 hours may lead to significant deficiencies, as with potassium. In all instances, the possibility of misleading laboratory data is eliminated by steady administration. Use of the following scheme in calculating electrolyte and mineral additives will help avoid omissions and errors.

1. Determine the desired amount of sodium, potassium, phosphate, calcium, and magnesium in milliequivalents or millimoles to be given over the next 24 hours. Divide each by the number of bottles or bags (not liters) of parenteral nutrition solution to be infused.
2. Subtract the amount of electrolytes and minerals contributed by the amino acid solution from the calculations of Step 1 to determine the amount of each ion to be added per bottle or bag.
3. Add phosphate as potassium phosphate in the amount determined from serum phosphate concentration, and add the remaining potassium as the chloride salt.
4. Determine the total chloride ion in each bottle by the following formula: Add that contributed by potassium chloride to the chloride from the amino acid solution. Subtract the sodium present in the amino acid solution, and add the difference as sodium acetate or sodium lactate. This will balance sodium and chloride ion concentrations.
5. Add the balance of desired sodium as the chloride salt. At this point, phosphate, potassium, and sodium have been added, and the sodium ion concentration will equal chloride ion concentration.
6. Add magnesium as magnesium sulfate.
7. Add calcium as calcium gluconate.
8. Add vitamins, heparin, and, if necessary, albumin and regular insulin to each bottle.

At Duke University Medical Center a standard order form for parenteral nutrition is used (Fig. 7–8). The first formula written for a patient is designated "Formula A," and each subsequent formula change designated B, C, and so forth. Bags mixed under each formula are numbered consecutively. We have found this standard form to be helpful in avoiding omissions of electrolytes or minerals and in assuring clarity in transmission of orders to pharmacy for preparation. If no changes in solution formulation are necessary, subsequent solution orders refer only to the solution letter and bag number (Fig. 7–9). Solution orders are written daily and based on collected metabolic data.

MAJOR BUSINESS FORMS, INC.
HILLSBOROUGH, N. C. 27278

14140

| | | | | | | | | | |
|---|---|---|---|---|---|---|---|---|---|
| | | | | DUKE UNIVERSITY<br><br>MEDICAL CENTER<br><br>DOCTORS' ORDERS | (PATIENT IDENTIFICATION) | | | | |
| DATE | TIME | SEQ. ORD.# | PROCEDURE NUMBER | DOCTORS' ORDERS | ENT. BY | SINGLE AND STAT ORDERS CARRIED OUT | TIME GIVEN | DATE GIVEN |
| | | 1. | | New TOTAL PARENTERAL NUTRITION Solution Orders | | | | |
| | | | | Formula | | | | |
| | | | | (FREAMINE) (SPECIAL MIXTURE-see below) | | | | |
| | | | | FreAmine ___ ml; D50W ___ ml; Distilled Water ___ ml | | | | |
| | | | | ___ ml MVI Conc. ___ mEq KCl | | | | |
| | | | | ___ ml B-Complex + C ___ mEq K as Phosphate | | | | |
| | | | | 300 mg Ascorbic Acid ___ mEq Ca Gluconate | | | | |
| | | | | 300 mcg Folic Acid ___ mEq Mg Sulfate | | | | |
| | | | | ___ mEq NaCl ___ ml Salt Poor Albumin | | | | |
| | | | | ___ mEq Na Lactate ___ units Heparin | | | | |
| | | | | ___ units Regular Insulin | | | | |
| | | | | To run at ___ ml/hour ( ___ ml/day) at IVAC setting | | | | |
| | | 2. | | Check each TPN bag label for formula code letter. All | | | | |
| | | | | bags on this order to hang in numerical order. | | | | |
| | | 4. | | Use MACRODRIP ADMINISTRATION SET with IVAC pump. | | | | |
| | | 5. | | Mark I&O with EXACT time each new bag is hung. | | | | |
| | | 6. | | FORMULA ___ BAG ___ to run from ___ to ___ on unit | | | | |
| | | | | FORMULA ___ BAG ___ to run from ___ to ___ | | | | |
| | | | | FORMULA ___ BAG ___ to run from ___ to ___ | | | | |
| | | | | FORMULA ___ BAG ___ to run from ___ to ___ | | | | |
| | | | | FORMULA ___ BAG ___ to run from ___ to ___ | | | | |
| | | 7. | | Have H.O. cosign please | | | | |
| | | 8. | | Thank you. | | | | |
| | | | | | | | | |

FORM MO5 B
1M 2 PART 10/75

**Figure 7–8**   Standard form used to order parenteral nutrition.

13927

MAJOR BUSINESS FORMS, INC.
HILLSBOROUGH, N. C. 27278

| | | | | | | | | | |
|---|---|---|---|---|---|---|---|---|---|

DUKE UNIVERSITY

MEDICAL CENTER

DOCTORS' ORDERS

| DATE | TIME | SEQ. ORD. # | PROCEDURE NUMBER | DOCTORS' ORDERS | ENT. BY | SINGLE AND STAT ORDERS CARRIED OUT | TIME GIVEN | DATE GIVEN |
|---|---|---|---|---|---|---|---|---|
| | | | | CONTINUATION OF PARENTERAL NUTRITION SOLUTION ORDERS | | | | |
| | | | | | | | | |
| | | | | Parenteral Nutrition Solution _____ to continue: | | | | |
| | | | | Bag No. _____ from _____ to _____ | | | | |
| | | | | Bag No. _____ from _____ to _____ | | | | |
| | | | | Bag No. _____ from _____ to _____ | | | | |
| | | | | Bag No. _____ from _____ to _____ | | | | |
| | | | | | | | | |
| | | | | at IVAC setting of _____ (approximately _____ ml/hour) | | | | |
| | | | | | | | | |
| | | | | | | | | |
| | | | | | | | | |
| | | | | | | | | |
| | | | | | | | | |
| | | | | | | | | |
| | | | | | | | | |
| | | | | | | | | |

FORM M05 B

**Figure 7–9**  Standard form for continuation of parenteral nutrition formula orders.

## INFUSION OF PARENTERAL NUTRITION SOLUTIONS

*Rate.* All patients but those with fluid intolerance should initially receive two bottles of parenteral nutrition solution infused over the first 24 hours. This is well within the range of normal water metabolism (2000 to 2500 ml/day) and carbohydrate utilization (0.3 to 0.4 gm/kg/hour). After 24 hours, the volume may be increased in increments of 1000 ml per day until the desired infusion volume is obtained (usually 2400 to 3000 ml/day). This is true even in the presence of glucose intolerance, in which case regular insulin should be added. No attempt should be made to accommodate patients gradually to increased carbohydrate loads in hopes of avoiding use of insulin. Patients with normal pancreatic function and insulin sensitivity will tolerate rapid increases in carbohydrate infusion. Patients with deficient pancreatic function or insulin resistance may require a week or more before carbohydrate tolerance improves (some never become tolerant), and a significant delay in nutritive support might occur.

There need be no concern about cardiac toxicity resulting from infusion of solutions containing high concentrations of dextrose and electrolytes into the superior vena cava. The solution is rapidly diluted by the high blood flow, and blood in the atrium has a normal composition. To demonstrate this, a central venous catheter was inserted via an antecubital vein and positioned 2 to 3 cm beyond the tip of a subclavian catheter. While the parenteral nutrition solution was infused at 125 ml/hour, multiple blood samples were drawn from the central venous catheter and compared to samples drawn simultaneously from a peripheral vein. No significant increase in electrolyte or mineral concentration or serum osmolality was detected in the blood from the long catheter (Table 7–7).

It is important that the parenteral nutrition solution be infused at a steady rate. Large changes in the infusion rate (± 15 per cent or more) can result in significant hypoglycemia or hyperglycemia and, if marked, in coma, convulsions, and even death. If

**Table 7–7** DILUTION OF PARENTERAL NUTRITION SOLUTION DELIVERED INTO THE SUPERIOR VENA CAVA*†

| SUBSTANCE | CONCENTRATION IN PERIPHERAL BLOOD | CONCENTRATION AT TIP OF CENTRAL VENOUS CATHETER |
|---|---|---|
| Na | 136 mEq/liter | 137 mEq/liter |
| K | 3.2 mEq/liter | 3.5 mEq/liter |
| Cl | 101 mEq/liter | 100 mEq/liter |
| $CO_2$ | 21 mEq/liter | 22 mEq/liter |
| Blood urea nitrogen | 13 mg/100ml | 13 mg/100ml |
| Blood sugar | 260 mg/100ml | 278 mg/100ml |
| Ca | 4.8 mEq/liter | 4.8 mEq/liter |
| Inorganic phosphate | 4.5 mg/100ml | 4.5 mg/100ml |
| Mg | 1.5 mEq/liter | 1.5 mEq/liter |
| Protein | 7.0 grams/100ml | 7.0 grams/100ml |
| Hematocrit | 38 per cent | 41 per cent |
| Osmolality | 289 mOsm | 288 mOsm |

*Solution infused at steady rate of 125 ml/hour via subclavian line. Concentrations of substances in the parenteral nutrition solution per liter: Na = 48 mEq, K = 61 mEq, Cl = 42 mEq, protein = 39 grams, N = 6.1 grams, glucose = 200 grams, Ca = 3.6 mEq, phosphate ion = 8.4 mmoles, Mg = 4.5 mEq.

†Unpublished data from author.

solution administration gets ahead or behind schedule, the drip rate should not be accelerated or slowed down to meet the ordered daily volume. Instead, the drip rate should be adjusted to the correct hourly infusion rate and continued at that rate thereafter. IVAC positive-pressure infusion pumps* with automatic empty-bottle cutoff circuits are used at Duke University Medical Center to aid in steady infusion. Other pumps are available, and selection depends on personal preference. In addition to assuring constant solution infusion, the pump helps prolong catheter life by preventing occlusion of the catheter tip by clot or fibrin sheaths (see Chapter 4 concerning subclavian vein thrombosis).

Orders should include the correct IVAC setting, expected time each bottle or bag is to be hung, and the approximate rate of infusion per hour (see Figs. 7–8 and 7–9). In the chance that the parenteral nutrition solution might have to be interrupted, standing orders should be written for administration of a 5 per cent dextrose solution at the same rate, either through the subclavian line, or if that line is removed, through a peripheral line. Five per cent dextrose will prevent sud-

*IVAC Corporation, 11353 Sorrento Valley Road, San Diego, Calif. 92121.

den hypoglycemia due to the high endogenous insulin secretion that is associated with the infusion of hypertonic dextrose. Higher concentrations of dextrose are not necessary and should not be given. When possible, all fluid and electrolyte additions should be incorporated into the parenteral nutrition solution, and peripheral lines removed. This will improve patient mobility and eliminate sources of sepsis. In patients with large variations in external drainage, however, it is preferable to replace those losses as they occur, through peripheral intravenous lines with appropriate solutions (see Table 7–1).

*Cyclic Parenteral Nutrition.* Continuous administration of hypertonic dextrose solutions during parenteral nutrition induces elevated levels of serum insulin. Insulin in turn blocks lipolysis and stimulates lipogenesis, particularly in the liver. As a consequence, a proportion of infused calories may be diverted from essential metabolic processes and deposited in body stores as glycogen, which will contribute to the development of an enlarged, fatty liver.

Studies are in progress to determine the metabolic effects of cyclical parenteral nutrition, in which dextrose is withheld for eight to ten hours each day, and only 3 per cent amino acids or 3 per cent amino acids and fat emulsions are given.[64-66] Theoretically, the withholding of dextrose should allow for development of a postabsorptive state that more nearly reflects normal nutrition. Calories stored as fat during hypertonic dextrose infusion might be mobilized and utilized for energy. The infused amino acids, with insulin reduced, might be more efficiently utilized for visceral protein synthesis instead of being forced into muscle compartments. Preliminary data demonstrate equal or slightly fewer calories are necessary to maintain nitrogen balance during cyclic nutrition. Serum insulin levels fall from a mean of 143 microunits per milliliter to 29, and blood glucose concentrations fall. No significant changes are seen after three hours, however, in free fatty acids, ketone bodies, alanine, or lactate. There is some suggestion that serum albumin, transferrin, and total lymphocyte counts recover more rapidly during cyclic

nutrition. Finally, fatty livers do not develop, and those previously induced by continuous nutrition slowly resolve during cyclical nutrition. Further studies are necessary, but cyclic nutrition may well prove preferable to continuous parenteral nutrition.

*Use of In-Line Filters.* In a 1974 survey of parenteral nutrition as practiced in 86 hospitals, Kaminski and Stolar[67] found in-line filters being used by slightly more than half of the hospitals. Those employing filters said they reduced risks of sepsis secondary to solution contamination during mixing and also of embolization caused by glass, protein aggregate, rubber, plastic, or microprecipitate. The standard filter (0.45 micron) allows gravity flow and removes particulate matter and most bacteria, but it does not remove some pleomorphic forms of Pseudomonas and Staphylococcus, both of which are common contaminants under unsterile mixing conditions. The 0.22 micron filter removes all bacteria and fungi but requires the use of a positive-pressure pump. Rubber, glass, and plastic particles are not unique to parenteral nutrition solutions but are found in peripheral intravenous solutions as well. Although particulate matter is a theoretical problem, no clinical symptoms of embolization have been reported (for a review of this subject, see reference 68).

As for prevention of septic complications in non-ideal situations where solutions are mixed on the ward by nursing or hospital staff without laminar air flow or sepsis control, in-line filters might be advantageous. Miller and Grogan,[69] working with infants in an intensive care unit, reported a 23 per cent incidence of positive cultures on the bottle side of 0.22 micron filters in-line with parenteral nutrition solutions. The fluids and added vitamins and minerals were mixed in the intensive care unit by personnel using gloves, an iodine preparation, and standard bacterial precautions, but not a laminar flow hood. The organisms cultured included diphtheroids, *Staphylococcus epidermidis*, coliforms, non-beta Streptococcus species, Candida species, and *Staphylococcus aureus*, in that order of frequency. Yet, when solutions are mixed under strict aseptic conditions by pharmacists employing closed transfer systems and laminar flow air systems, bottle contamination is negligible and in-line filters are unnecessary. In the absence of good solution preparation facilities, hospitals should perhaps not attempt parenteral nutrition rather than rely on in-line filters.

Miller and Grogan[69] further studied the effects of multiple filters in the intravenous line. They found that increasing the number of filters increased the incidence of contamination, especially between the filters and suggested that the contamination was due to the extra breaks in the closed system. Collin et al.[70] found no significant reduction of thrombophlebitis or bacterial contamination of cannulae in a prospective study using 0.45 micron filters during peripheral intravenous fluid administration. MacLean[71] found a decreased incidence of infectious complications after abandoning use of filters during parenteral nutrition. Finally, there is evidence to suggest that catheter and fluid contamination by organisms from the patient's body may be of greater importance than solution contamination. Ashcraft and Leape,[72] who investigated cultures of parenteral nutrition solutions passing through administration sets that were fitted with in-line filters, discovered no contaminating fungi above the filter but found positive cultures in the solution between the filter and the patient. This could occur because of reflux of fungi from the patient's bloodstream into the intravenous line, growth of skin organisms down the catheter and back up the intravenous line, or contamination at the connection between the filter and the catheter.

In-line filters are not used at Duke University Medical Center, and we have yet to detect an infection secondary to bottle contamination after infusion of more than 207,000 bottles. With properly prepared solutions (which can nearly guarantee sterility), proper care of the subclavian catheter, and optimal metabolic management, the use of an in-line filter is unnecessary and perhaps harmful. Finally, if it is necessary to add albumin to the parenteral nutrition solution, filters cannot be used because of rapid blockage by albumin molecules.

## STANDING CHEMISTRY ORDERS

To administer parenteral nutrition solutions safely, it is necessary to monitor certain serum chemistries closely. During the first week, concentrations of serum sodium, potassium, chloride, carbon dioxide, blood urea nitrogen, and glucose should be measured daily, and appropriate alterations made in solution formulation. Critically ill patients may need to be monitored more closely, with chemistries every 6 to 12 hours. Measurements of serum albumin, protein, calcium, phosphorus, and magnesium (usually obtained with a battery of tests, such as a Chem 12), as well as complete blood counts, should be done twice a week. Serum prothrombin time should be measured once a week to determine the adequacy of vitamin K administration. Likewise, serum copper levels should be assessed prior to beginning parenteral nutrition and at bi-weekly intervals, with oral or intravenous supplementation if necessary. After the desired infusion rate of parenteral nutrition has been attained and blood chemistries are stable, studies can be reduced to twice and then once a week but should never be omitted. All laboratory values and metabolic data should be recorded daily on flow sheets for easy reference. Figures 7–10 and 7–11 show forms in use at Duke University Medical Center.

In some centers, facilities are available to monitor serum trace element concentrations. These elements may indeed be critical for achievement of maximal metabolic benefits. (See Chapter 10 for further discussion.)

## STANDING NURSING ORDERS

To assure proper patient monitoring, nurses should be well informed of signs of metabolic derangements and pending sepsis. The following are suggested standing orders for nursing care.
1. Frequent weights: No more than 0.2 to 0.5 kg/day weight gain can be attributed to lean body mass accumulation. Greater daily gains usually indicate excessive

PAGE_____

PATIENT_____     HISTORY NUMBER _____

DIAGNOSIS_____
_____

| DAY/DATE | NORMAL VL. | | | | | | | | |
|---|---|---|---|---|---|---|---|---|---|
| NA | 135–145 | | | | | | | | |
| K | 3.5–5.3 | | | | | | | | |
| CL | 98–108 | | | | | | | | |
| CO2 | 24–33 | | | | | | | | |
| BUN | 8–23 | | | | | | | | |
| FBS | 75–110 | | | | | | | | |
| T.P. | 6.0–8.0 | | | | | | | | |
| ALB | 3.5–5.0 | | | | | | | | |
| CA | 8.5–10.5 | | | | | | | | |
| PO4 | 2.5–4.5 | | | | | | | | |
| CHOL | 120–290 | | | | | | | | |
| U/A | 3–7 | | | | | | | | |
| CREAT | 0.7–1.2 | | | | | | | | |
| BILI | / 1 | | | | | | | | |
| ALK.P | 30–110 | | | | | | | | |
| LDH | 90–200 | | | | | | | | |
| SGOT | 10–50 | | | | | | | | |
| SGPT | 5–30 | | | | | | | | |
| MG | 1.6–2.2 | | | | | | | | |
| HCT/HGB | | | | | | | | | |
| WBC | | | | | | | | | |
| PT RATIO | | | | | | | | | |
| NH4 | 10–61 | | | | | | | | |
| CU | 80–120 | | | | | | | | |
| | | | | | | | | | |
| WEIGHT | KG | | | | | | | | |
| TPN VOLUME(BAGS) | | | | | | | | | |
| IV VOLUME (PERI) | | | | | | | | | |
| PO VOLUME (DIET) | | | | | | | | | |
| TOTAL INTAKE | | | | | | | | | |
| TOTAL OUTPUT | | | | | | | | | |
| BALANCE +/- | | | | | | | | | |
| FISTULA OUTPUT | | | | | | | | | |
| | | | | | | | | | |
| NA | mEq | | | | | | | | |
| K | mEq | | | | | | | | |
| CL | mEq | | | | | | | | |
| CA | mEq | | | | | | | | |
| MG | mEq | | | | | | | | |
| PHOS | mM | | | | | | | | |
| CHO | GM | | | | | | | | |
| PROTEIN | GM | | | | | | | | |
| NITROGEN | GM | | | | | | | | |
| MVI/B+C | ML | | | | | | | | |
| FA/AA | UG /MG | | | | | | | | |
| ALBUMIN | | | | | | | | | |
| HEPARIN | | | | | | | | | |
| REGULAR INS. | U | | | | | | | | |
| BLD/RBC | ML | | | | | | | | |
| PLASMA | ML | | | | | | | | |
| HCO3 | mEq | | | | | | | | |
| GLUCOSURIA | | | | | | | | | |
| MAX. TEMP | | | | | | | | | |
| COMMENTS: | | | | | | | | | |

**Figure 7–10**  Standard form for recording metabolic data.

Patient Information PAGE_____

| | | | | | | | | | |
|---|---|---|---|---|---|---|---|---|---|
| DATE | | | | | | | | | |
| FORMULA | | | | | | | | | |
| NA | | | | | | | | | |
| K | | | | | | | | | |
| CL | | | | | | | | | |
| CA | | | | | | | | | |
| MG | | | | | | | | | |
| PHOS | | | | | | | | | |
| CHO | | | | | | | | | |
| PROTEIN | | | | | | | | | |
| NITROGEN | | | | | | | | | |
| MVI | | | | | | | | | |
| B + C | | | | | | | | | |
| VIT. C /FA | | | | | | | | | |
| ALBUMIN | | | | | | | | | |
| HEPARIN | | | | | | | | | |
| R. INSULIN | | | | | | | | | |
| BAG VOL: | | | | | | | | | |
| CARRY: | | | | | | | | | |
| TPN: | | | | | | | | | |
| OLD: | | | | | | | | | |
| NEW: | | | | | | | | | |
| D5W | | | | | | | | | |
| NS | | | | | | | | | |
| D5 1/4 NS | | | | | | | | | |
| D5 1/2 NS | | | | | | | | | |
| D5NS | | | | | | | | | |
| D50W | | | | | | | | | |
| LR(5%) | | | | | | | | | |
| PLASMA SPA | | | | | | | | | |
| BLOOD RBC | | | | | | | | | |
| KCL | | | | | | | | | |
| RI | | | | | | | | | |
| INTAKE: | | | | | | | | | |
| PO: | | | | | | | | | |
| TF: | | | | | | | | | |
| IV: | | | | | | | | | |
| TPN: | | | | | | | | | |
| OUTPUT: | | | | | | | | | |
| URINE: | | | | | | | | | |
| FISTULA: | | | | | | | | | |
| GASTRIC: | | | | | | | | | |
| BILE: | | | | | | | | | |
| OTHER: | | | | | | | | | |
| STOOL: | | | | | | | | | |
| TIME: | | | | | | | | | |
| BAG: | | | | | | | | | |
| IVAC: | | | | | | | | | |
| COMMENT: | | | | | | | | | |

**Figure 7–11** Standard form for recording laboratory values.

water retention. In patients who are not critically ill, weights should be measured at least three times a week. In critically ill patients, daily weights may be needed.

2. Vital signs: Frequent measurements of temperature, blood pressure, pulse, and respirations are routinely done on seriously ill patients and seldom need to be emphasized. In patients who are not critically ill, it is still important to monitor vital signs initially every four hours to detect possible fluid overload or septic complications. After one to two weeks, if the patient has been stable, monitoring of vital signs can be reduced to two or three times a day. Nurses should be instructed to notify the physician of any change in the vital signs.

3. Urine samples for sugar and acetone: Monitoring of urine for sugar and acetone every four to six hours will detect not only glucose intolerance but also impending sepsis, with glucosuria secondary to hormonal responses. (For a further discussion of glucosuria, see Chapter 9.)

4. Mouth care: Patients should maintain normal oral hygiene and periodically suck on sour balls or lemon slices to maintain salivary secretion.

5. Solution infusion: The parenteral nutrition solution should be infused at the ordered IVAC drip rate or by drip chamber at a steady, even rate. The formula, bottle number, and time each new bottle is hung should be marked on the patient's intake and output sheet. Only by accurately recording the time bottles are hung can the total volume received over each 24-hour period be determined.

6. Solution interruption: If the parenteral nutrition solution must be interrupted at any time, 5 per cent dextrose in quarter strength normal saline should be infused either through the same catheter or through a peripheral intravenous line at a rate equal to that of the discontinued nutrition solution until the parenteral nutrition solution is restarted.

7. Catheter care: Catheter dressings are changed routinely every Monday, Wednesday, and Friday and as necessary if soiled. The nurses should notify the parenteral nutritional team if the dressing becomes soiled or if it is wet or loose. Each new bottle should be administered through a new IV administration set. No blood may be drawn from the subclavian vein catheter. No stopcocks may be placed in the line, and no injections may be given through the line.

8. Physical therapy: Each patient should be evaluated by a physical therapist to determine exercise tolerance. Exercise programs should begin on the first day of parenteral nutrition therapy.

9. Finally, in the standing orders, each parenteral nutrition team member should be identified so that the proper person can be notified for questions or complications.

## CONVERSION TO ORAL INTAKE

The effects of parenteral nutrition on appetite during and after therapy remain to be determined. Grinker et al.[73] reported a reduction in hunger in normal-weight human volunteers with the administration of intravenous glucose, although no decrease in food intake was observed. Jordan et al.[74] studied appetite and food ingestion in patients receiving total parenteral nutrition and found no relationship between hunger and the amount or duration of parenteral nutrition. Only 10 of 50 patients reported the absence of hunger during parenteral nutrition, while the remaining patients experienced normal hunger sensations. Half of the patients noted an increase in appetite as they were weaned from parenteral nutrition, while the other half experienced fullness and early satiety with resumption of an oral diet. Hansen et al.[75] measured changes in oral intake and gastric motility in rhesus monkeys during and following intravenous nutrition. They found provision of less than calculated caloric requirements often was associated with overeating and accelerated weight gain, while provision of normal or excessive caloric support decreased oral intake to nearly zero.

Discontinuation of total parenteral nutrition was followed by depressed oral intake for one to three weeks. Gastric motility studies during parenteral nutrition in the monkeys showed a complete absence of large amplitude contractions, which are associated with hunger pains in humans. In addition to loss of appetite and early satiety, other factors may delay resumption of an adequate oral diet. Some patients may have a loss of taste acuity, perhaps due to zinc deficiency (see Chapter 10). Others may have a psychological aversion to eating related to their initial disease.

When patients are to resume an oral diet, parenteral nutrition solution should be reduced by 1000 ml increments per day to 1500 or 2000 ml/day to decrease any effect a dextrose load might have on appetite. Abrupt withdrawal of hypertonic dextrose solutions after pancreatic adaptation, in the absence of oral intake, has resulted in hypoglycemia and should be avoided (see Chapter 9). Parenteral nutrition should be continued at 1500 to 2000 ml/day until the patient is able to take 1500 to 1800 kcal per day orally. At that point an overnight infusion of 5 per cent dextrose at 100 ml/ hour should be given and the catheter removed the following morning.

Food should initially be offered as frequent small feedings with nutritious snacks at the bedside. If adaptation to an oral diet is prolonged, especially when due to psychological factors, a small feeding tube (No. 8 French or smaller) may be passed into the stomach or duodenum via the nose, and tube feeding supplements given with discontinuation of parental nutrition. Occasionally, patients develop significant diarrhea upon resumption of an oral diet, especially if that diet contains excessive fat or has high osmolarity. This may be due in part to mucosal atrophy and loss of absorptive function of the gastrointestinal tract following prolonged parenteral nutrition.[76, 77] In addition, deficiences of the intestinal disaccharidases, maltase, sucrase, and lactase, are often found in patients with protein-calorie malnutrition or diseases affecting the intestinal mucosa.[78-80] Lactase deficiency is especially common in adult patients, even in the absence of intestinal mucosal disease. As many as 5 to 15 per cent of American whites, 70 per cent of blacks, and 70 per cent of persons of Jewish descent develop lactose intolerance during adulthood.[81-84] The reduced level of these enzymes, whether induced by disease or inanition or inherited, results in incomplete hydrolysis of ingested disaccharides and leads to cramps, bloating, and diarrhea with abnormally high amounts of sugar and lactic acid in the stool. Therefore, patients who have some difficulty resuming an oral diet because of diarrhea should be given diets of frequent small feedings containing little fat, milk, or complex sugars. Low-residue, lactose-free diets often work well. During recovery of intestinal function and until the diarrhea resolves, parenteral nutrition should be continued.

This chapter has dealt with writing of parenteral nutrition solution orders and techniques of solution administration. For a more detailed discussion of the role played by various minerals, trace elements, and vitamins in human metabolism and the clinical signs of various deficiency states, refer to Chapters 9, 10, and 11.

## REFERENCES

1. Elwyn, D. H., Bryan-Brown, C. W., and Shoemaker, W. C.: Nutritional aspects of body water dislocations in postoperative and depleted patients. Ann. Surg., 182:76–84, 1975.
2. Spanier, A. H., and Shizgal, H. M.: Caloric requirements of the critically ill patient receiving intravenous hyperalimentation. Am. J. Surg., 133:99–104, 1977.
3. Vogel, C. M., Kingsbury, R. J., and Baue, A. E.: Intravenous hyperalimentation. A review of two and one-half years experience. Arch. Surg., 105:414–419, 1972.
4. Hartley, T. F., and Lee, H. A.: Investigations into the optimal nitrogen and caloric requirements and comparative nutritive value of three intravenous amino acid solutions in the postoperative period. Nutr. Metabol., 19:201–211, 1975.
5. Long, C. L., Crosby, F., Geiger, J. W., and Kinney, J. M.: Parenteral nutrition in the septic patient: Nitrogen balance, limiting plasma amino acids, and caloric to nitrogen ratios. Am. J. Clin. Nutr., 29:380–391, 1976.
6. Munro, H. N.: General aspects of the regulation of protein metabolism by diet and hormones. *In*

Monroe, H. N., and Allison, J. B. (eds.): Mammalian Protein Metabolism, Vol. 1. New York, Academic Press, Inc., 1964, pp. 381–481.

7. Kinney, J. M.: Energy requirements of the surgical patient. *In* American College of Surgeons, Committee on Pre- and Postoperative Care: Manual of Surgical Nutrition. Philadelphia, W. B. Saunders Company, 1975, pp. 233–234.

8. Blackburn, G. L., and Bistrian, B. R.: Nutritional care of the injured and/or septic patient. Surg. Clin. North Am., 56(5):1195–1224, 1976.

9. Kinney, J. M., Duke, J. H., Jr., Long, C. L., and Gump, F. E.: Tissue fuel and weight loss after injury. J. Clin. Pathol., 23(Suppl. 4):65–72, 1970.

10. DuBois, E. F.: Basal Metabolism in Health and Disease. Philadelphia, Lea & Febiger, 1924.

11. Caldwell, M. D., O'Neill, J. A., Jr., Meng, H. C., and Stahlman, M. H.: Evaluation of a new amino acid source for use in parenteral nutrition. Ann. Surg., 185:153–161, 1977.

12. Heuckenkamp, R. U., and Zolliner, N.: The comparative metabolism of carbohydrate administration intravenously. Nutr. Metab., 14(Suppl.):58–73, 1972.

13. Dudrick, S. J., and Rhoads, J. E.: Metabolism in surgical patients: Protein, carbohydrates, and fat utilization by oral and parenteral routes. *In* Sabiston, D. C., (ed.): Davis-Christopher Textbook of Surgery, 11th Edition. Philadelphia, W. B. Saunders Company, 1977, p. 160.

14. Cooper, D. R., Iob, V., and Coller, F. A.: Response to parenteral glucose of normal kidneys and of kidneys of postoperative patients. Ann. Surg., 129:1–13, 1949.

15. Geyer, R. P.: Parenteral nutrition. Physiol. Rev., 40:150–186, 1970.

16. Dudrick, S. J., Wilmore, D. W., Vars, H. M., and Rhoads, J. E.: Can intravenous feeding as the sole means of nutrition support growth in the child and restore weight loss in an adult? An affirmative answer. Ann. Surg. 169:974–984, 1969.

17. Hansen, L. M., Hardie, W. R., and Hidalgo, J.: Fat emulsion for intravenous administration: Clinical experience with Intralipid 10%. Ann. Surg., 184:80–88, 1976.

18. Long, J. M., III, Wilmore, D. W., Mason, A. D., Jr., and Pruitt, B. A., Jr.: Effect of carbohydrate and fat intake on nitrogen excretion during total parenteral feeding. Ann. Surg., 185:417–422, 1977.

19. Long, J. M., Wilmore, D. W., Masson, R. D., Jr., and Pruitt, B. A., Jr.: Fat-carbohydrate interaction: Nitrogen sparing effect of varying caloric sources for total intravenous feeding. Surg. Forum, 25:61–63, 1974.

20. Paradis, C., Spanier, A. H., Calder, M., and Shizgal, H. M.: Total parenteral nutrition with lipid. Am. J. Surg., 135:164–171, 1978.

21. Daniel, A. M., Pierce, C. H., Shizgal, H. M., and MacLean, L. D.: Protein and fat utilization in shock. Surgery, 84:588–594, 1978.

22. Jeejeebhoy, K. N., Anderson, G. H., Nakhooda, A. F., Greenberg, G. R., Sanderson, I., and Marliss, E. B.: Metabolic studies in total parenteral nutrition with lipid in man. J. Clin. Invest., 57:125–136, 1976.

23. Belin, R. P., Bivins, B. A., Jona, J. Z., and Young, V.

L.: Fat overload with 10% soybean oil emulsion. Arch. Surg., 111:1391–1393, 1976.

24. van der Linden, W., and Nakayama, F.: Effect of intravenous fat emulsion on hepatic bile. Acta Chir. Scand., 142:401–406, 1976.

25. Shils, M. E.: Guidelines for total parenteral nutrition. J.A.M.A., 220:1721–1729, 1972.

26. Chang, S., and Silvis, S.E.: Fatty liver produced by hyperalimentation of rats. Am. J. Gastroenterol., 62:410–418, 1974.

27. Sheldon, G. F., Petersen, S. R., and Sanders, R.: Hepatic dysfunction during hyperalimentation. Arch. Surg., 113:504–508, 1978.

28. Long, C. L., Crosby, F., Geiger, J. W., and Kinney, J. M.: Parenteral nutrition in the septic patient: Nitrogen balance, limiting plasma amino acids, and calorie to nitrogen ratios. Am. J. Clin. Nutr., 29:380–391, 1976.

29. Rutten, P., Blackburn, G. L., Flatt, J. P., Hallowell, E., and Cochran, O.: Determination of optimal hyperalimentation infusion rate. J. Surg. Res., 18:477–483, 1975.

30. Blackburn, G. L., Bistrian, B. R., Maini, H. T., Schlamm, H. T., and Smith, M. F.: Nutritional and metabolic assessment of the hospitalized patient. J. Parenteral Enteral Nutr., 1:11–22, 1977.

31. Soroff, H. S., Pearson, E., and Artz, C. P.: An estimation of the nitrogen requirements for equilibrium in burned patients. Surg. Gynecol. Obstet., 112:877–883, 1971.

32. Oyama, J. H., Kark, R. M., McElain, R., Berryman, G. H., and Macalaiad, F. V.: Ultra-rapid nitrogen balances in man. Proc. Soc. Exp. Biol. Med., 137:877–883, 1971.

33. Anderson, G. H., Patel, D. G., and Jeejeebhoy, K. N.: Design and evaluation by nitrogen balance and blood aminograms of an amino acid mixture for total parenteral nutrition of adults with gastrointestinal disease. J. Clin. Invest., 53:904–912, 1974.

34. Bozzetti, F.: Parenteral nutrition in surgical patients. Surg. Gynecol. Obstet., 142:16–20, 1976.

35. Loirat, Ph., Rohan, J. E., Chapman, A., Beaufils, F., David, R., and Nedey, R.: Positive nitrogen balance in hypercatabolic states: Results obtained with parenteral feeding after major surgical procedures. Europ. J. Intensive Care Med., 1:11–17, 1975.

36. Bland, J. H.: Clinical Metabolism of Body Water and Electrolytes. Philadelphia, W. B. Saunders Company, 1963, pp. 42–43.

37. Rudman, D., Millikan, W. J., Richardson, T. J., Bixler, T. J., II, Stackhouse, W. J., and McGarrity, W. C.: Elemental balances during intravenous hyperalimentation of underweight adult subjects. J. Clin. Inves., 55:94–104, 1975.

38. Condon, R. E., and Nyhus, L. M.: Manual of Surgical Therapeutics, 2nd Edition. Boston, Little, Brown & Company, 1972, p. 200.

39. Hull, R. L.: Physiochemical considerations in intravenous hyperalimentation. Am. J. Hosp. Pharm., 31:236–243, 1974.

40. Shils, M. E.: Minerals in Total Parenteral Nutrition. *In* Symposium on Total Parenteral Nutrition. Chicago, American Medical Association, 1972.

41. Conn, J.: Hypertension, the potassium ion and

impaired carbohydrate tolerance. N. Engl. J. Med., 273:1135–1142, 1965.

42. Beal, J. M., Frost, P. M., and Smith, J. L.: The influence of caloric and potassium intake on nitrogen retention in man. Ann. Surg., 138:842–845, 1953.

43. Bernard, R. W., and Stahl, W. M.: Total body potassium measurements as a guide to intravenous alimentation. Ann. Surg., 178:559–562, 1973.

44. Dietary Allowances Committee and Food and Nutrition Board: Recommended Dietary Allowances, 8th Edition. Washington, D.C., National Academy of Sciences, 1974.

45. Wittine, M. F., and Freeman, J. B.: Calcium requirements during total parenteral nutrition in well-nourished individuals. J. Parenteral Enteral Nutr., 1:152–155, 1977.

46. McLean, F. C., and Hastings, A. B.: Clinical estimation and significance of calcium–ion concentrations in the blood. Am. J. Med. Sci., 189:601–613, 1935.

47. Hellman, D. E., Au, W. Y. W., and Bartier, F. C.: Evidence for a direct effect of parathyroid hormone on urinary acidification. Am. J. Physiol., 209:643–650, 1965.

48. Manson, R. R.: Acute pancreatitis secondary to iatrogenic hypercalcemia: Implications of hyperalimentation. Arch. Surg., 108:213–215, 1974.

49. Adelman, R. D., Abern, S. B., and Halstead, C. H.: Nephrolithiasis in a patient on total parenteral nutrition. J. Clin. Nutr., 28:420, 1975. (abstract)

50. Jones, J. E., Manalo, R., and Flink, E. B.: Magnesium requirements in adults. Am. J. Clin. Nutr., 20:632–635, 1967.

51. Harken, A. H., and Woods, M.: The influence of oxyhemoglobin affinity on tissue oxygen consumption. Ann. Surg., 183:130–135, 1976.

52. Craddock, P. R., Yawata, Y., Van Santen, L., Gilberstadt, S., Silvis, S., and Jacob, H. S.: Acquired phagocyte dysfunction. A complication of the hypophosphatemia of parenteral hyperalimentation. N. Engl. J. Med., 290:1403–1407, 1974.

53. Sheldon, G. F., and Grzyb, S.: Phosphate depletion and repletion: Relation to parenteral nutrition and oxygen transport. Ann. Surg., 182:683–689, 1975.

54. Cahill, G. F., Jr.: Physiology of insulin in man. Diabetes, 20:785–799, 1971.

55. Dudrick, S. J., Long, J. M., Steiger, E., and Rhoads, J. E.: Intravenous hyperalimentation. Med. Clin. North Am., 54:577–589, 1970.

56. Dennis, C., and Grosz, C. R.: A quarter century of intracaval feeding. Surg. Gynecol. Obstet., 135:883–889, 1972.

57. FreAmine. Information Brochure 560. Glendale, Calif., McGaw Company, 1971.

58. Sleasman, W. P.: Absorption of insulin to syringes and intravenous containers. Doctural thesis. School of Pharmacy, Duquesne University, Oct., 1973.

59. Weber, S. S., Wood, W. A., and Jackson, E. A.: Availability of insulin from parenteral nutrient solutions. Am. J. Hosp, Pharm., 34:353–357, 1977.

60. Oh, T. E., Dyer, H., Wall, B. P., Hall, R. A., and Jellett, L. B.: Insulin loss in parenteral nutrition systems. Anaesth. Intensive Care, 4:342–346, 1976.

61. Weisenfeld, S., Podolsky, S., Goldsmith, L., and Ziff, L.: Adsorption of insulin to infusion bottles and tubing. Diabetes, 17:766–771, 1968.

62. Binder, C.: Absorption of injected insulin; a clinical-pharmacological study. Acta Pharmacol. Toxicol., 27(Suppl. 2):1–87, 1969.

63. Alberti, K. G. M. M., Hockaday, T. D. R., and Turner, R. C.: Small doses of intramuscular insulin in the treatment of diabetic "coma." Lancet, 2:515–525, 1976.

64. Blackburn, G. L.: Nitrogen conservation using fat as a non-protein calorie source. Proceedings, A.M.A. Symposium on Fat Emulsions in Parenteral Nutrition, Chicago, 1975.

65. Benotti, P. N., Bothe, A., Jr., Miller, J. D. B., and Blackburn, G. L.: Cyclic hyperalimentation. Compr. Ther., 2:27–36, 1976.

66. Maini, B., Blackburn, G. L., Bistrian, B. R., Flatt, J. P., Page, J. G., Bothe, A., Benotti, P., and Rienhoff, H. Y.: Cyclic hyperalimentation: An optimal technique for preservation of visceral protein. J. Surg. Res., 20:515–525, 1976.

67. Kaminski, M. V., Jr., and Stolar, M. H.: Parenteral hyperalimentation — A quality of care survey and review. Am. J. Hosp. Pharm., 31:228–235, 1974.

68. Avis, K. E.: Chemicals and particulate matter. In Symposium on Total Parenteral Nutrition. Chicago, American Medical Association, 1972, pp. 147–158.

69. Miller, R. C., and Grogan, J. B.: Efficacy of inline bacterial filters in reducing contamination of intravenous nutritional solutions. Am. J. Surg., 130:585–589, 1975.

70. Collin, J., Tweedle, D. E. F., Venables, C. W., Constable, F. L., and Johnston, I. D. A.: Effect of a millipore filter on complications of intravenous infusions: A prospective clinical trial. Br. Med. J., 4:456–458, 1973.

71. MacLean, L. D.: Discussion. Ann. Surg. 176:271, 1972.

72. Ashcraft, K. W., and Leape, L. L.: Candida sepsis complicating parenteral feeding. J.A.M.A., 212:454–456, 1970.

73. Grinker, J., Cohn, C., and Hirsh, J.: The effect of intravenous administration of glucose, saline, and mannitol on meal regulation in normal weight human subjects. Comm. Behav. Biol., 6:203–208, 1971.

74. Jordan, H. A., Moses, H., MacFadyen, B. V., Jr., and Dudrick, S. J.: Hunger and satiety in humans during parenteral hyperalimentation. Psychosom. Med., 36:144–155, 1974.

75. Hansen, B. W., DeSomery, C. H., Hagedorn, P. K., and Kalnasy, L. W.: Effects of enteral and parenteral nutrition on appetite in monkeys. J. Parenteral Enteral Nutr., 1:83–88, 1977.

76. Green, H. L., Stifel, F. B., Hagler, L., and Herman, R. H. L.: Comparison of the adaptive changes in disaccharidase, glycolytic enzyme and fructosediphosphatase activities after intravenous and oral glucose in normal men. Am. J. Clin. Nutr., 28:1122–1125, 1975.

77. Koga, Y., Ikeda, K., Inokuchi, K., Watanbe, H.,

and Hashimoto, N.: The digestive tract in total parenteral nutrition. Arch. Surg., *110*:742–745, 1975.

78. Bowie, M. D., Brinkman, G. L., and Hansen, J. D. L.: Acquired disaccharide intolerance in malnutrition. J. Pediatr., *66*:1083–1091, 1965.

79. Cook, G. C., and Lee, F. D.: The jejunum after kwashiorkor. Lancet, *2*:1263, 1966.

80. Welsh, J. D.: Isolated lactase deficiency in humans: Report on 100 patients. Medicine, *49*:257–277, 1970.

81. Cook. G. C.: Intestinal enzyme deficiencies and their nutritional implications. Symposia of the Swedish Nutrition Foundation, *11*:52, 1973.

82. Newcomer, A. D., and McGill, D. B.: Disaccharidase activity in the small intestine: Prevalence of lactase deficiency in 100 healthy subjects. Gastroenterology, *53*:881–889, 1967.

83. Cuatrecasas, P., Lockwood, D. H., and Caldwell, J. R.: Lactase deficiency in the adult: A common occurrence. Lancet, *1*:14–18, 1965.

84. Littman, A., and Hammond, J. B.: Diarrhea in adults caused by deficiency in intestinal disaccharidases. Gastroenterology, *48*:237–249, 1965.

# Chapter 8

# PREPARATION OF PARENTERAL NUTRITION SOLUTIONS

## SOLUTION PREPARATION

Studies at the Center for Disease Control have demonstrated that certain common hospital pathogens proliferate rapidly at room temperature in parenteral nutrition solutions prepared from casein hydrolysates and dextrose.[1] In particular, *Candida albicans, Torulopsis glabrata, Serratia marcescens, Klebsiella pneumoniae*, and some strains of *Staphylococcus aureus* increased more than three log concentrations in 24 hours. Solutions prepared from synthetic amino acids and dextrose, however, did not support bacterial growth, although Candida and Torulopsis did proliferate. These studies have been confirmed by other investigators.[2, 3] A protocol for safe administration of parenteral nutrition solutions must, therefore, include aseptic solution preparation. Solutions should not be prepared on the ward near high-traffic areas or contaminated areas but rather in the clean-air environment provided by laminar flow hoods. All manipulations and additions should be performed by trained personnel using aseptic techniques.

To aid in sterile preparation of nutritional solutions in hospitals with limited facilities and small demand, parenteral nutrition kits have been developed. These kits contain a bottle of concentrated amino acids, either as protein hydrolysates or as crystalline amino acids, and a partially filled bottle of hypertonic dextrose in water. The solutions are mixed together just before use by transferring the amino acid solution into the dextrose bottle through a sterile transfer set. Electrolytes, minerals, vitamins, and other components are added as needed. The mixing is best performed in a laminar air-flow unit by personnel using strict aseptic techniques. These kits are convenient and effective for most patients.

Larger hospitals, where the demand for both standard and individually tailored solutions is high, have found plastic bags quite useful in solution preparation and administration. Not only do they readily expand to hold up to 1.3 liters and accommodate large volumes of additives, but they also allow fluid administration without an air inlet system, thus decreasing the possibility of airborne contamination. Plastic bags, which can be stacked, have the further advantage of requiring less storage space than glass bottles after solution preparation.

At Duke University Medical Center, solutions are mixed in batches of 50 to 100 liters in a ratio of 250 grams carbohydrate to 39 grams crystalline amino acids. The solution is prepared in a large stainless steel tank and sterilized by passage through a 0.22 micron millipore filter. Viaflex* plastic bags are filled to a predetermined weight to provide 1 liter. Samples at the beginning, middle, and end of the bagging procedure

---

*PL–146, Travenol Laboratories, Deerfield, Ill. 60015.

are cultured and the batch lot held in quarantine until these cultures confirm sterility. A 30-day expiration date is assigned to each batch, and the solution is stored in the dark under 3° C refrigeration.

When orders are received, bags of parenteral nutrition solution are withdrawn from the refrigerator and additives injected from single-dose vials. Again, all additions are performed by aseptic technique under a laminar air-flow hood. Using the range of additives discussed in Chapter 7, we have had no difficulty with precipitations in our solutions. The exact order of mixture does not appear to be important except that phosphate should be added before calcium. We currently use the following sequence:

To a bag of 500 ml D50W and 500 ml crystalline amino acids add:

1. Multivitamin solution
2. Folic acid
3. Ascorbic acid
4. Sodium chloride (4 mEq/ml)
5. Sodium lactate (5 mEq/ml)
6. Potassium phosphate (4.4 mEqK$^+$ and 3 mmoles phosphate/ml)
7. Potassium chloride (2 mEq/ml)
8. Calcium gluconate (0.5 mEq/ml)
9. Magnesium sulfate (0.8 mEq/ml)
10. Heparin (1000 units/ml)
11. Regular insulin (U-100)
12. Salt-poor albumin
13. Copper, zinc, chromium, and other trace elements as indicated

Following each addition, the solution is thoroughly mixed and inspected for precipitants against both a light and dark background. After final inspection, the solution is sent to the floor where it is refrigerated until used. An expiration date of 24 hours is placed on each bag once additives have been injected. In addition to the above routine solution, special formulations for pediatric patients, renal failure patients, and cardiac patients are prepared on an individual basis in the Viaflex bags.

Lot numbers of all solutions used are maintained in the pharmacy. Different formulas utilized in individual patients are designated with alphabetical letters. Bags mixed under each formula are numbered consecutively. Each bag is labeled clearly

```
NAME                    WARD
#                       FORMULA
BASIC FreAmine II HYPERALIMENTATION SOLUTION
1000 ml.                CONTAINING
——ml. MVI CONC.         ——mEq. KCL
——ml. BEROCCA-C         ——mEq. K PHOSPHATE
300 mg. ASCORBIC ACID   ——mEq. Ca GLUCONATE
300 mcg. FOLIC ACID     ——mEq. Mg SULFATE
——mEq. NaCl             ——ml. ALBUMIN
——mEq. Na LACTATE       ——UNITS HEPARIN
——UNITS REGULAR INSULIN
TOTAL VOLUME IN BAG——
IVAC SETTING            ——
***USE MACRODRIP SET ONLY ***
DO NOT BEGIN ADMINISTRATION AFTER: 2 PM
```

**Figure 8–1** Bag label. Each liter of parenteral nutrition solution must be clearly labeled with the patient's name and ward, the formula letter, and bottle number. It is also helpful to state the infusion rate and date of expiration.

with the patient's name, ward, formula letter, and bag number, along with infusion rate and IVAC pump setting (Fig. 8–1). The bags must be clearly marked to avoid confusion with routine solutions or administration in the wrong vein or to the wrong patient.

## AMINO ACID SOURCES

Amino acids for parenteral nutrition are commercially available either from acid or from enzymatic hydrolysis of casein, fibrin, or meat, or as synthetic crystalline amino acids. Acid hydrolysis denatures tryptophan, an essential amino acid, and occasionally cystine. In commercial production, therefore, hydrolysis is stopped before it is complete.[4] When given intravenously, the few remaining large peptides are taken up by the reticuloendothelial system, where they are metabolically unavailable.[5] In addition to the few large peptides, many small peptides are present after acid and enzymatic hydrolysis of various proteins and represent up to 40 per cent of the nitrogen content. When infused intravenously, some of these smaller peptides are metabolized by the liver. Some pass into the glomerular filtrate and are degraded in the renal tubules to free amino acids, reabsorbed into the blood stream and utilized as metabolic substrates, or excreted in the urine unaltered.[6] In patients with renal disease, a significant renal loss of infused amino aicds as small peptides can occur. Of the single amino acids present in hydrolysates, a variable amount is present as dextro-isomers; except for D-methionine and D-phenylalanine, they are not utilized by the body.[7] As much as 11 per cent of the infused protein can be excreted unchanged in the urine as D-amino acids.[8]

Development of synthetic crystalline L-amino acid solutions permitted various peptides and D-amino acids to be eliminated. Metabolic studies comparing protein hydrolysates to crystalline amino acid solutions have, in general, shown more efficient utilization of nitrogen from crystalline amino acids.[9, 10] Anderson et al.[11] found that patients with various gastrointestinal diseases needed only 64 mg/kg/day nitrogen intravenously to support positive nitrogen balance when crystalline amino acid solutions were used but 128 mg/kg/day when protein hydrolystates were infused along with comparable carbohydrate support. Because of these advantages and improved availability, use of crystalline amino acids is preferable.

Administration of either protein hydrolysates or crystalline amino acid solutions significantly alters the normal serum amino acid pattern,[4, 12-15] as might be expected from comparison of the respective amino acid concentrations (Table 8–1). Similar changes have been observed at Duke University Medical Center when a crystalline amino acid solution (FreAmine II) is used (Table 8–2). The significant increase in serum glutamic and aspartic acids following administration of amino acid solutions containing large amounts of each is of some concern in that both can cause brain damage[16-18] and retinal damage[19] in experimental animals. To date, no evidence for such injury has been observed in human beings. Crystalline amino acids solutions, unlike protein hydrolysates, can be formulated to reflect normal serum amino acid patterns, to meet intravenous amino acid requirements as they become better known, and to provide special amino acid profiles known to stimulate anabolism. For example, low concentrations of glycine seem to be favorable for obtaining positive nitrogen balance.[20, 21] Alanine, which is the main transport form of amino-nitrogen between tissues, should be a major part of the non-essential amino acids given. Alanine, proline, glutamic acid, and leucine have all been shown to play important roles in the utilization of amino acid solutions by enhancing their protein-sparing effect.[22, 23] Finally, patients with renal failure[24, 25] and hepatic failure[26] require special amino acid profiles during parenteral nutrition that can be obtained only through crystalline amino acids.

In general, although protein hydrolysate solutions work satisfactorily in many patients requiring parenteral nutrition, the future solutions will certainly be formulated from crystalline amino acids. The current crystalline amino acid solutions are highly efficient sources of nitrogen but do not yet represent the optimal amino acid composition.[27] Recent work suggests that some non-essential amino acids become essential during illness and stress, and future amino acid solutions should be altered to meet these requirements. For example, the adult human being can synthesize cystine from methionine, and cystine is normally not considered an essential amino acid. The ability to synthesize cystine is, however, limited,[15] and patients with moderate or greater surgical stress are unable to synthesize adequate cystine during intravenous nutrition. As cystine is important in metabolic pathways involving other amino acids,[28] it should be provided in greater quantities to patients with stress.

In a similar manner, phenylalanine is normally hydroxylated in the liver to form tyrosine. During metabolic stress the efficiency of this pathway is impaired, with the accumulation of phenylalanine in the serum and depression of tyrosine.[28, 29] In stressful situations tyrosine supplementation may need to be increased and phenylalanine decreased. Arginine, normally not an essential amino acid, plays a critical role in the Krebs urea cycle, which is important in the metabolism of ammonia. Yet, the body's ability to synthesize arginine is limited. Neonates and stressed adults have de-

Preparation of Parenteral Nutrition Solutions**  **121**

**Table 8-1**  AMINO ACID CONTENT OF AMINO ACID SOLUTIONS (grams/liter)

| | NORMAL SERUM CONCEN-TRATION (mg/liter) | MDR* (Rose) | AMIGEN 5% | AMIGEN 10% | AMINOSOL 5% | CPH 5% | HYPROTOGEN 5% | AMINOSYN 7% | FREAMINE II 8.5% | TRAVASOL 5.5% | TRAVASOL 8.5% | VEINAMINE 8.0% |
|---|---|---|---|---|---|---|---|---|---|---|---|---|
| **Essential Amino Acids** | | | | | | | | | | | | |
| Lysine | 28.5 | 0.8 | 3.1 | 6.2 | 4.0 | 3.5 | 3.5 | 5.1 | 8.7 | 3.2 | 4.9 | 5.4 |
| Tryptophan | 4.7 | 0.25 | 0.35 | 0.7 | 0.5 | 0.5 | 0.4 | 1.2 | 1.3 | 1.0 | 1.5 | 0.8 |
| Phenylalanine | 11.1 | 1.1 | 2.0 | 4.0 | 1.0 | 2.3 | 2.0 | 3.1 | 4.8 | 3.4 | 5.3 | 4.0 |
| Methionine | 2.5 | 1.1 | 1.3 | 2.6 | 1.0 | 2.2 | 1.6 | 2.8 | 4.5 | 3.2 | 4.9 | 4.3 |
| Threonine | 18.0 | 0.5 | 1.9 | 3.8 | 2.3 | 1.8 | 1.9 | 3.7 | 3.4 | 2.3 | 3.6 | 1.6 |
| Leucine | 17.3 | 1.1 | 4.1 | 8.2 | 6.4 | 4.1 | 4.1 | 6.6 | 7.7 | 3.4 | 5.3 | 3.5 |
| Isoleucine | 11.0 | 0.7 | 2.6 | 5.2 | 2.2 | 2.4 | 2.5 | 5.1 | 5.9 | 2.6 | 4.1 | 4.9 |
| Valine | 28.8 | 0.8 | 3.1 | 6.2 | 1.6 | 3.0 | 3.0 | 5.6 | 5.6 | 2.5 | 3.9 | 2.5 |
| **Non-Essential Amino Acids** | | | | | | | | | | | | |
| Histadine | 14.4 | | 1.3 | 2.6 | 1.2 | 1.2 | – | 2.1 | 2.4 | 2.4 | 3.7 | 2.4 |
| Glutamate | 71.1 | | 13 | 26 | 1.4 | – | – | – | – | – | – | 4.3 |
| Proline | 23.0 | | 4.5 | 9.0 | 3.2 | – | – | 6.1 | 9.5 | 2.3 | 3.6 | 1.1 |
| Aspartate | 7.6 | | 3.5 | 7.0 | 0.5 | – | – | – | – | – | – | 4.0 |
| Serine | 14.6 | | 3.0 | 6.0 | 3.4 | – | – | 3.0 | 5.0 | – | – | – |
| Arginine | 10.3 | | 1.8 | 3.6 | 2.9 | 1.5 | – | 6.9 | 3.1 | 5.7 | 8.8 | 7.5 |
| Alanine | 32.4 | | 1.5 | 3.0 | 2.2 | – | – | 9.0 | 6.0 | 11 | 18 | – |
| Glycine | 22.3 | | 1.1 | 2.2 | 2.1 | – | – | 9.0 | 18 | 11 | 18 | 34 |
| Tyrosine | 9.8 | | 0.6 | 1.2 | 5.6 | – | – | 0.44 | – | 0.22 | 0.34 | – |
| Cysteine | 1.0 | | – | – | 0.3 | – | – | – | 0.2 | – | – | – |
| Ornithine | 11.1 | | – | – | – | – | – | – | – | – | – | – |
| Hydroxyproline | 2.0 | | – | – | – | – | – | – | – | – | – | – |

*MDR = minimal daily requirement, see Table 6–2.

**Table 8-2**  ALTERATION OF SERUM AMINO ACID PATTERN DURING PARENTERAL NUTRITION USING FREAMINE II 8.5% (39 grams/liter)*

| AMINO ACID | NORMAL SERUM CONCEN-TRATION $\mu$moles/liter | PT. 1 | PT. 2 | PT. 3 | PT. 4 | PT. 5 | PT. 6 | PT. 7 |
|---|---|---|---|---|---|---|---|---|
| Lysine | 19.5 | 26.6 | 23.5 | 21.4 | 19.4 | 18.5 | 35.9 | 20.4 |
| Tryptophan | 2.3 | 2.4 | 1.3 | 1.7 | 1.1 | 2.8 | 0.7 | 3.8 |
| Phenylalanine | 6.7 | 13.8 | 9.7 | 11.2 | 13.0 | 14.3 | 19.2 | 9.2 |
| Methionine | 1.7 | 22.3 | 23.0 | 10.0 | 21.0 | 9.9 | 9.7 | 2.7 |
| Threonine | 15.1 | 25.2 | 17.6 | 20.4 | 22.4 | 20.2 | 28.5 | 9.4 |
| Leucine | 13.2 | 22.2 | 8.4 | 15.4 | 18.6 | 13.9 | 19.7 | 16.0 |
| Isoleucine | 8.4 | 14.2 | 5.4 | 8.8 | 13.0 | 7.6 | 11.1 | 9.6 |
| Valine | 24.6 | 41.4 | 17.0 | 24.7 | 35.8 | 24.3 | 36.6 | 36.2 |
| Histadine | 9.3 | – | – | – | – | – | – | – |
| Glutamic Acid | 48.4 | 71.3 | 37.6 | 52.9 | 59.0 | 45.6 | 65.4 | 54.6 |
| Proline | 20.0 | 62.5 | 95.3 | 59.1 | 53.7 | 40.6 | 64.6 | 26.1 |
| Aspartic Acid | 5.7 | 8.7 | 3.4 | 7.6 | 7.3 | 6.0 | 10.5 | 2.2 |
| Serine | 13.9 | 35.8 | 20.4 | 19.8 | 26.9 | 21.9 | 29.9 | 11.0 |
| Arginine | 5.9 | 8.5 | 2.5 | 3.2 | 2.0 | 8.2 | 13.6 | 6.4 |
| Alanine | 36.4 | 88.1 | 40.2 | 37.4 | 43.6 | 30.1 | 47.1 | 28.0 |
| Glycine | 29.7 | 112.6 | 85.6 | 41.6 | 75.6 | 62.6 | 88.6 | 30.6 |
| Tyrosine | 5.4 | 1.8 | 1.0 | 6.4 | 4.4 | 7.3 | 5.5 | 4.4 |
| Cysteine | 0.8 | 0.9 | 7.5 | 2.3 | 2.9 | 0.3 | 1.7 | 0.3 |
| Ornithine | 8.4 | 6.7 | 6.8 | 9.8 | 6.1 | 4.9 | 11.6 | 10.3 |
| Hydroxyproline | 1.5 | 0.4 | 2.0 | 1.5 | 1.6 | 1.4 | 2.3 | 1.4 |
| Cystine | 1.65 | 1.7 | 5.0 | 6.0 | 0.9 | 1.2 | 5.7 | 3.0 |

*The amino acid solution was infused at a steady rate of 117 grams per day with an IVAC pump.

veloped marked hypoargininemia, and subsequently, hyperammonemia, during parenteral nutrition with solutions containing little or no arginine. Because of the role of arginine in ammonia metabolism and its ability to counteract the toxic effects associated with infusion of large amounts of glycine, it is recommended that arginine be supplemented during parenteral nutrition (0.5 to 1.0 mmoles/kg/day) (see Chapter 10). Finally, histidine appears to augment utilization of amino acid mixtures in patients with uremia.[30, 31]

Further research on intravenous amino acid requirements, including the ratio of essential to non-essential amino acids, the ratio of non-protein to protein calories, and the utilization of intravenously administered amino acids, will lead to more nearly ideal amino acid solutions. Some work along these lines has been published and appears promising.[32]

## ADDITIVE COMPATIBILITY

To provide all nutrients intravenously, parenteral nutrition solutions must contain a large number of different components in a relatively small volume of fluid. The possibility of component interactions and microprecipitation is quite high and must be considered with each bottle mixed. The final solution should be inspected against both black and white backgrounds with proper lighting, and all bottles with precipitates must be discarded. The bottles should be reinspected by the nursing staff just before they are administered to a patient.

Although precise solubility studies with parenteral nutrition solutions are practically impossible because of their complex nature,[33] some limitations have been observed:

*pH.* Sterilized hydrochloric acid (1 mEq/ml) may be added to all amino acid–dextrose solutions in nearly any amount. Care should be taken, however, to keep the pH between 3.0 and 6.8.

*Calcium and phosphorus.* These two ions readily combine to form a precipitate.

However, by adding the phosphate ion first, with thorough mixing, and then slowly adding the calcium ion, with constant swirling, up to 15 mEq calcium and 10 mmoles phosphate can be added to one liter without precipitate formation.[34] We have found additions of up to 17 mmoles phosphate per liter possible when only 5 mEq calcium ion were present. These concentrations are ample for all but the exceptional patient (see Chapter 7 for electrolyte and mineral requirements). When additional supplementation is necessary, it should be given through a separate intravenous line.

*Magnesium.* In our experience, magnesium is compatible at concentrations up to 12 mEq per liter. The sulfate salt is preferred to provide the necessary sulfate ions. When magnesium sulfate is used, calcium should not be given as the chloride salt, as calcium sulfate precipitates rather quickly. The glucoheptonate salt of calcium reacts more slowly, requiring several days before calcium sulfate precipitates.

*Insulin.* Insulin is not stable in the presence of sodium bicarbonate. It can be added to parenteral nutrition solutions in any amount.

*Albumin.* Though listed by manufacturers of amino acid solutions as incompatible or of unknown compatibility, albumin appears to be stable and clinically effective for at least 24 hours in concentrations up to 35.5 grams per liter.

*Heparin.* Heparin is compatible at all concentrations. It may be inactivated by vitamin C.

*Sodium hydrocortisone.* Hydrocortisone is compatible and stable at all concentrations.

*Vitamins.* Multiple vitamin preparations are compatible at all concentrations. Ascorbic acid may significantly deteriorate following storage for one or more weeks.[35] Ascorbic acid inactivates vitamins $B_{12}$ and K, and the latter two vitamins inactivate each other. Vitamin $B_{12}$ and K should be given in separate infusions or intramuscularly. Folic acid can precipitate in the presence of calcium salts. Vitamin A appears to bind rapidly to plastic and glass and is easily oxidized.

*Antibiotics.* Because of potential protein binding, antibiotics should not be added to parenteral nutrition solutions. The penicillins are rapidly degraded by FreAmine. In the presence of calcium or magnesium, insoluble complexes with tetracycline may form. To insure optimal effects, all antibiotics, as well as other pharmaceuticals, should be given by separate intravenous routes.

*Sodium, potassium,* and *chloride.* These electrolytes are compatible at all concentrations.

*Digitalis.* Digitalis is incompatible with parenteral nutrition solution and should not be added to it. To avoid serious complications associated with digitalization during excessive calcium ion administration, calcium should be eliminated from the parenteral nutrition solution and digitalization begun only after calcium has cleared from the plasma (serum calcium half-life is three hours).

## SOLUTION STABILITY

Amino acid solutions appear to be relatively stable except for the amino acid tryptophan, which decays in the presence of sodium bisulfite (a preservative in all commercially available solutions) and during light exposure with gradual yellowing of the solution.[36] Grant et al.[37] have correlated liver enzyme elevations and periportal fatty changes of the liver with the administration of solutions containing decayed tryptophan in patients and experimental rats. Use of yellowed solutions should be avoided. McGaw Laboratories, recognizing this potential problem, advised protection of crystalline amino acid solutions from light exposure in a letter dated December 12, 1975.

Once amino acid solutions are mixed with dextrose, they are stable in the dark for at least six months. Even when various electrolytes and minerals are added, the solutions remain relatively unchanged, except for significant loss of vitamins A and C, if refrigerated for about 21 days. To assure optimal safety, however, it is advised that

parenteral nutrition solutions be stored under continuous refrigeration at 3° C for no longer than 48 hours prior to use.[38]

## REFERENCES

1. Goldman, D. A., Martin, W. T., and Worthington, J. W.: Growth of bacteria and fungi in total parenteral nutrition solutions. Am. J. Surg., *126*:314–318, 1973.
2. Brennan, M. F., O'Connell, R. C., Rosol, J. A., and Kundsin, R.: The growth of *Candida albicans* in nutritive solutions given parenterally. Arch. Surg., *103*:705–708, 1971.
3. Flores, L. L.: Hyperalimentation and sepsis. Clinical Digest, McGaw Laboratories, *1*(2), Aug., 1972.
4. Jeejeebhoy, K. N., Langer, B., Tsallas, G., Chu, R. C., Kuksis, A., and Anderson, G. H.: Total parenteral nutrition at home: Studies in patients surviving 4 months to 5 years. Gastroenterology, *71*:943–953, 1976.
5. McFarlane, I. G., and von Holt, C.: Metabolism of amino acids in protein-calorie–deficient rats. Biochem. J., *111*:557–563, 1969.
6. Wochner, R. D., Strober, W., and Waldmann, T. A.: The role of the kidney in the catabolism of Bence Jones proteins and immunoglobulin fragments. J. Exp. Med., *126*:207–221, 1967.
7. Peaston, M. J. T.: A comparison of hydrolyzed L- and synthesized DL-amino acids for complete parenteral nutrition. Clin. Pharmacol. Ther., *9*:61–66, 1967.
8. Elman, R.: Amino acid mixtures as parenteral protein food. Am. J. Med., *5*:760–774, 1948.
9. Long, C. L., Zikria, B. A., Kinney, J. M., and Geiger, J. W.: Comparison of fibrin hydrolysates and crystalline amino acid solutions in parenteral nutrition. Am. J. Clin. Nutr., *27*:163–174, 1974.
10. Tweedle, D. E. F., Spivey, J., and Johnston, I. D. A.: A comparison of the effect of some currently available mixtures of amino acids on postoperative metabolism. Br. J. Surg. *58*:855, 1971.
11. Anderson, G. H., Patel, D. G., and Jeejeebhoy, K. N.: Design and evaluation by nitrogen balance and blood aminograms of an amino acid mixture for total parenteral nutrition of adults with gastrointestinal disease. J. Clin. Invest., *53*:904–912, 1974.
12. Ghadimi, H., Abaci, F., Kumar, S., and Rathi, M.: Biochemical aspects of intravenous alimentation. Pediatrics, *48*:955–965, 1971.
13. Stegink, L. D., and Baker, C. L.: Infusion of protein hydrolysates in the newborn infant: Plasma amino acid concentrations. J. Pediatr., *78*:595–602, 1971.
14. Dudrick, S. J., MacFadyen, B. V., Jr., VanBuren, C. T., Ruberg, R. L., and Maynard, A. T.: Parenteral hyperalimentation. Metabolic problems and solutions. Ann. Surg., *176*:259–264, 1972.
15. DenBesten, L., and Stegink, L. D.: Effect of parenteral alimentation mixtures on plasma amino acid levels in adult subjects: Comparison of

the route of administration. Fed. Proc., *31*:732, 1972.

16. Olney, J. W., and Sharpe, L. G.: Brain lesions in an infant rhesus monkey treated with monosodium glutamate. Science, *166*:386–388, 1969.

17. Olney, J. W., and Ho, O. L.: Brain damage in infant mice following oral intake of glutamate, aspartate, or cysteine, Nature, *227*:609–611, 1970.

18. Olney, J. W., Ho, O. L., and Rhee, V.: Brain-damaging potential of protein hydrolysates. N. Engl. J. Med., *289*:391–395, 1973.

19. Olney, J. W.: Glutamate-induced retinal degeneration in neonatal mice. Electron microscopy of the acutely evolving lesion. J. Neuropathol. Exp. Neurol., *28*:455–474, 1969.

20. Tuttle, S. G., Swendseid, M. E., Mulcare, D., Griffith, W. H., and Bassett, S. H.: Essential amino acid requriements of older men in relation to total nitrogen intake. Metabolism, *8*:61–72, 1959.

21. Johnston, I. D. A., Tweedle, D., and Spivey, J.: Intravenous feeding after surgical operation. *In*: Wilkinson, A. W. (ed.): Parenteral Nutrition. Baltimore, Williams & Wilkins Company, 1972, pp. 189–197.

22. Dolif, D., and Jurgens, P.: Die Bedeutung der nichtessentiellen Amino-sauren bei der parenteralen Ernahrung. *In* Berg, G. (ed.): Advances in Parenteral Nutrition. Symposium of the International Society of Parenteral Nutrition. Stuttgart, George Thieme Verlag, 1969.

23. Buse, M. G., and Reid, S. S.: Leucine. A possible regulator of protein turnover in muscle. J. Clin. Invest., *56*:1250–1261, 1975.

24. Dudrick, S. J., Steiger, E., and Long, J. M.: Renal failure in surgical patients. Treatment with intravenous essential amino acids and hypertonic glucose. Surgery, *68*:180–186, 1970.

25. Abel, R. M., Abbott, W. M., and Fischer, J. E.: Intravenous essential L-amino acids and hypertonic dextrose in patients with acute renal failure. Am. J. Surg., *123*:632–638, 1972.

26. Fischer, J. E., Funovics, J. M., Aguirre, A., James, J. H., Keane, J. M., Wesdorp, R. I. C.,Yoshimura, N., and Westman, T.: The role of plasma amino acids in hepatic encephalopathy. Surgery, *78*:276–290, 1975.

27. Tweedle, D. E. F.: Intravenous amino acid solutions. Br. J. Hosp. Med., *13*:81–85, 1975.

28. Dale, G., Young, G., Latner, A. L., Goode, A., Tweedle, D., and Johnston, I. D. A.: The effect of surgical operation on venous plasma free amino acids. Surgery, *81*:295–301, 1977.

29. Groves, A. C., Woolf, L. I., Allardyce, D. B., and Hasinoff, C.: Arterial plasma amino acids in patients receiving an elemental diet. Surg. Forum, *25*:54–56, 1974.

30. Bergstrom, J., Furst, P., Josephson, B., and Noree, L.-O.: Improvement of nitrogen balance in a uremic patient by the addition of histidine to essential amino acid solutions given intravenously. Life Sci., *9*:787–794, 1970.

31. Swendseid, M. E., Kopple, J. D., and Paniagua, M.: Effect of essential amino acid diets on nitrogen balance and amino acid levels in chronic uremia. Abst. Am. Soc. Nephrol., *5*:79, 1971.

32. Ghadimi, H.: Development of amino acid solutions for intravenous nutrition. J. Parenteral Enteral Nutr., *1*:7A, 1977. (abstract)

33. Cluxton, R. J., Jr.: Some complexities of making compatibility studies in hyperalimentation solutions. Drug Intelligence and Clinical Pharmacy, *5*:177–178, 1971.

34. Kaminski, M. V., Jr., Harris, D. F., Collin, C. F., and Sommers, G. A.: Electrolyte compatibility in a synthetic amino acid hyperalimentation solution. Am. J. Hosp. Pharm., *31*:244–246, 1974.

35. Williams. J. T., and Moravec, D. F.: Intravenous Therapy. Chicago, Clissold Books, Inc., 1967.

36. Kleinman, L. M., Tangrea, J. A., Gallelli, J. F., Brown, J., and Gross, E.: Stability of solutions of essential amino acids. Am. J. Hosp. Pharm., *30*:1054–1057, 1973.

37. Grant, J. P., Cox, C. E., Kleinman, L. M., Maher, M. M., Pittmann, M. A., Tangrea, J. A., Brown, J. H., Gross, E., Beazley, R. M., and Jones, R. S.: Serum hepatic enzyme and bilirubin elevations during parenteral nutrition. Surg. Gynecol. Obstet., *145*:573–580, 1977.

38. Rowlands, D. A., Wilkinson, W. R., and Yoshimura. N. N.: Storage stability of mixed hyperalimentation solutions. Am. J. Hosp. Pharm., *30*:436–438, 1973.

# Chapter 9

# SEPTIC AND METABOLIC COMPLICATIONS: RECOGNITION AND MANAGEMENT

## FEVER

Sepsis is a serious complication of parenteral nutrition. Patients who require parenteral nutrition are often predisposed to infectious complications as a result of malnutrition,[1-3] frequent use of broad-spectrum antibiotics,[2, 4] and the presence of concomitant infections in wounds, the urinary tract, or the lungs. The presence of Candida species in the urine or mouth is particularly prominent. In addition, the indwelling subclavian catheter can serve as a nidus for microbial growth, with the parenteral nutrition solution providing all necessary nutrients. The frequency of septic complications related to parenteral nutrition ranges from 2 to 33 per cent.[5, 6] In early experiences with parenteral nutrition, Candida species predominated.[7] More recently, gram-positive and gram-negative bacteria have become important.

With increasing experience, it has become evident that septic complications during parenteral nutrition are inversely related to the emphasis placed on aseptic techniques in catheter placement and maintenance and in solution preparation and administration. In 1972 the Center for Disease Control reported an incidence of catheter-associated sepsis of 7 per cent in 2078 patients receiving parenteral nutrition at 31 hospitals where protocols incorporating "adequate" infection control measures were followed.[8] In some medical centers where an intensive effort has been made to

provide safe parenteral nutrition, infection rates of less than 3 per cent have been reported.[9-11] Similar low rates have been reported even in patients highly susceptible to infection.[12] When optimal care is given, the incidence of primary catheter sepsis should be negligible. Primary catheter sepsis is defined as a septic episode in which no other site of infection is obvious, the complication resolves upon catheter removal, and cultures of the catheter tip and peripheral blood grow the same organism. Those septic complications that do occur should only follow seeding of the indwelling catheter by organisms from other infected sites. However, even with proven bacteremia, seeding of the catheter should occur in only 5 to 7 per cent of patients.

The incidence of septic complications at Duke University Medical Center has been 3.5 per cent. This rate is based on a total of 414 patients receiving infusions for 8694 patient-days through 462 catheters in place an average of 18.8 days (range: 1 day to 84 days). We have had seven primary infections attributed to the indwelling catheter (1.7 per cent). In four instances the cultured organisms were coagulase-negative *Staphylococcus aureus* and could be traced to line violations. In another case, a catheter contaminated with *Klebsiella pneumoniae* during insertion was not immediately removed, and a positive catheter culture was obtained two days later during a febrile episode. In these cases, therefore, contamination was documented, and sepsis could have been avoided if the catheter had been removed. We have had two asymptomatic primary fungal catheter infections, which were detected by routine culture during catheter removal. The organism in each case was *Candida parapsilosis*. The significance of these cultures is not known. We have had no instances of symptomatic primary fungal catheter infections even though a large proportion of our patients are critically ill and on broad-spectrum antibiotics during parenteral nutrition. For this reason we, along with others,[11] do not subscribe to the "amphotericin flush" once advocated by Brennan et al.[13] We have had five instances (1.2 per cent) of secondary catheter infections, in which the indwelling catheter was infected by organisms from other sites of infection. In two cases, *Klebsiella pneumoniae* was cultured from the catheter as well as from either a wound or the urine. In two other cases, *Candida albicans* septicemia was documented before and at the time of subclavian catheter insertion and was cultured later on the catheter. In one case, *Staphylococcus aureus* was cultured first in a wound infection and 48 hours later on the subclavian catheter. The rate of catheter sepsis has not increased with prolonged catheter maintenance, in agreement with the findings of others.[11, 14, 15] The risk of catheter infection may well be greatest during the first three to five days following catheter placement while a fibrin sheath is forming about it (see Chapter 4 on subclavian vein thrombosis). After the sheath is fully organized, bacterial and fungal colonization is difficult. The changing of catheters at regular intervals is therefore discouraged. Catheter removal should be reserved for such cases as termination of therapy, mechanical malfunction (cracked or kinked catheter or catheter occlusion by a fibrin sheath), and suspected catheter sepsis.

The differential diagnosis of febrile reactions in patients receiving parenteral nutrition must include not only the usual causes, such as wound infections, pneumonia, urinary tract infections, thrombophlebitis, and gram-negative septicemia, but also reactions to pyrogens in the parenteral nutrition solution and allergic reactions to vitamin solutions containing thiamine.[16] Allergic reactions to casein derivatives in casein hydrolysates have been reported, but no such reactions have been observed to result from fibrin or protein hydrolysates or crystalline amino acid solutions. Allergic reactions to casein hydrolysates and thiamine are usually characterized by an elevation of temperature and a minimal elevation of the white blood count, with a normal differential count or indications of mild eosinophilia.

Septic complications related to the subclavian catheter are often not difficult to detect, as fevers (usually greater than 38.5° C) and shaking chills occur every four to eight hours and glucose intolerance often develops (see next section). A leukocytosis with increased polymorphonuclear cells and band formation is often seen early. Patients with pre-existing fevers may demonstrate superimposed acute temperature elevations and chills. If sepsis is suspected, the subclavian catheter should be removed and cultures of the patient's blood, the catheter tip, and the solution obtained.

In some patients, however, it is very difficult to diagnose catheter sepsis. Cultures from the intravenous line may be helpful if performed aseptically, as described by Macht.[17] At the end of an infusion the bottle is lowered below the patient to allow blood to reflux into half of the connecting tubing. The entire set-up of parenteral nutrition solution and tubing is then changed according to the usual routine, and infusion is resumed with 5 per cent dextrose in quarter normal saline with 10 mEq potassium per liter. Three cultures are taken: one of the blood in the intravenous tubing, one of a mixture of the blood and parenteral nutrition solution, and one of the parenteral nutrition solution alone. Negative cultures are good indication that neither the parenteral nutrition solution nor the catheter is the source of sepsis. Positive cultures must be interpreted with caution, as the catheter, tubing, parenteral nutrition solution, or patient's blood may be responsible.

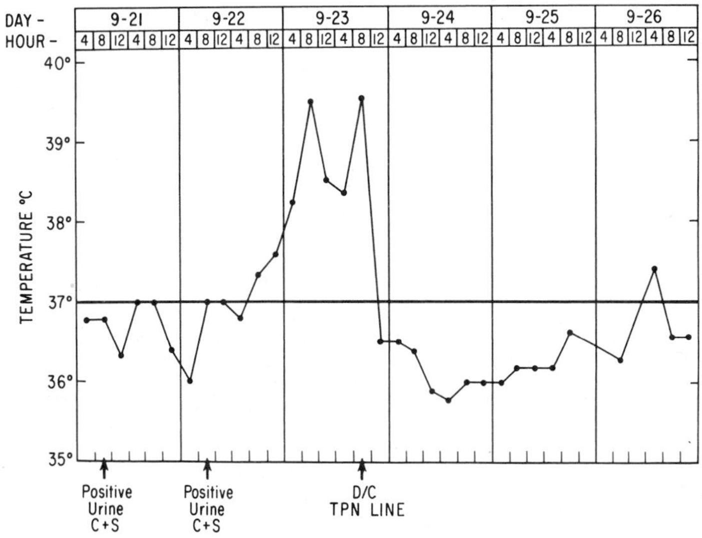

**Figure 9–1** Catheter-related sepsis during parenteral nutrition is often characterized by recurring fevers and shaking chills as in this patient. Removal of the catheter should result in rapid improvement (see text for patient history).

After the above cultures have been taken, the patient must be closely observed and temperatures recorded hourly. If the temperature returns to normal and remains so for 12 hours, the parenteral nutrition solution may be infused again through the same catheter while the cultures are incubating. If the temperature does not return to normal and the source of the fever is not found within 6 to 12 hours, the subclavian catheter should be removed and appropriate cultures taken. A cardinal principle that must be observed is that the subclavian catheter must be implicated, and the entire system, including the solution, intravenous tubing, and catheter removed, when any doubt exists as to the cause of a febrile episode. No attempt should be made to clear a suspected catheter infection with antibiotics because of the risk of significant morbidity.[6]

The clinical course of a patient who developed secondary infection of the subclavian catheter is illustrated in Figure 9–1.

M.S. had been on parenteral nutrition for 15 days without complication and had a normal temperature. A routine urine culture taken on the thirteenth day was found on the fifteenth day to be growing greater than 100,000 colonies of *Klebsiella pneumoniae*. No treatment was initiated at that time. A repeat urine culture 24 hours later

again demonstrated a heavy growth of *Klebsiella pneumoniae*. As noted in Figure 9–1, the patient experienced shaking chills and a temperature of 39.5° C 12 hours later. At the second temperature elevation, a blood culture was drawn through the subclavian catheter, and the catheter was removed. Antibiotic therapy was instituted. The patient's temperature rapidly returned to normal, and he remained afebrile. A new subclavian catheter was inserted after 24 hours, and parenteral nutrition resumed without further complication. Final culture results demonstrated *Klebsiella pneumoniae* from the blood drawn through the catheter and from the catheter tip, while the peripheral blood culture was sterile.

This patient's clinical course demonstrates several points. First, fever associated with shaking chills must always be considered as evidence of catheter-related sepsis. Second, temperatures and shaking chills continue intermittently until the catheter is removed. Finally, upon removal of the catheter the fever should abate over the next 8 to 12 hours, and there should be little morbidity and no mortality. (A note of caution: Although the above clinical findings are often present, catheter-related sepsis can occur with low-grade temperature elevations and no shaking chills.)

The following steps should be taken if a febrile reaction occurs during parenteral nutrition in which the source of infection is not obvious or in which catheter sepsis is suspected:

1. A routine fever work-up, including physical examination, chest x-ray, and appropriate cultures, should be done.
2. The parenteral nutrition solution should be discontinued and sent to the laboratory for fungal and routine cultures.
3. A blood sample should be drawn through the catheter prior to its removal, and that sample and the catheter tip (which must be removed aseptically) sent for fungal and routine cultures. Blood from a peripheral vein should also be sent for fungal and routine cultures.
4. All intravenous and intra-arterial lines should be removed and a peripheral intravenous line inserted. A 5 per cent dextrose and salt solution should be infused at the same rate as the previous parenteral nutrition solution to prevent rebound hypoglycemia until the fever resolves. Use of more concentrated dextrose solutions is unnecessary.
5. After 24 to 48 hours, if intravneous nutrition is still indicated, a new subclavian catheter may be placed and parenteral nutrition resumed at the previous rate. There is no need to accommodate patients to the high dextrose load again if the solution is started within 48 hours.

If the patient's fever resolves following removal of the subclavian catheter and discontinuation of parenteral nutrition, no antibiotic therapy is needed in primary catheter-associated sepsis. This is true whether a bacterial or fungal organism was the causal agent. If the temperature remains elevated and the patient continues a septic course, however, appropriate antibiotic therapy should be given, based on the cultured organism. Delay of 24 to 48 hours before restarting parenteral nutrition as mentioned in Step 5 is well advised. Not only does this allow for clearing of any bacteremia or fungemia, but it also eliminates concern over the catheter as a possible source of continuing sepsis. After 24 to 48 hours the etiology of the sepsis will likely be known, and if it is other than the subclavian catheter, specific therapy can be investigated. At no time should one feel obligated to resume parenteral nutrition immediately, as starvation for 24 to 48 hours will not materially alter a patient's course.

## GLUCOSURIA

The normal adult can tolerate infusion of up to 400 to 500 grams of glucose over 24 hours with little difficulty. By gradually increasing glucose infusion over several days, up to 1500 grams a day can be metabolized. However, patients with severe stress, malnutrition, septicemia, or diabetes, and the very young or very old, are often quite intolerant of glucose and can develop marked hyperglycemia and glucosuria even with minimal glucose infusion. If allowed to spill 2 grams glucose per 100 ml urine (4+ nitroprusside reaction), an osmotic diuresis will follow, leading to the development of hyperglycemic, hyperosmolar, non-ketotic acidosis with an overall death rate of 40 to 50 per cent.[18, 19] If the syndrome develops within 2 to 4 hours, it is often associated with headache and convulsions. If it develops within 8 to 24 hours, it is usually accompanied by stupor, confusion, and coma. In both cases, dry skin, excessive urinary output, and massive glucosuria are present. Metabolic acidosis is always present, although the blood pH is usually not less than 7.2 in the presence of normal renal, hepatic, and pulmonary function. Acidosis with a pH of less than 7.2 is associated with a very poor prognosis.

Survival is greatly improved by early diagnosis. Treatment should initially be directed toward rapid fluid replacement. One-half normal saline plus 10 to 20 mEq potassium per liter should be administered at about 250 cc/hour. Regular insulin should be added to the intravenous fluid to administer 15 to 20 units per hour. Acidosis should be corrected with sodium bicarbonate, the amount of which can be calculated:

$$\text{mEq HCO}_3^= = (\text{body weight in kg}) \times (24 - \text{HCO}_3 \text{ plasma}) \times (0.6)$$

Half of the calculated bicarbonate should be given rapidly intravenously and the other half added to the intravenous solution and given over four to six hours. During treatment, serum glucose and electrolytes, arterial blood gases, and urine dextrose must be monitored hourly. Plasma osmolality (Posm) can be estimated by the formula:

$$Posm = (Na + K) + \frac{Sugar}{18} + \frac{BUN}{2.8}$$

As blood dextrose returns to normal, urinary output decreases. A precipitious fall in blood glucose should be avoided, as cerebral edema may develop because of the delay in equilibrium between blood and cerebral spinal fluid dextrose. Rapid de-crease in blood dextrose concentrations may also result in contraction of intravascular volume and hypotension.

Blood glucose concentrations during parenteral nutrition will normally be less than 130 or 140 mg/100 ml with no more than 2+ glucosuria. Any episode of hyperglycemia with concentrations greater than 200 mg/100 ml or 4+ glucosuria must be evaluated immediately and treated appropriately. The following is a list of considerations for evaluating hyperglycemia and glucosuria.

1. *Check medications*: There are many medications that interfere with determination of urinary sugar by either the Clini-test or Tes-Tape techniques (Table 9–1). In addition to interfering with the meas-

**Table 9–1**   DRUG INTERFERENCE WITH URINE GLUCOSE DETERMINATIONS

| DRUG | EFFECT ON COPPER REDUCTION (CLINITEST) | EFFECT ON GLUCOSE OXIDASE (TES-TAPE) | DEALING WITH POTENTIAL INTERFERENCES |
|---|---|---|---|
| Cephalosporins | False positive (black-brown color) | No effect | Use glucose oxidase test. |
| Keflin | " | " | " |
| Keflex | " | " | " |
| Kefzol, Ancef | " | " | " |
| Kafocin | " | " | " |
| Loridine | " | " | " |
| Vitamin C (in large doses) | False positive | False negative | See note below. Also may monitor blood glucose. |
| Aspirin and other salicylates (in very large doses) | False positive | False negative | See note below. Also may monitor blood glucose. |
| Aldomet (methyldopa) (in very large doses) | False positive | No effect | Use glucose oxidase test. |
| Benemid (probenecid) | False positive | No effect | Use glucose oxidase test. |
| Achromycin (tetracycline) (inj. only) | False positive | False negative | See note below. Also may monitor blood glucose. |
| Pyridium (phenazopyridine) | No effect | False positive & false negative | Use copper reduction method. |
| Chloromycetin (chloramphenicol) | False positive (potentially) | No effect | If in doubt, use glucose oxidase test. |
| Levodopa (in large doses) | False positive | False negative | See note below. Also may monitor blood glucose. |

Note: Potential interferences with glucose oxidase tests (Tes-Tape) can be eliminated by careful testing. While interfering substances will prevent color development in the part of the paper actually dipped into the urine sample, they will not prevent accurate development in a band across the very highest portion of the wetted tape. A true negative test occurs when the band remains the same color as the rest of the tape, and a true positive test occurs when the band changes to one of the colors shown on the color chart.

urement of glucose in the urine, some drugs have a significant influence on glucose metabolism, and their administration may lead to hyperglycemia. Serum glucose concentration should always be obtained to document hyperglycemia. Corticosteroids enhance gluconeogenesis and may induce hyperglycemia directly. Diuretics may also be responsible for elevated blood sugars. The benzothiadiazides, by depleting body potassium or by some unknown mechanism, may induce a diabetic state, especially in patients with "latent diabetes" or hypertension.[20-22] Furosemide[23] and ethacrinic acid[24] may also impair glucose tolerance. Phenytoin, when given in large doses, delays insulin secretion in response to glucose administration, resulting in hyperglycemia and glucosuria.[25, 26] Finally, the phenothiazines, especially chlorpromazine, induce hyperglycemia after prolonged administration.[27]

2. *Check rate of administration*: A sudden increase in the infusion rate is the most common cause of glucosuria. The infusion should be readjusted to the correct rate and urinary glucose followed closely for four to six hours to assure prompt resolution of glucosuria.

3. *Check serum and urinary potassium*: The potassium ion is an essential activator of intracellular enzymatic reactions, particulary those involved in the transfer of high-energy phosphate in carbohydrate metabolism.[28, 29] Potassium deficiency has been shown to result in glucose intolerance and glucosuria in many clinical settings.[30-33] The exact mechanism remains to be determined, but there is some suggestion that in addition to activating enzymes, potassium is required for the rapid release of insulin from the pancreas in response to a glucose load. If glucosuria occurs during parenteral nutrition, serum and urinary potassium should be determined. Urinary potassium concentration during normal renal function should be equal to, or in excess of, 40 mEq/liter, and serum concentration should be normal or high normal. If serum or urinary potassium concentrations are low, potassium should be added to the parenteral nutrition solution in greater amounts. Glucosuria, if due to hypokalemia, corrects rapidly as serum potassium returns to normal. Serum potassium levels must always be determined prior to administration of insulin to avoid severe hypokalemia.

4. *Check for sepsis-stress-steroid syndrome*: Sepsis, stress, and steroids initiate gluconeogenesis and glycogenolysis by stimulating release of ACTH and catecholamines. The outpouring of glucose can occur rapidly with stress. It is accompanied by an efflux of potassium from the intracellular to the extracellular compartment and results in hyperkalemia. Administration of parenteral nutrition during surgical procedures has been associated with serum glucose concentrations ranging from 40 to 400 mg/100 ml with no change in the rate of administration. Potassium shifts accompanying the glucose fluctuations increase anesthetic risks. It is suggested, therefore, that parenteral nutrition be tapered and discontinued before surgery. It should be replaced with 5 per cent dextrose in one-quarter to one-half strength saline, with potassium chloride added as indicated. In stressful situations other than surgery, patients receiving parenteral nutrition must be carefully observed, as insulin supplementation will likely be necessary — sometimes in rather large amounts. Glucosuria and hyperkalemia can occur up to 12 hours before a temperature elevation or other sign of developing sepsis. The appearance of glucosuria in patients previously tolerant of carbohydrate infusion therefore suggests the possibility of sepsis, and a thorough evaluation should be begun even in the absence of other clinical symptoms.

5. *Check for insulin needs*: Finally, the use of insulin should be considered. The serum glucose concentration during parenteral nutrition should remain about normal, although a level of 130 to 140 mg/100 ml is often observed and accepted. The pan-

creatic beta cell gradually produces increased quantities of insulin in response to increasing glucose loads. There is, however, a time lag and limit. At the beginning of therapy and beyond the patient's maximal response, insulin supplementation may be necessary. Regular insulin should not be given as intermittent subcutaneous or intramuscular doses but added directly to the parenteral nutrition solution in order to maintain serum glucose at less than 130 mg/100 ml. (A discussion of insulin recoverability from solutions containing amino acids was presented in Chapter 7.) The importance of maintaining normal serum glucose concentrations is emphasized because it is thought that hyperglycemia contributes to infectious complications and, in particular, to fungal infections.

Occasionally a patient will demonstrate insulin resistance and maintain elevated blood sugar concentrations and glucosuria in spite of high doses of exogenous insulin. In such cases two possibilities must be considered: (1) the formation of antibodies to insulin, and (2) resistance of peripheral tissues to the effects of insulin due to the depression of glucose tolerance with chromium deficiency (see Chapter 10). (Note: Manganese deficiency has also been indirectly implicated in insulin resistance).

Antibodies to insulin usually form after prolonged exposure to insulin, as in the insulin-dependent diabetic patient. These are typically IgG antibodies, and treatment consists of steroid therapy or utilization of pork or fish insulin.[34]

## HYPOGLYCEMIC SYNDROME

Serum insulin concentrations have been measured before, during, and after intravenous nutrition.[35, 36] A rise in serum insulin occurs rapidly with carbohydrate infusion, reaching a steady state of four to six times basal secretion within six hours. Initial insulin secretion is proportional to infused glucose load. With time, both blood sugar and serum insulin concentrations decline, perhaps as a result of less insulin resistance in peripheral tissues. Interruption of carbohydrate infusion, even after prolonged administration, is associated with a fall in serum insulin to normal levels within 60 minutes. A fall in blood sugar below previous basal levels has been demonstrated, but the level is seldom below 60 mg/100 ml. In the author's experience, assays in six patients (Fig. 9–2) demonstrated the following sequence: a rapid rise in serum insulin with carbohydrate infusion, establishment of a new baseline secretion having fairly large daily variations, and a rapid fall over 6 to 24 hours with termination of infusion.

In spite of the rapid decrease in serum insulin with cessation of hypertonic dextrose infusion, instances of reactive hypoglycemia are not uncommon.[37, 38] Hypoglycemia may occur when the infusion is interrupted for as little as 15 to 30 minutes. Symptoms of hypoglycemia include tingling sensations in the extremities and mouth, posterior occipital headaches, cold clammy skin, thirst, dizziness, rapid pulse, and infrequently, convulsions. Central nervous system injury and death have been reported in severe cases. In the interest of safety, even though experimental data show a rapid decrease in serum insulin, it is advised that patients receiving more than 2000 ml/day parenteral nutrition be tapered to 2000 ml by daily decrements of 1000 ml and then given 5 per cent dextrose at 100 to 125 ml/hour for 12 to 24 hours before the subclavian catheter is removed. If parenteral nutrition must be discontinued abruptly, a bottle of 5 per cent dextrose with one-quarter or one-half normal saline and appropriate potassium should be administered at the previous parenteral nutrition rate until insulin secretion decreases (approximately 12 to 24 hours) or until parenteral nutrition is restarted.

## HYPOPHOSPHATEMIA

The adult body contains about 700 grams of phosphorus, of which about 80 per cent is located in bones and teeth and 9

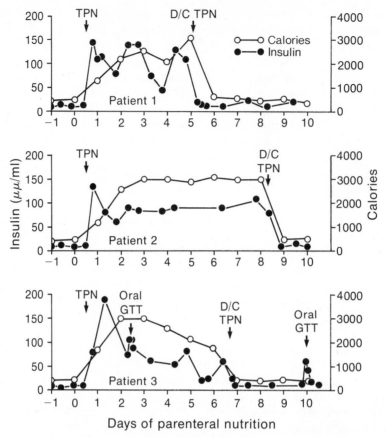

**Figure 9–2** Serum insulin concentration during parenteral nutrition. There is a rapid rise in serum insulin as carbohydrate infusion begins, establishing a new base-line concentration with fairly large fluctuations. If parenteral nutrition is suddenly stopped, a rapid fall in serum insulin to normal concentrations occurs over 6 to 24 hours. In patient 3, a standard glucose tolerance test was performed during parenteral nutrition. It showed increased insulin secretion, suggesting that pancreatic reserves existed despite steady high carbohydrate infusion.

per cent in skeletal muscle. Plasma inorganic phosphorus concentration ranges from 2.5 to 4.3 mg/100 ml. In normal states it is inversely related to serum calcium, so that the product of plasma calcium and phosphorus (measured in mg/100 ml) is constant and ranges between 30 and 40. The estimated daily oral intake of phosphorus in a 2000 kcal diet is 10 to 12 mmoles. Serum phosphate is regulated by the kidneys, with both excessive phosphate intake and greater parathormone secretion increasing renal clearance of phosphate ions.

Phosphate depletion, which may heighten hypophosphatemia associated with parenteral nutrition, has been reported in several clinical settings.[39] Alkalosis is known to stimulate glycolysis, which in-

creases phosphorylation of carbohydrate compounds within cells.[40] The subsequent intracellular movement of phosphate results in hypophosphatemia. Respiratory alkalosis appears to induce hypophosphatemia more readily than metabolic alkalosis because of the more rapid diffusion of carbon dioxide, rather than bicarbonate ions, into cells.[41] Gram-negative bacteremia and acute salicylate intoxication may also cause hypophosphatemia, which results, at least in part, from the associated hyperventilation.[42]

Likewise, impaired phosphate absorption may result in phosphate depletion. The link between chronic administration of phosphate-binding antacids, such as magnesium and aluminum hydroxide, and subsequent hypophosphatemia was first reported in 1960.[43, 44] Phosphate depletion may also occur with sustained vomiting and malabsorption diseases.[45]

In addition, diseases associated with increased renal phosphate clearance, such as hyperparathyroidism, vitamin D deficiency, Fanconi syndrome, and congenital renal tubular disorders, can lead to hypophosphatemia. Renal injury due to severe hypokalemia is associated with marked phosphaturia and phosphate depletion, reversible by potassium supplementation.[46] Similarly, hypomagnesemia may prompt large losses of phosphorus in the urine and lead to phosphate depletion, although serum phosphate levels may remain normal.[39] Marked hypophosphatemia may occur during correction of magnesium deficiencies if adequate phosphorus supplementation is not given.

Metabolic acidosis of various etiologies results in the decomposition of intracellular organic compounds and the release of inorganic phosphate, which may be lost in the urine. Hypophosphatemia becomes evident only after correction of the acidosis.

Finally, acute and chronic alcoholism is often associated with phosphate depletion due to both decreased phosphate intake and increased losses.[47, 48] The phosphate depletion may augment hepatic coma.[49]

Development of marked hypophosphatemia during administration of parenteral nutrition solutions lacking phosphate supplementation has been well documented in humans and may occur early in therapy, even within the first 24 hours.[37, 50, 51] The mechanism by which serum phosphate concentration is lowered is only partially understood. Measured renal losses are minimal,[52, 53] amino acid binding of phosphate appears insignificant, and serum phosphorus concentrations rapidly return to normal upon termination of parenteral nutrition. Glucose administration, by stimulating insulin secretion, promotes the transport of both glucose and phosphate into liver and skeletal muscle. It is estimated that 1 to 2 mmoles of phosphate are required per gram of nitrogen incorporated during tissue synthesis. Hill et al.,[54] using radiolabeled phosphorus in rat studies, found that radiophosphorus was rapidly incorporated into skeletal muscles of previously starved rats during parenteral nutrition and that uptake by the liver and gut was less than that of nonstarved animals. They concluded that the early hypophosphatemia seen with parenteral nutrition was due to a rapid influx of phosphorus into the body muscle mass at the initiation of anabolism after a period of catabolism.

Clinical symptoms of hypophosphatemia usually appear after inorganic phosphate concentrations fall below 1.0 mg/100 ml and are always present when concentrations fall below 0.5 mg/100 ml. Patients characteristically show progressive weakness in use of muscles of the extremities and neck, and of mastication, articulation, and respiration, with tremors or ballismic movements of the upper extremities. Serum muscle enzymes may be elevated, and an electromyogram may be abnormal. There may be circumoral and peripheral-extremity paresthesias, and deep tendon reflexes may be absent. Anisocoria, mental obtundity, anorexia, and hyperventilation may also be present.[44, 50, 51, 53] Exquisite pain of long bones may occur, and syndromes mimicking ankylosing spondylitis and other rheumatic symptoms may be present.[55] Laboratory studies[56-58] have demonstrated that there is a depletion of red blood cell and platelet ATP that is associated with membrane conformational changes. These changes lead to rigid spherocyte formation (limiting perfusion of tissue capillaries). The studies have also shown that when the serum phosphorus concentration falls below 0.5 mg/100 ml, red cell and platelet survival is reduced. Platelet dysfunction resulting in an abnormal bleeding tendency has been demonstrated in phosphate-depleted dogs[58] but not yet in man. Changes in the oxyhemoglobin dissociation curve occur with an increase in hemoglobin oxygen affinity,[50, 59, 60] which decreases tissue oxygen transfer.[61] There is experimental evidence that white blood cell chemotaxis and phagocytosis are impaired during hypophosphatemia, resulting in lowered resistance to infection.[62] Finally, there is some preliminary evidence that hypophosphatemia may diminish myocardial stroke work. The condition is corrected by phosphate replacement.[63]

Treatment of hypophosphatemia should primarily be preventive. Maintenance phosphate may be administered in routine parenteral nutrition solutions by substituting the phosphate salt for the chloride salt of potassium. Sheldon and Grzyb[64] have suggested that 7 to 9 mmoles of phosphate as potassium dihydrogen phosphate be given per 1000 kcal, while others have proposed amounts ranging from 3 to 17 mmoles per 1000 kcal.[37, 65, 66] Some disparity in recommended phosphate supplementation arises from these uses of amino acid solutions containing different amounts of inorganic phosphate. Review of phosphate requirements of patients at Duke University Medical Center suggests no standard phosphate administration applicable to all patients (see Fig. 7–5). Phosphate requirements are determined by basal maintenance, total body depletion, degree of stress, and measurable and unmeasurable losses. In general, patients started on parenteral nutrition should be given a minimum of 7 to 9 mmoles of phosphate per 1000 kcal until serum inorganic phosphate concentrations have been measured and phosphate administration adjusted accordingly. To avoid a precipitous fall in serum calcium and possible tetany, additions of phosphate should be accompanied by calcium supplementation given as calcium gluconate at 0.2 to 0.3 mEq calcium per liter.

## HYPOMAGNESEMIA

The adult human body contains approximately 2000 mEq of magnesium.[67] Sixty per cent is firmly bound to bone. The remainder is distributed in the soft tissues, with only 1.4 to 2.2 mEq/liter circulating in the blood.[68] Of soft tissues, liver and striated muscle have the highest concentrations.[69] Balance studies have indicated that 0.30 to 0.35 mEq/kg/day magnesium is re-

quired orally to maintain positive balance in normal persons.[70] It is absorbed by the entire small intestine[71] and at least part of the colon.[72, 73] Excess dietary intake is excreted by the kidneys, with only small amounts lost in the feces.[74] During magnesium deprivation, renal losses decrease markedly to less than 1 mEq per day.[75]

Magnesium ion is important metabolically in the activation of many enzyme systems critical to cellular metabolism.[76] It is a cofactor for oxidative phosphorylation,[77, 78] stabilizes macromolecular structures such as DNA, RNA, and ribosomes,[79, 80] assists in the binding of messenger RNA to the 70S ribosome in protein synthesis,[81] and is active in the transfer of high-energy phosphate radicals to and from ATP. Magnesium ions are also important in cardiac physiology, decreasing cardiac irritability in ischemic disease and improving coronary artery blood flow. Deficiency of magnesium has been associated with early mitochondrial and sarcosomal damage and frank myocardial necrosis and calcification (see review by Seelig and Heggtveit[82]). Hypomagnesemia accentuates digitalis toxicity much as hypokalemia does.[83]

Clinical symptoms of hypomagnesemia are present when the serum concentration falls below 1.0 mEq/liter.[76] The most common manifestation is a positive Trousseau's sign.[84] Less frequently, Chvostek's sign is positive or overt tetany is present with painful carpopedal spasm. Other signs include muscle fasciculations, tremors, generalized muscle spasticity, hyporeflexia, ataxia, vertigo, muscular weakness, depression, irritability, psychotic behavior, apathy, and nausea and vomiting.[84, 85] The symptoms of magnesium deficiency, therefore, are indistinguishable from those of hypocalcemia. The two syndromes can be distinguished by measurement of serum magnesium and serum calcium concentrations and, if more rapid differentiation is necessary, by changes in the electrocardiogram. Magnesium deficiency is associated with depression of ST segments and inversion of T waves in the precordial leads, while prolongation of the QT interval is seen with hypocalcemia. The differentiation between hypocalcemia and hypomagnesemia is important, as each deficiency must be treated with its specific replacement. Infusion of either ion in the presence of the other's deficiency will only reduce symptoms temporarily and may be misleading.

In addition to producing neuromuscular symptoms, magnesium deficiency has a significant effect on potassium, calcium, and phosphorus metabolism. Urinary potassium losses can increase markedly (to as high as 100 to 300 mEq per day), resulting in significant and progressive hypokalemia.[84] The etiology of urinary potassium loss is poorly understood, although glomerular and tubular structural changes have been described in studies of magnesium deficiency.[83] In addition, as magnesium ions are necessary for normal activity of transport ATPase, magnesium deficiency may depress the sodium pump, resulting in the entry of sodium into cells and the loss of potassium, which is subsequently excreted in the urine.[86] Magnesium replacement reverses potassium loss. Calcium balance studies indicate a positive balance during hypomagnesemia and decreased urinary losses. Nevertheless, many patients develop hypocalcemia even with adequate calcium and vitamin D intake.[87-89] Infusion of excessive amounts of calcium only increases serum calcium concentration, while magnesium replacement results in a rapid and sustained correction. An explanation of the effect of magnesium on calcium remains theoretical. Perhaps magnesium depletion hinders the conversion of parathyroid hormone to an active form or produces a peripheral resistance to parathyroid hormone as a result of magnesium-dependent vitamin D metabolic steps.[89] Urinary phosphate excretion may be greatly increased during hypomagnesemia, although serum phosphate concentrations are usually normal.[39] Significant phosphate depletion can occur but not become obvious until magnesium replacement is begun.

Two instances of incomplete distal renal tubular acidosis related to magnesium deficiency have been reported.[89] In each case there was an inability to secrete an acid load, but neither patient lost bicarbonate or amino acids in their urine. It was suggested that since magnesium deficiency decreased ATP production,[76] the sodium-potassium-hydrogen pump of the distal renal tubule was weakened, and the steep $H^+$ gradient could not be maintained.

Symptomatic hypomagnesemia has been reported most commonly in malnourished patients with gastrointestinal disorders or certain endocrine disorders, alcoholics, and patients with renal disease or on chronic diuretic therapy. Gastrointestinal disorders most commonly associated with magnesium depletion include various malabsorption syndromes,[90, 91] extensive small bowel resection,[92, 93] intestinal and biliary tract fistulas,[94] prolonged nasogastric suction with administration of magnesium-free parenteral fluids,[95] acute pancreatitis,[96] and alcoholic cirrhosis.[97] Endocrine disorders that alter magnesium metabolism include both hyperparathyroidism[98, 99] and hypoparathyroidism,[100] hyperaldosteronism,[101] and uncontrolled diabetes.[102] High-dose insulin administration can also lower serum magnesium. Various renal diseases, including glomerulonephritis, pyelonephritis, hydronephrosis, nephrosclerosis, and renal tubular acidosis, produce hypomagnesemia due to renal magnesium losses.[102] Depletion of magnesium is also likely to occur as a result of diuretic therapy, especially with mercurials, ammonium chloride, and thiazides.[103, 104] Finally, excessive intake of vitamin D can lower serum magnesium concentrations.[105]

Losses of magnesium need not be large to produce hypomagnesmia. Clinical symptoms can occur with a total loss of as little as 35 to 100 mEq.[76] All clinical symptoms are reversible with magnesium replacement and can be avoided by maintenance administration. Because of new tissue synthesis (0.5 mEq magnesium is required for each gram of nitrogen retained), maintenance magnesium requirements are higher during parenteral nutrition than during normal oral nutrition and range from 0.35 to 0.45 mEq/kg/day plus estimated excessive urinary and gastrointestinal losses. Convulsive episodes must be treated vigorously with 33 mEq magnesium intravenously as a 10 per cent magnesium sulfate solution over a period of 10 minutes. This administration is followed by a slower intravenous or intramuscular replacement program.[104, 106]

## HYPERMAGNESEMIA

Clinical symptoms of excessive magnesium administration occur with impairment of neuromuscular transmission.[102, 107] Hypotension, nausea, and vomiting are often seen when serum concentrations reach 3 to 5 mEq/liter. With 5 and 10 mEq/liter, drowsiness, hyporeflexia, and muscular weakness occur, and cardiac conduction becomes abnormal. Prolongation of the QT interval, AV block, and even cardiac arrest in diastole may occur. When serum concentrations reach 12 to 15 mEq/liter, coma and respiratory arrest are common, and cardiac arrest is certain at concentrations greater than 25 mEq/liter.

Hypermagnesemia most often occurs in patients with renal failure when the creatinine clearance is less than 30 ml/minute.[108] Complications can be avoided by monitoring serum magnesium levels twice a week initially and once a week during prolonged infusion and making appropriate alterations in magnesium supplementation. Intravenous administration of 10 per cent calcium gluconate will temporarily reverse severe symptoms of hypermagnesemia, but peritoneal dialysis or hemodialysis may be required.

## SERUM LIPID CONCENTRATIONS

Long-term parenteral nutrition with fat-free, hypertonic dextrose–amino acid solutions might be expected to lower serum cholesterol and elevate triglyceride concentrations. To the contrary, however, in 414 patients at Duke University Medical Center, no change in triglyceride concentration was seen during parenteral nutrition, but there were marked decreases in serum cholesterol, sometimes to less than

half the original concentration. The lowest concentrations occurred during the second to fourth week. Occasionally, a gradual recovery of cholesterol was seen in spite of continued fat restriction. In a similar study by Abbott, Abel, and Fischer,[109] intravenous nutrition with fat-free solutions was found to have no effect on serum triglyceride levels. Cholesterol levels, however, decreased rapidly during the first 10 days and then slowly to 55 to 60 per cent normal by the third to fourth week. The esterified fraction of serum cholesterol remained normal. DenBesten et al.[110] fed healthy volunteers a fat-free diet containing a casein hydrolysate and hypertonic glucose. When the diet was given orally, serum triglyceride values increased significantly. When the identical diet was given intravenously, no elevation in serum triglyceride was seen. No harmful metabolic effects of cholesterol depression are known. Perhaps a beneficial effect might be anticipated in patients with severe familial hypercholesterolemia, as suggested by Torsvik et al.[111]

## ESSENTIAL FATTY ACID DEFICIENCY

It has been recognized since 1929 that certain fatty acids cannot be synthesized by mammals and are, therefore, essential in the diet.[112] Of the three polyunsaturated fatty acids that cannot be synthesized by man (linoleic, arachidonic, and linolenic), only linoleic appears to be required in the diet. Arachidonic acid can be synthesized *in vivo* if linoleic acid is present, and the role of linolenic acid as an essential fatty acid is unclear. Deficiencies of essential fatty acids have been produced in a wide variety of experimental animals and, with prolonged administration of fat-free parenteral nutrition, in human beings as well.[113-115] The average daily adult oral intake of fat is 100 to 180 grams, which include approximately 12 to 125 grams of essential fatty acids. The minimal daily requirement has not been established for oral intake, but 10 to 15 ml of safflower oil (containing 60 to 70 per cent linoleic acid) appears to be adequate. Estimates of intravenous requirements for essential fatty acids ranges from 1 to 4 per cent of the total caloric intake or 25 to 100 mg/kg/day linoleic acid.[114, 116-119] Jeejeebhoy et al.,[120] however, reported that up to 25 grams linoleic acid were required daily to maintain normal serum levels in a patient with massive small bowel resection. Topical application of linoleic acid has also been shown effective in meeting essential fatty acid requirements. Press et al.[121] and Skolnik et al.[122] reported that as little as 2 to 3 mg/kg/day linoleic acid applied to the skin could reverse fatty acid deficiencies and maintain normal serum and tissue levels of essential fatty acids during prolonged parenteral nutrition.

Essential fatty acids account for a substantial proportion of the fatty acids of cholesterol esters and phospholipids in plasma and mitochondrial lipoproteins; as such, they play a critical role in membrane structure and transport processes.[123, 124] Fatty acid deficiencies decrease the efficiency of caloric utilization[125] and, in rats, result in dissociation of oxidative phosphorylation, decreasing the production of high-energy phosphate bonds.[126] Clinical symptoms of essential fatty acid deficiency include mild diarrhea, dryness, thickening, and desquamation of the skin (Fig. 9–3), coarsening of the hair and hair loss, impaired wound healing, and brittle and osteoporotic

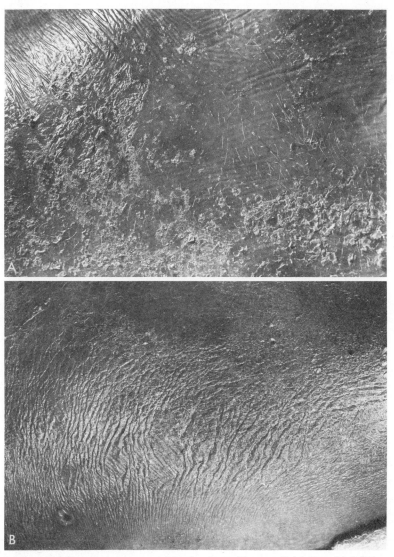

**Figure 9–3**　Typical appearance ot skin changes with essential fatty acid deficiency.

bones.[116-119, 127] It should be noted that high humidity diminishes the severity of the skin lesions and may prevent early diagnosis.

Chemical changes include decreased cholesterol, thrombocytopenia, increased platelet aggregation, increased red blood cell fragility and anemia, and increased capillary permeability. Hepatomegaly, elevations of serum glutamic-oxaloacetic transaminase (SGOT), serum glutamic-pyruvic transaminase (SGPT), and lactic dehydrogenase (LDH) with fatty infiltration of hepatocytes (particularly in the region of the central veins), and enlarged spherical mitochondria have been reported after four to six weeks of fat-free parenteral nutrition.[114, 125, 128] Two members of the linoleic acid family are essential for the synthesis of prostaglandin $E_1$ and $E_2$. Decreased serum prostaglandin concentrations[129] and decreased platelet prostaglandin levels[130] have been reported in newborn infants during fat-free parenteral nutrition. A markedly abnormal plasma lipid pattern develops with accumulation of 5,8,11-eicosatrienoic acid, which is present only in trace amounts in normal subjects, and a concomitant decrease in arachidonic acid.[113-115] The ratio of eicosatrienoic acid to arachidonic acid reflects the severity of essential fatty acid deficiency, with normal values being less than 0.4.[116, 131] Also noted are increases in palmitoleic and oleic acids.

For patients developing symptoms consistent with essential fatty acid deficiency, blood studies should be done to determine the 5,8,11-eicosatrienoic:arachidonic acid ratio, if this study is available. All symptoms of essential fatty acid deficiency can be reversed with administration of linoleic acid.[127, 132] The eicosatrienoic:arachidonic acid ratio corrects after seven to ten days, while the clinical symptoms of essential fatty acid deficiency remain for two to three weeks.[130] Administration of only linolenic and arachidonic acids, without linoleic acid, offers some improvement but does not entirely correct the clinical symptoms.[133] Oleic acid, with its single double bond, and unsaturated fatty acids cannot correct symptoms of essential fatty acid deficiency.[134, 135]

Blood or plasma transfusions, even in large amounts, are inadequate to meet daily essential fatty acid requirements. If small amounts of oral fluids can be tolerated, essential fatty acid requirements may be met by the ingestion of oils containing high concentrations of linoleic acid, such as 5 cc corn oil or safflower oil, two to three times a day. If oral fluids are not tolerated, 10 to 15 ml corn oil or safflower oil can be applied topically three times a day.[121, 136] A third alternative is to administer 25 to 100 mg/kg/day linoleic acid intravenously as a 10 per cent fat emulsion.[137] Since serum fatty acid abnormalities can be detected within the first three days of a fat-free diet[138] and the clinical syndrome of essential fatty acid deficiency can occur as early as two to three weeks,[130] linoleic acid should be administered orally, topically, or intravenously to all patients requiring parenteral nutrition, beginning with the first day of nutritional support.

## SERUM ALBUMIN

Serum albumin is present in the plasma at concentrations between 3.5 and 5.0 grams/100 ml. The exchangeable albumin pool is about 4.0 grams/kg in women and 4.5 to 5.0 grams/kg in men.[139] According to isotope tracing, 31 to 42 per cent of the exchangeable albumin pool is located in plasma, 20 to 26 per cent in the skin, and the remainder distributed in muscle, viscera, tears, bile, sweat, gastric juice, exudates, and various interstitial fluids. Less than 1 per cent of the exchangeable albumin pool is located within the liver.[140] In the plasma, albumin serves to maintain osmotic pressure and acts as a carrier of metals, ions, fatty acids, amino acids, metabolites, bilirubin, enzymes, drugs, and hormones.

Albumin is synthesized by the liver and constitutes as much as 50 per cent of the liver's total protein production. The rate of production averages 130 to 200 mg/kg/day but may be as high as 860 mg/kg/day during maximal production. The half-life of albumin is approximately 20 days.[141] Degradation occurs in sites yet unknown, although the intestine may play an important role.[142]

Depressed serum albumin concentration has been associated with both decreased albumin synthesis and increased albumin degradation. Conditions associated with decreased albumin synthesis include malnutrition, cirrhosis, carcinoma, hypothyroidism, and acute stress arising from surgery, trauma, burns, and infection. It may also follow exposure to various hepatic toxins, including alcohol and carbon tetrachloride.[139] The reduction in albumin synthesis associated with starvation is one of the initial adaptive mechanisms to lowered nitrogen intake and occurs even in the presence of proteolysis, which supplies the necessary amino acids for albumin synthesis. When animals are deprived of food or placed on protein-deficient diets, albumin synthesis decreases by as much as 50 per cent within the first 24 hours and remains depressed as long as protein restriction continues.[143-146] The main conditions associated with increased albumin degradation are those leading to marked catabolism. Active proteolysis may reduce the plasma half-life of albumin to 50 per cent of normal.[147]

Because of redistribution of extravascular albumin into the plasma pool, serum albumin concentration falls slowly during decreased albumin production or increased degradation. When serum albumin concentration falls below 2.5 mg/100 ml, the total exchangeable albumin pool may be one third or less its normal level. As the albumin pool decreases, the fractional and absolute degradation rates decline, thus conserving the remaining albumin. In experimental animals, if an adequate oral diet is resumed, or if parenteral nutrition is given, the exchangeable albumin pool and plasma albumin concentrations rise, reflecting a net increase in albumin synthesis.[148-151] In one study, infusion of isotonic amino acids and dextrose into catabolic patients increased albumin synthesis to 237 mg/kg/day from 157 mg/kg/day when only dextrose was given.[152] The effect of parenteral nutrition on albumin synthesis in human beings has yet to be examined.

In agreement with others[153] the experience at Duke University Medical Center has shown that hypoalbuminemia is reversible with administration of amino acids and adequate calories but may require four to eight weeks. There are specific priorities in protein synthesis during treatment of protein-calorie malnutrition. Generally, retinol-binding protein, prealbumin, and the vitamin K–dependent coagulation factors, prothrombin and proconvertin, diminish early during starvation but respond quickly to nutritional support. Hemoglobin, serum transferrin, $\beta$-lipoprotein apopeptide, the $C_3$ component of complement, and serum albumin decrease later and respond more slowly and only with high protein infusion.[154] It has been estimated that albumin synthesis during oral feeding of malnourished patients progresses at the rate of 1 gram albumin for every 30 grams body protein synthesized or about 2 to 3 grams albumin per day.[155] This represents only a small fraction of the normal 240 to 300 grams of total body albumin and further explains the slow recovery of serum albumin concentrations during parenteral nutrition.

Hypoalbuminemia has been associated with impaired healing of soft[156-160] and bony[161] tissues, decreased resistance to infection,[162-164] depressed gastric and intestinal motility,[165-167] and impaired intestinal absorption of water and electrolytes.[168] Albumin also plays a major role in body water distribution through its osmotic properties.[169] Consequently, normal serum albumin concentration should be re-established early in catabolic, malnourished patients. The addition of up to 25 grams salt-poor albumin per liter of parenteral nutrition solution will result in gradual replenishment of the exchangeable albumin pool. This is in contrast to the undernourished, catabolic patient, in whom intravenously administered plasma protein fractions or albumin is rapidly broken down as a caloric substrate. Within three to seven days normal serum albumin concentration is usually re-established (Fig. 9–4). If albumin supplementation is discontinued at this point, a progressive decrease in serum albumin will be observed, reflecting

| PATIENT | | -1 | 0 | 1 | 2 | 3 | 4 | 5 | 6 | 7 | 8 | 9 | 10 | 11 | 12 | 13 | 14 | 15 |
|---|---|---|---|---|---|---|---|---|---|---|---|---|---|---|---|---|---|---|
| | | | | | | | DAYS OF PARENTERAL NUTRITION | | | | | | | | | | | |
| 1 | IV albumin | 0 | 0 | 29 | 27 | 19 | 38 | 39 | 37 | 42 | 33 | 25 | 25 | 25 | 69 | 0 | 0 | |
| | Serum albumin | | 2.1 | | | | 2.9 | | 3.3 | | | | 4.0 | 3.8 | 3.8 | | 3.9 | |
| 2 | IV albumin | 0 | 0 | 0 | 0 | 0 | 22 | 35 | 25 | 32 | 9 | 0 | 0 | | | | | |
| | Serum albumin | | 2.5 | | 2.4 | | 2.2 | 2.5 | 2.9 | 2.7 | 3.8 | 3.5 | 3.5 | | | | | |
| 3 | IV albumin | 0 | 0 | 16 | 19 | 9 | 26 | 31 | 32 | 23 | 8 | | | | | | | |
| | Serum albumin | | 1.6 | | 2.2 | 2.1 | 2.3 | 2.6 | 3.9 | | 3.7 | | | | | | | |
| 4 | IV albumin | 0 | 0 | 22 | 32 | 36 | 38 | 24 | 35 | 12 | 0 | 0 | 0 | 0 | 0 | | | |
| | Serum albumin | 2.0 | | | | | | 3.6 | | | 3.7 | | | 3.3 | 3.3 | | | |
| 5 | IV albumin | 0 | 0 | 0 | 0 | 0 | 6 | 28 | 21 | 30 | 35 | 24 | 25 | 15 | 0 | 0 | 0 | |
| | Serum albumin | 2.2 | | | | 2.2 | 2.3 | 2.8 | 3.1 | | 2.9 | | 3.4 | 3.5 | | 3.2 | | |
| 6 | IV albumin | 0 | 0 | 0 | 10 | 34 | 36 | 35 | 38 | 38 | 22 | 0 | 0 | 0 | | | | |
| | Serum albumin | | 2.9 | | | | 3.7 | | | | 4.9 | | | 4.4 | | | | |
| 7 | IV albumin | 0 | 0 | 0 | 0 | 14 | 33 | 34 | 37 | 37 | 20 | 0 | 0 | 0 | 0 | 0 | 0 | |
| | Serum albumin | | 2.9 | | 1.8 | 2.0 | 2.2 | | 3.0 | | 3.5 | 3.4 | 3.0 | | | | 2.8 | |
| 8 | IV albumin | 0 | 0 | 23 | 25 | 30 | 35 | 32 | 33 | 33 | 34 | 35 | 25 | 0 | 0 | 0 | | |
| | Serum albumin | | 2.4 | | 2.9 | | | 3.5 | | 3.8 | | | 4.7 | | | 3.3 | | 3.5 |
| 9 | IV albumin | 0 | 0 | 16 | 9 | 15 | 16 | 12 | 8 | 16 | 14 | 14 | 15 | 15 | 17 | 16 | 17 | |
| | Serum albumin | | 2.2 | | | 3.1 | | | | 3.4 | | | 3.1 | | | | 3.7 | |
| 10 | IV albumin | 0 | 0 | 44 | 37 | 42 | 42 | 42 | 42 | | | | | | | | | |
| | Serum albumin | | 1.1 | 1.2 | | | | 3.2 | | | | | | | | | | |

IV albumin in grams per day; Serum albumin in grams per 100 cc.

**Figure 9–4**  Infusion of salt-poor albumin during parenteral nutrition is effective in correcting serum albumin depletion. An abrupt discontinuation of albumin infusion after attainment of a normal serum concentration is often followed by a rapid fall in serum albumin due to a redistribution of the body pool. Gradual tapering of albumin infusion permits replenishment of the body pool, after which endogenous albumin production should be adequate to maintain normal serum albumin concentrations.

redistribution of the albumin into the extravascular and tissue pools. To replace the exchangeable albumin pool completely, 25 to 75 grams salt-poor albumin should be administered daily until serum values reach 4.0 grams/100 ml and then given at 12.5 to 25 grams per day for five to seven more days. At this point the albumin pool will be replenished, and the endogenous production of albumin should be adequate, allowing discontinuation of intravenous albumin administration.

It should be noted that administration of albumin to patients in whom a breakdown in capillary integrity has occurred may be associated with a "leakage" of the albumin into the perivascular tissues, causing a detrimental reversed osmotic gradient.[170] Whenever pulmonary capillary integrity is impaired, as in shock lung or sepsis, albumin may not be recommended. This subject is still controversial.

## HYPERAMMONEMIA

Hyperammonemia during parenteral nutrition was initially reported in newborn infants receiving casein or fibrin hydrolysates.[171] The elevated blood ammonia concentrations were attributed to free ammonia present in hydrolysate solutions, reported to be between 250 and 43,000 $\mu$g/100 ml,[171-173] an amount thought to exceed the metabolic capacity of the Krebs urea cycle. However, administration of crystalline amino acids containing very low quantities of free ammonia also led to blood ammonia elevations in infants.[174]

Hyperammonemia is not a common complication of parenteral nutrition in adults. Dudrick et al.[37] reported elevations of blood ammonia in adult patients in direct proportion to the rate of infusion of crystalline amino acids. Plasma aminoacidograms demonstrated that virtually no ar-

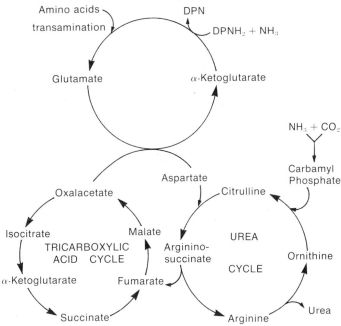

**Figure 9–5**   Krebs urea cycle — interactions with the tricarboxylic acid cycle.

ginine was present in the serum of those patients with hyperammonemia, and the authors related its absence to the relatively low arginine content of the infused crystalline amino acid solution. Because arginine plays a critical role in the Krebs urea cycle, in which ammonia is converted to urea (Fig. 9–5),[175] deficiencies of arginine might contribute to the development of hyperammonemia. Heird et al.[174] corrected hyperammonemia by adding 2 to 3 mmoles/kg/day arginine as the hydrochloride or glutamate salt. They reported that they could prevent development of hyperammonemia by administering 0.5 to 1.0 mmoles/kg/day arginine.

The first symptom of hyperammonemia in infants is decreased responsiveness. Approximately 24 hours later, twitching of the eyes and extremities may be seen. Finally, frank grand mal seizures occur.[174] Clinical symptoms of hyperammonemia in adult patients during parenteral nutrition have yet to be described.

The above data suggest that arginine is an essential amino acid in neonates and seriously ill, malnourished adults. In these patients serum ammonia should be monitored, and arginine administered as indicated. The operation of the Krebs urea cycle (Fig. 9–5) suggests that deficiencies of orni-thine and aspartic acid might also be related to the development of hyperammonemia.

## ACID-BASE EQUILIBRIUM

Acid-base disturbances during parenteral nutrition in adults have been observed occasionally at Duke University Medical Center and elsewhere.[175] Because many metabolic processes are pH sensitive, the acid-base status of patients receiving parenteral nutrition should be monitored.

Usually, metabolic acidosis can be attributed to excessive fluid losses, particularly pancreatic, biliary, or small intestine fluids, or to low cardiac output syndromes with lactic acidosis. Yet there are at least three other potential causes that should be considered:

1. Protein hydrolysates are acidic solutions and have a very high buffering capacity.[176, 177] Infusion of 2.5 to 3.5 liters in adults, especially in the presence of pulmonary or renal insufficiency, can result in significant metabolic acidosis, which will be affected by the duration and quantity of infusion.

2. Synthetic L-amino acids contain a third to a fifth the titratable acidity of pro-

tein hydrolysates. Yet, they too induce metabolic acidosis. Heird et al.[178] attributed the acidosis to the increased amounts of cationic amino acids (arginine, histidine, and lysine) compared to anionic amino acids. Metabolism of cationic amino acids releases free hydrogen ion. Again, the degree of metabolic acidosis is related to the duration and quantity of infusion. In addition, acidosis is more likely in patients with pulmonary or renal insufficiency.

3. Frequently not considered is the acidosis associated with abnormal chloride ion loads.[179, 180] Excessive chloride infusion, with or without hyperchloremia, increases the glomerular filtration of chloride ion, which provides more chloride ions to be reabsorbed with sodium in the renal tubules. Less than normal amounts of hydrogen ion are secreted into the tubules in exchange for sodium ion and metabolic acidosis follows.

Alkalosis during parenteral nutrition is most often due to aspiration of large volumes of acidic gastric secretions, which results in loss of both hydrogen ion and chloride ion. Instances of isolated hypochloremia are uncommon but can occur if insufficient chloride ion is administered. Metabolic alkalosis occurs when chloride ion depletion leads to less chloride being filtered by the renal glomerulus and greater than normal quantities of hydrogen ion being secreted by the renal tubules in exchange for sodium.

To avoid acid-base disturbances due to chloride ion abnormalities, the infused sodium:chloride ratio should be adjusted to 1:1 by using acetate, lactate, or phosphate salts instead of chloride (see Chapter 7). There is some suggestion that acetate ions compete with chloride ions for renal tubular absorption, thereby decreasing renal reabsorption of chloride ion and further preventing hyperchloremic acidosis.[181] Losses from nasogastric aspirations should be replaced with appropriate saline solutions containing adequate chloride ion (Table 7–1). In some cases it may be necessary to infuse diluted hydrochloric acid solutions intravenously to replace large acid losses. A solution of 5N hydro-

chloric acid can be added to parenteral nutrition solutions of crystalline amino acids (not protein hydrolysates) or to standard dextrose solutions and administered through a central venous line. The amount of acid needed can be calculated from the formula: $mEqH^+ = $ (body weight in kg) $\times$ ($HCO_3$ plasma-24) $\times$ (0.6). Generally, only half the calculated acid is given over the first eight hours and then the acid-base status is reassessed.

The acidity of parenteral nutrition solutions can be titrated with sodium hydroxide (providing that pH is maintained at less than 6.8 to avoid additive incompatibilities). Bicarbonate solutions should not be used, as precipitates with calcium or magnesium can occur.

## LIVER ENZYME ELEVATIONS

At Duke University Medical Center we have seen a high percentage of patients receiving parenteral nutrition develop elevations of serum hepatic enzymes or bilirubin in a biphasic pattern.[182] Only a few reports document similar elevations. Ghadimi et al.[183] and Wigger[184] reported serum hepatic enzyme elevations and fatty changes in livers of infants receiving parenteral nutrition. Shils[185] reported serum hepatic enzyme elevations in a young patient undergoing prolonged therapy. Parsa[186, 187] noted liver enzyme elevations and occasional hepatomegaly among adults during the second week of therapy whenever blood sugar concentrations were between 180 and 200 mg/100 ml. Host et al.[188] observed hepatic enzyme elevations in 6 of 19 patients who were receiving parenteral nutrition and had no prior history of hepatic disease, blood transfusions, or alcoholism. They found alkaline phosphatase levels were 2 times, SGPT 18.4 times, and SGOT 4 times baseline levels after five to ten days. Liver biopsies performed on all six patients during maximal enzyme elevations showed mild fatty change, glycogen deposition, and very mild periportal inflammation in contrast to normal biopsies in two patients receiving parenteral nutrition but not showing enzyme elevations.

Grant et al.[182] studied serial hepatic enzyme concentrations and bilirubin levels in 100 patients receiving parenteral nutrition between July 1972, and April, 1976. Patients with hepatocellular disease or malignant disease involving the liver and those receiving hepatotoxic drugs were excluded from the study. SGPT, measured in 89 patients, became transiently elevated in 79 (89 per cent) after 10 ± 4 days of parenteral nutrition. These elevations averaged 5.4 times baseline levels and returned to baseline 4 to 10 days after peak elevation (Fig. 9–6). In patients receiving parenteral nutrition for more than 20 days, 35 per cent demonstrated a second elevation after 30 ± 11 days. This elevation remained for several weeks after parenteral nutrition was discontinued. SGOT elevations were somewhat less, averaging 2.8 times baseline in 93 per cent of the patients, and occurred after 8 ± 4 days of parenteral nutrition (Fig. 9–7). A second elevation after 36 ± 13 days

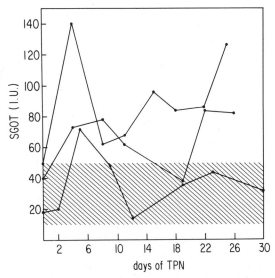

**Figure 9–7** Serum SGOT concentrations during parenteral nutrition for three representative patients. Peak elevations occurred after 8±4 days and 16±13 days of infusion. Normal range is within the shaded area. (By permission of Surgery, Gynecology & Obstetrics.)

of therapy was seen in 34 per cent of the patients receiving prolonged intravenous nutrition. These elevations rapidly returned to normal after parenteral nutrition was discontinued.

Alkaline phosphatase, measured in 94 patients, remained normal during the first 20 days. Of patients receiving parenteral nutrition for more than 20 days, 56 per cent demonstrated elevations, which averaged 2.2 times baseline. Bilirubin rose to 2.3 times baseline in 26 per cent of patients after 8 ± 3 days of therapy and gradually returned to normal with no second elevation observed. LDH rose in 69 per cent of the patients to an average 1.5 times baseline after 8 ± 4 days of parenteral nutrition. These elevations tended to remain high. Half of the patients receiving therapy longer than 20 days demonstrated a second, higher elevation of LDH after 28 ± 10 days of therapy.

Attempts to correlate early and late enzyme elevations with various parameters were unsuccessful. Elevations were seen with equal frequency when casein or protein hydrolysates or crystalline amino acids were used as protein sources. Patients

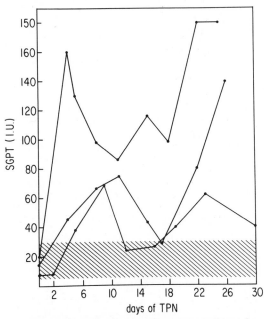

**Figure 9–6** Serum SGPT concentrations during parenteral nutrition for three representative patients. Peak elevations occurred after 10 ± 4 days and 30 ± 11 days of infusion. Normal range is within shaded area. (By permission of Surgery, Gynecology & Obstetrics.)

given either MVI or B-complex vitamin supplements did not demonstrate distinguishable differences. Enzyme elevations occurred in preoperative, postoperative, and nonoperative patients and in those who received blood products and those who did not. Elevations could not be correlated with average daily caloric input per kilogram, average blood glucose concentration, or insulin administration.

In patients demonstrating no enzyme elevations after eight days of parenteral nutrition, liver biopsies demonstrated no histological abnormalities. In one patient a liver biopsy was taken after six days of parenteral nutrition, just as SGOT and SGPT were rising. It demonstrated patchy areas of mild periportal fatty changes (Fig. 9–8). In four patients liver biopsies were taken when early enzyme elevations were highest. All showed marked periportal fatty change with no evidence of periportal inflammation or other abnormality (Fig. 9–9). In each case, centrolobular architecture was unaltered and no fatty change was present about central veins.

From studies with laboratory rats, the authors concluded that early liver enzyme elevations and histological changes were likely due to toxic "conversion products" of the amino acid tryptophan, which is unstable in the presence of sodium bisulfite, a

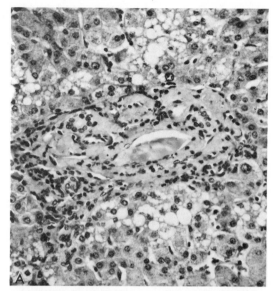

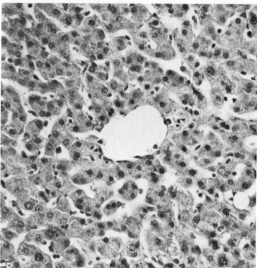

**Figure 9–9**   Liver biopsy after 13 days of parenteral nutrition, during maximal liver enzyme elevations. A marked fatty change is present about each portal triad (A) with complete sparing of the hepatocytes about the central vein (B). No periportal inflammation or portal triad bridging is present. Hematoxylin-eosin × 125. (By permission of Surgery, Gynecology & Obstetrics.)

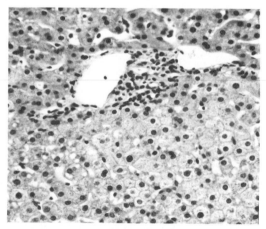

**Figure 9–8**   Liver biopsy from a patient after six days of parenteral nutrition, just as SGOT and SGPT values were beginning to rise. Mild fatty change is present near several of the portal triads. Hematoxylin-eosin × 125. (By permission of Surgery, Gynecology & Obstetrics.)

preservative added to all amino acid preparations available commercially. Light was shown to act as a catalyst. Whether the liver changes were transient or marked the onset of progressive hepatic damage was not determined.

The cause of enzyme and bilirubin changes during prolonged parenteral nutrition (more than 20 days) remains to be determined. Sheldon et al.[189] found evidence of progressive intrahepatic cholestasis, bile duct proliferation, and bile plugs in liver biopsies of adult patients having increasing serum concentrations of alkaline phosphatase and bilirubin (SGOT was normal) after 20 days of parenteral nutrition. Other investigators have found similar changes in neonates or young infants.[190-192] These authors have suggested that the late hepatic dysfunction might be due to a hypersensivity-type reaction or a toxic effect involving amino acid solutions. Popper[193] suggested that a deficit of an essential amino acid might lead to inadequate conjugation of bile acids and interfere with normal bile salt formation and flow. Sheldon et al.[189] found that resolution of the liver function abnormalities occurred over two weeks when dextrose infusion was decreased from a 25 per cent solution to a 15 per cent solution and amino acid infusion maintained at previous levels. We have found a similar gradual resolution of all abnormal liver functions without altering the carbohydrate:amino acid ratio.

Because of the possible hepatotoxic effects of solutions, parenteral nutrition may not be recommended for some patients with known hepatic disease, contrary to recent suggestions.[194] Caution is necessary because of the possibility of inducing further hepatic damage and perhaps liver failure. Patients with suspected hepatic disease should undergo liver function tests prior to infusion of parenteral nutrition. Premature and newborn infants may be especially susceptible to hepatic toxicity and should be observed carefully during parenteral nutriton. In all these cases parenteral nutrition should be interrupted if signs of hepatic decompensation become evident. On the other hand, no adverse side effects of prolonged parenteral nutrition in adult patients with normal hepatic function have been observed. In these patients serum enzyme elevations do not mandate discontinuing solution infusion.

Packaging of amino acid solutions without the commonly utilized antioxidant, sodium bisulfite, and protection of the solution from light would prevent tryptophan decay even after six months of storage at room temperature.[195] If amino acid solutions were prepared in this manner, they could be administered to patients with suspected or proven borderline hepatic function (within limits of protein tolerance) with little risk of inducing hepatic failure. On December 12, 1975, McGaw Laboratories notified its customers of the photosensitivity of their amino acid solution and advised protecting it from light until ready for use. The decay of tryptophan occurs rapidly however, and significant changes may occur during manufacturing. To be effective, the solution must be thoroughly protected from light exposure.

## FAILURE TO INDUCE ANABOLISM

Occasionally, a patient will not achieve positive nitrogen balance, weight gain, and potassium retention despite administration of calculated caloric and nitrogen requirements. Some of these patients are simply hypercatabolic and need only to have their caloric and nitrogen intake increased. If this fails and nutritional depletion demands immediate attention, one can attempt to stimulate anabolism by manipulating the hormonal milieu.

Human growth hormone is the most potent anabolic agent known. Wilmore et al.[196] demonstrated a marked improvement in nitrogen retention following growth hormone administration to patients with large thermal injuries. Yet, in each case the serum insulin concentration also increased, and improved nitrogen balance could be attributed to the effects of insulin alone. As discussed in Chapter 6, the molar insulin: glucagon ratio plays a primary role in determination of metabolic processes. A high ratio favors glycogenesis, tissue synthesis, and nitrogen retention, while a low ratio results in marked catabolism. Artificial elevation of insulin concentration by exogenous insulin administration may therefore aid significantly in establishing anabolism.[197]

Insulin acts on three target tissues. In muscle it increases transport of glucose

$$N_{Bal} = -3.83 + 0.6072\ N_{In} - 0.006599\ MR + 0.004376\ NPC + 0.0557\ BI$$

$N_{Bal}$ = Nitrogen balance ($N_{In} - N_{Out}$) in kcal/sq m/day
$N_{In}$  = Nitrogen intake in kcal/sq m/day
MR   = Metabolic rate in kcal /sq m/day
NPC = Non-protein caloric intake in kcal/sq m/day
BI    = Basal insulin in microunits per milliliter

**Figure 9–10**   Relationship between nitrogen balance, energy production, food intake, and basal insulin. (From Wilmore, D. W., et al.: Catecholamines: Mediator of the hypermetabolic response following thermal injury. Ann. Surg., *180*:653–669, 1974.)

across the cell membrane, by a mechanism that remains unknown. The increased intracellular glucose concentration stimulates hexokinase production and thereby increases glycolysis. The liver cell membrane is freely permeable to glucose, and insulin does not act on the cell membrane but stimulates synthesis of glucokinase and uridine diphosphoglucose (UDPG)–glucosyl transferase. These two enzymes act to phosphorylate glucose and increase the rate of glycogen synthesis. They may also affect glucose uptake by the liver. In addition, insulin decreases the activity of both pyruvate carboxylase, a key enzyme in gluconeogenesis, and phosphorylase, which is necessary for glycogen breakdown. In fat cells, insulin acts as it does in muscle, aiding in transport of glucose across the cell membrane. In addition, it stimulates the synthesis of glycogen synthetase and tryglyceride within the fat cell.

Wilmore et al.[198] formulated a mathematical relationship for nitrogen balance that emphasizes the effect of insulin (Fig. 9–10). The formula points out the greater effect achieved by increasing nitrogen infusion rather than non-protein calorie infusion. It supports the developing idea that an ideal nitrogen-to-calorie ratio may be between 1:100 and 1:150 instead of 1:250 as previously thought, especially during stress and hypercatabolism.[199]

## MISCELLANEOUS COMPLICATIONS

*Lethargy.*   It is not unusual for patients to become lethargic after one or two days of parenteral nutrition. The lethargy may last for six to ten days and, in rare instances, may render the patient semicomatose. One pa-

tient in the author's experience became incontinent of urine and feces. In most instances, however, the patient will only remark that he feels weaker or more tired than normal. The cause of lethargy is unknown. Perhaps the provision of adequate calories after significant starvation causes metabolic changes that induce sleep, or possibly a psychological factor of relief from starvation plays a role. It may be that acute changes in the serum amino acid profile in some way induce lethargy (see Chapter 8). For example, reduction in branch-chain amino acids enhances passage of tryptophan into the brain, leading to serotonin production and lethargy. In any event, there is no specific therapy. Patients should be stimulated to continue active exercise. Perhaps if the lethargy is severe and results in near coma, the rate of parenteral nutrition solution infusion should be temporarily decreased.

*Allergic Reactions.*   In addition to febrile reactions to casein hydrolysates and thiamine as discussed earlier in this chapter, skin rashes during infusion of casein hydrolysates have also been reported.[15, 200] The rash is macular-papular and erythematous and is predominantly located on the trunk. It resolves rapidly with discontinuance of hydrolysate infusion.

*Prolonged Tachycardia.*   After being placed on parenteral nutrition, patients will occasionnaly manifest a moderate to marked tachycardia that cannot be explained by an infectious process, fluid overload, pain, anxiety, or other common cause. Measurement of the basal metabolic rate shows moderate or greater elevation. Reduction in the caloric and nitrogenous input, but not in the volume of the solution, results in a return to normal cardiac rate. It is suggested that high cardiac output follows conversion to positive nitrogen balance because of increased metabolic demands. The syndrome, which is rare, occurs mainly in wasted patients given excessively high caloric infusions. The caloric load should be reduced to calculated requirements. At any sign of cardiac decompensation the parenteral nutrition solution should be temporarily discontinued and then slowly resumed after normal cardiac function returns.

*Headache.* Occasionally, a patient receiving parenteral nutrition will experience a throbbing generalized or frontal headache, the severity of which is directly related to the rate of infusion. Whether the headache is due to amino acid infusion or to hypertonic dextrose is unknown. Usually symptoms occur during the first few days of therapy and can be relieved by slowing the infusion rate temporarily. After 24 to 36 hours a tolerance develops, and the rate can be increased with no further headaches. Headaches have also occurred following rapid infusion of a bolus of solution either accidentally or during an ill-advised attempt to "catch up" a bottle that is behind time. In these instances the headache resolves over four to six hours after infusion is reset at the proper rate.

*Elevation of Blood Urea Nitrogen.* Nearly all patients will have an increase in blood urea nitrogen during parenteral nutrition. With normal renal function the elevations seldom exceed normal limits. However, an occasional patient with normal renal function, and most patients with impaired renal function, will have a progressive elevation in blood urea nitrogen to above-normal ranges. In those patients with normal renal function blood urea nitrogen usually plateaus at concentrations below 80 mg/100 ml, and it is rarely necessary to reduce amino acid infusion. Part of the elevation can often be attributed to dehydration in the face of normal nitrogen intake, and the blood urea nitrogen concentration gradually decreases toward normal with rehydration. In some patients with previously unsuspected renal impairment, however, blood urea nitrogen concentrations will progressively increase and become clinically significant. If the creatinine clearance is 20 ml/minute or more, patients will usually tolerate 9 or more grams of nitrogen a day. If renal function is more severely impaired, a renal failure formula with severe nitrogen restriction (3 to 5 grams or less) is often required (see Chapter 3 concerning renal failure).

*Anemia.* Anemia is common in protein-calorie malnutrition with a depression of both hematocrit and hemoglobin.[201] The anemia is often associated with deficiencies in iron, folate, vitamin $B_{12}$, and vitamin E (see Chapter 11), but it also appears that protein-calorie malnutrition decreases production of factors stimulating erythropoietin.[202] Provision of adequate nutritional support, including vitamins, copper, and iron, usually results in a rapid reticulocyte response. There should be no hesitancy, however, to give blood transfusions to malnourished patients early during nutritional support to establish a normal blood volume and hematocrit.

*Alopecia.* There are three phases of normal hair growth. The anagen phase consists of intense mitotic activity, formation of the hair root, and growth of the hair shaft. After a variable period of growth (two to six years), mitosis suddenly ceases, and the follicle regresses to a state similar to the embryologic follicle germ. This phase, called the catagen phase, is short-lived. The final stage is a resting phase, telogen, with the keratinized hair shaft and hair bulb lying within the resting follicle. After about three months, the folilicles reactivate and enter the anagen phase with shedding of the old hairs. At any one time, an average of 85 per cent of hairs in the scalp are in the anagen phase, while 15 per cent are in the telogen phase.

With stressful events, whether trauma, infection, acute malnutrition, or acute psychiatric disease, the normal hair cycle is interrupted with precipitation of anagen follicles into the telogen phase. Approximately three months later, if the stressful event has resolved, the hair follicles reactivate, resulting in a sudden and marked loss of old hairs as new shafts grow. This process has been termed telogen effluvium by Klingman.[203]

Patients requiring parenteral nutrition

frequently develop telogen effluvium as a result of the stress of their primary illness. The diagnosis of telogen effluvium can easily be made by plucking hairs from the scalp and examining their roots with a hand lens or dissecting microscope to determine the ratio of anagen to telogen hairs. If nearly all hairs are in the telogen phase, the patient can be reassured that hair will grow back within one to two months after hair loss began and that regeneration will be complete.

Other etiologies for hair loss include chronic diseases, especially those associated with protein depletion, and zinc deficiency (see Chapter 10).

## CONCLUSION

The provision of nutrient requirements solely by intravenous fluids bypasses natural regulatory mechanisms of the gastrointestinal tract. In addition, the requirements for electrolytes and minerals are markedly altered when patients are converted to an anabolic state with parenteral nutrition. To provide effective and safe parenteral nutrition, therefore, it is necessary to become knowledgeable of requirements for protein, carbohydrate, vitamins, and some relatively unfamiliar electrolytes and minerals. Previous chapters have covered most of the nutrients, and the next two chapters will review trace element and vitamin requirements.

This chapter has dealt with recognition and treatment of usually avoidable metabolic complications. Although one must be familiar with symptoms of these complications and their treatment, the major purpose of this chapter is to reinforce the importance of providing all nutritive substances in maintenance amounts to avoid nutritional deficiencies. Other complications discussed, if recognized early, should not cause significant morbidity. Adequate interest, knowledge, and supervision by an individual or a parenteral nutrition team are essential in the administration of parenteral nutrition.

## REFERENCES

1. McGovern, B.:, Intravenous hyperalimentation. Milit. Med., *135*:1137–1145, 1970.
2. Louria, D. B., Stiff, D. P., and Bennett, B.: Disseminated moniliasis in the adult. Medicine, *41*:307–337, 1962.
3. Neumann, C. G., Lawlor, G. J., Jr., Stiehm, E. R., Swendseid, M. E., Newton, C., Herbert, J., Ammann, A. J., and Jacob, M.: Immunologic responses in malnourished children. Am. J. Clin. Nutr., *28*:89–104, 1975.
4. Seelig, M. S.: The role of antibiotics in the pathogenesis of Candida infections. Am. J. Med., *40*:887–917, 1966.
5. Editor's Note, N. Engl. J. Med., *286*:3, 1972.
6. Curry, C. R., and Quie, P. G.: Fungal septicemia in patients receiving parenteral hyperalimentation. N. Engl. J. Med., *285*:1221–1225, 1971.
7. Ashcraft, K. W., and Leape, L. L.: Candida sepsis complicating parenteral feeding. J.A.M.A., *212*:454–456, 1970.
8. Guidelines for Infectious Control in Hyperalimentation Therapy. National Nosocomial Infections Study Quarterly Report, May, 1972, p. 22.
9. Parsa, M. H., Habif, D. V., and Ferrer, J. M.: Techniques for Placement of Long-Term Indwelling Superior Vena Cava Catheters. New York, Dept. of Surg., Columbia University, College of Physicians and Surgeons, and the Surgical Service, Harlem Hospital Center, 1972. (pamphlet)
10. Sanderson, I., and Deitel, M.: Intravenous hyperalimentation without sepsis. Surg. Gynecol. Obstet., *136*:577–585, 1973.
11. Ryan, J.A., Jr., Abel, R. M., Abbott, W. M., Hopkins, C. C., Chesney, T. McC., Colley, R., Phillips, K., and Fischer, J. E.: Catheter complications in total parenteral nutrition. A prospective study of 200 consecutive patients. N. Engl. J. Med., *290*:757–761, 1974.
12. Copeland, E. M., MacFadyen, B. V., McGown, C., and Dudrick, S. J.: The use of hyperalimentation in patients with potential sepsis. Surg. Gynecol. Obstet., *138*:377–380, 1974.
13. Brennan, M.F., Goldman, M. H., O'Connell, R. C., Kundsin, R. B., and Moore, F. D.: Prolonged parenteral alimentation: Candida growth and the prevention of candidemia by amphotericin instillation. Ann. Surg., *176*:265–272, 1972.
14. Bernard, R. W., Stahl, W. M., and Chase, R. M., Jr.: Subclavian vein catheterizations: A prospective study. II. Infectious complications. Ann. Surg., *173*:191–200, 1971.
15. Sanders, R. A., and Sheldon, G. F.: Septic complications of total parenteral nutrition. Am. J. Surg., *132*:214–220, 1976.
16. Wyrick, W. J., Jr., Rea, W. J., and McClelland, R. N.: Rare complications with intravenous hyperosmotic alimentation. J.A.M.A., *211*:1697–1698, 1970.
17. Macht, S. D.: A technique for evaluating sepsis in TPN patients. J. Parenteral Enterol Nutr. *1*:97–99, 1977.

18. McCurdy, D. K.: Hyperosmolar hyperglycemic nonketotic diabetic coma. Med. Clin. North Am., *54*:683–699, 1970.

19. Flanigan, W. J., Thompson, B. W., Casali, R. E., and Caldwell, F. T.: The significance of hyperosmolar coma. Am. J. Surg., *120*:652–659, 1970.

20. Chazan, J. A., and Boshell, B. R.: Etiological factors in thiazide-induced or aggravated diabetes mellitus. Diabetes, *14*:132–136, 1965.

21. Runyan, J.W., Jr.: Influence of thiazide diuretics on carbohydrate metabolism in patients with mild diabetes. N. Engl. J. Med., *267*:541–543, 1962.

22. Shapiro, A. P., Benedek, T. G., and Small, J. L.: Effects of thiazides on carbohydrate metabolism in patients with hypertension. N. Engl. J. Med., *265*:1028–1033, 1961.

23. Toivonen, S., and Mustala, O.: Diabetogenic action of furosemide. Br. Med. J., *1*:920–921, 1966.

24. Jones, I.G., and Pickens, P. T.: Diabetes mellitus following oral diuretics. Practitioner, *199*:209–210, 1967.

25. Peters, B. H., and Samaan, N. A.: Hyperglycemia with relative hypoinsulinemia in diphenylhydantoin toxicity. N. Engl. J. Med., *281*:91–92, 1969.

26. Dahl, J. R.: Diphenylhydantoin toxic psychosis with associated hyperglycemia. Calif. Med., *107*:345–347, 1967.

27. Thonnard-Neumann, E.: Phenothiazines and diabetes in hospitalized women. Am. J. Psychiatry, *124*:978–982, 1968.

28. Conn, J. W.: Hypertension, the potassium ion and impaired carbohydrate intolerance. N. Engl. J. Med., *273*:1135–1143, 1965.

29. Hastings, A. B., and Buchanan, J. M.: Role of intracellular cations in liver glycogen formation in vitro. Proc. Natl. Acad. Sci. U.S.A., *28*:478–482, 1942.

30. Gardner, L. T., Talbot, N. B., Cook, C. D., Berman, H., and Uribe, R.: The effect of potassium deficiency on carbohydrate metabolism. J. Lab. Clin. Med., *35*:592–602, 1950.

31. Golden, P.: Glucose intolerance with hypokalemia. Diabetes, *22*:544–551, 1973.

32. Rappaport, M. I., and Hurd, H. F.: Thiazide-induced glucose intolerance treated with potassium. Arch. Intern. Med., *113*:405–412, 1964.

33. Glazier, W. B., and Silen, W.: Acute potassium deficit. Its relationship to polyuria in the postoperative period. Arch. Surg., *112*:1165–1168, 1977.

34. Patterson, R., O'Rourke, J., Roberts, M., and Suszko, I.: Immunologic reactions against insulin. J. Immunol., *110*:1126–1134, 1973.

35. Sanderson, I., and Deitel, M.: Insulin response in patients receiving concentrated infusions of glucose and casein hydrolysate for complete parenteral nutrition. Ann. Surg., *179*:387–394, 1974.

36. Genuth, S.: Insulin response to intravenous alimentation. N. Engl. J. Med., *289*:107, 1973.

37. Dudrick, S. J., MacFadyen, B. V., Jr., Van Buren, C. T., Rubert, R. L., and Maynard, A. T.: Parenteral hyperalimentation. Metabolic problems and solutions. Ann. Surg., *176*:259–264, 1972.

38. Kaplan, M. S., Mares, A., Quintana, P., Strauss, J., Huxtable, R. F., Brennan, P., and Hays, D. M.: High caloric glucose-nitrogen infusions. Postoperative management of neonatal infants. Arch. Surg., *77*:567–571, 1969.

39. Knochel, J. P.: The pathophysiology and clinical characteristics of severe hypophosphatemia. Arch. Intern. Med., *137*:203–220, 1967.

40. Okel, B. B., and Hurst, J. W.: Prolonged hyperventilation in man. Associated electrolyte changes and subjective symptoms. Arch. Intern. Med., *108*:757–762, 1961.

41. Mostellar, M. E., and Tuttle, E. P., Jr.: The effects of alkalosis on plasma concentration and urinary excretion of inorganic phosphate in man. J. Clin. Invest., *43*:138–149, 1964.

42. Riedler, G. F., and Scheitlin, W. A.: Hypophosphatemia in septicemia: Higher incidence in gram-negative than gram-positive infections. Br. Med. J., *1*:753–756, 1969.

43. Boelens, P. A., Norwood, W., Kjellstrand, C., and Brown, D. M.: Hypophosphatemia with muscle weakness due to antacids and hemodialysis. Am. J. Dis. Child., *120*:350–353, 1970.

44. Bloom, W. L., and Flinchum, D.: Osteomalacia with pseudofractures caused by the ingestion of aluminum hydroxide. J.A.M.A., *174*:1327–1330, 1960.

45. Betro, M. G., and Pain, R. W.: Hypophosphatemia and hyperphosphatemia in a hospital population. Br. Med. J., *1*:273–276, 1972.

46. Vianna, N. J.: Severe hypophosphatemia due to hypokalemia. J.A.M.A., *215*:1497–1498, 1971.

47. Stein, J. H., Smith, W. O., and Ginn, H. E.: Hypophosphatemia in acute alcoholism. Am. J. Med. Sci., *252*:78–83, 1966.

48. Roberts, K. E., Vanamee, P., Poppell, J. W., Rubin, A., Braveman, W., and Randall, H. T.: Electrolyte alterations in liver disease and hepatic coma. Med. Clin. North Am., *40*:901–914, 1956.

49. Frank, B. W., and Kern, F., Jr.: Serum inorganic phosphorus during hepatic coma. Arch. Intern. Med., *110*:865–871, 1962.

50. Travis, S. F., Sugerman, J. H., Ruberg, R. L., Dudrick, S. J., Delivoria-Papadopoulos, M., Miller, L. D., and Oski, F. A.: Alterations of red cell glycolytic intermediates and oxygen transport as a consequence of hypophosphatemia in patients receiving intravenous hyperalimentation. N. Engl. J. Med., *285*:763–768, 1971.

51. Silvis, S. E., and Paragas, P. D., Jr.: Paresthesias, weakness, seizures, and hypophosphatemia in patients receiving hyperalimentation. Gastroenterology, *62*:513–520, 1972.

52. Ruberg, R. L., Allen, T. R., Goodman, M. J., Long, J. M., and Dudrick, S. J.: Hypophosphatemia with hypophosphaturia in hyperalimentation. Surg. Forum, *22*:87–88, 1971.

53. Lotz, M., Zisman, E., and Bartter, F. C.: Evidence for a phosphorus depletion syndrome in man. N. Engl. J. Med., *278*:409–415, 1968.

54. Hill, G. L., Guinn, E. J., and Dudrick, S. J.: Phos-

phorus distribution in hyperalimentation induced hypophosphatemia. J. Surg. Res., *20*:527–531, 1976.

55. Moser, C. R., and Fessel, W. J.: Rheumatic manifestations of hypophosphatemia. Arch. Intern. Med., *134*:647–678, 1974.

56. Jacob, H. S., and Amsden, T.: Acute hemolytic anemia with rigid red cells in hypophosphatemia. N. Engl. J. Med., *285*:1446–1450, 1971.

57. Nakao, K., Wada, T., Kamiyama, T., Nakao, M., and Nagano, K.: A direct relationship between adenosine triphosphate level and *in vivo* viability of erythrocytes. Nature (London), *194*:877–878, 1962.

58. Yawata, Y., Hebbel, R. P., Silvis, S., Howe, R., and Jacob, H.: Blood cell abnormalities complicating the hypophosphatemia of hyperalimentation: Erythrocyte and platelet ATP deficiency associated with hemolytic anemia and bleeding in hyperalimented dogs. J. Lab. Clin. Med., *84*:643–653, 1974.

59. Lichtman, M. A., Miller, D. R., Cohen, J., and Waterhouse, C.: Reduced red cell glycolysis, 2, 3-diphosphoglycerate and adenosine triphospate concentration, and increased hemoglobin-oxygen affinity caused by hypophosphatemia. Ann. Intern. Med., *74*:562–568, 1971.

60. Chanutin, A., and Crunish, R. R.: Effect of organic and inorganic phosphates on the oxygen equilibration of human erythrocytes. Arch. Biochem., *121*:96–102, 1967.

61. Harken, A. H., and Woods, M.: The influence of oxyhemoglobin affinitiy on tissue oxygen consumption. Ann. Surg., *183*:130–135, 1976.

62. Craddock, P. R., Yawata, Y., VanSanten, L., Gilberstadt, S., Silvis, S., and Jacob, H. S.: Acquired phagocyte dysfunction. A complication of the hypophosphatemia of hyperalimentation. N. Engl. J. Med., *290*: 1043–1047, 1974.

63. O'Conner, L. R., Wheeler, W. S., and Bethune, J. E.: Effect of hypophosphatemia on myocardial performance in man. N. Engl. J. Med., *297*:901–903, 1977.

64. Sheldon, G. F., and Grzyb, S.: Phosphate depletion and repletion: Relation to parenteral nutrition and oxygen transport. Ann. Surg., *182*:683–689, 1975.

65. Sedgwick, C. E., and Viglotti, J.: Hyperalimentation. Surg. Clin. North Am., *51*:681–686, 1971.

66. Sheldon, G. F.: Defective hemoglobin function: A complication of hyperalimentation. J. Trauma, *13*:971–979, 1973.

67. Widdowson, E. M., McCance, R. A., and Spray, C. M.: Chemical composition of the human body. Clin. Sci., *10*:113–125, 1951.

68. Aikawa, J. K.: The Role of Magnesium in Biologic Processes. Springfield, Ill., Charles C Thomas, Publisher, 1963.

69. Aikawa, J. K.: Effect of glucose and insulin on magnesium metabolism in rabbits. A study with Mg-28. Proc. Soc. Exp. Biol. Med., *103*:363–366, 1960.

70. Jones, J. E., Manalo, R., and Flink, E. B.: Magnesium requirements in adults. Am. J. Clin. Nutr., *20*:632–635, 1967.

71. Aikawa, J. K.: Gastrointestinal absorption of Mg-28 in rabbits. Proc. Soc. Exp. Biol. Med., *100*:293–295, 1959.

72. Stevens, A. R., Jr., and Wolff, H. G.: Magnesium intoxication: Absorption from intact gastrointestinal tract. Arch. Neurol. Psychiatr. *63*:749–759, 1950.

73. Fawcett, D. W., and Gens, J. P.: Magnesium poisoning following enema of epson salt solution. J.A.M.A., *123*:1028–1029, 1943.

74. Silver, L., Robertson, U. S., and Dahl, L. K.: Magnesium turnover in the human studied with Mg-28. J. Clin. Invest., *39*:420–425, 1960.

75. Shils, M. E.: Experimental human magnesium depletion. I. Clinical observations and blood chemistry alterations. Am. J. Clin. Nutr., *15*:133–143, 1964.

76. Wacker, W. E. C., and Parisi, A. F.: Magnesium metabolism. N. Engl. J. Med., *278*:658–662, 712–717, 772–776, 1968.

77. Vitale, J. J., Nakamura, M., and Hegsted, D. M.: The effect of magnesium deficiency on oxidative phosphorylation. J. Biol. Chem., *228*:573–576, 1957.

78. Beechey, R. B., Alcock, N. W., and MacIntyre, I.: Oxidative phosphorylation in magnesium and potassium deficiency in the rat. Am. J. Physiol., *201*:1120–1122, 1961.

79. Venner, H., and Zimmer, C.: Studies on nucleic acids. VIII. Changes in the stability of DNA secondary structure by interaction with divalent metal ions. Biopolymers, *4*:321–335, 1966.

80. Rodgers, A.: Magnesium ions and the structure of *Escherichia coli* ribosomal ribonucleic acid. Biochem. J., *100*:102–109, 1966.

81. Brenner, S., Jacob, F., and Meselson, M.: An unstable intermediate carrying information from genes to ribosomes for protein synthesis. Nature (London), *190*:576–581, 1961.

82. Seelig, M. S., and Heggtveit, H. A.: Magnesium interrelationships in ischemic heart disease: A review. Am. J. Clin. Nutr., *27*:59–79, 1974.

83. Seller, R. H., Cangiano, J., Kim, K. E., Mendelssohn, S., Brest, A. N., and Swartz, C.: Digitalis toxicity and hypomagnesemia. Am. Heart J., *79*:57–68, 1970.

84. Shils, M. E.: Experimental human magnesium depletion. Medicine, *48*:61–81, 1969.

85. Vallec, B. L., Wacher, W. E.C., and Ulmer, D. D.: The magnesium-deficiency tetany syndrome in man. N. Engl. J. Med., *262*:155–161, 1960.

86. Whang, R., and Welt, L. G.: Observations in experimental magnesium depletion. J. Clin. Invest., *42*:305–313, 1963.

87. Woodard, J. C., Webster, P. D., and Carr, A. A.: Primary hypomagnesemia with secondary hypocalcemia, diarrhea, and insensitivity to parathyroid hormone. Am. J. Dig. Dis., *17*:612–618, 1972.

88. Gitelman, H. J., and Welt, L. G.: Magnesium

deficiency. Annu. Rev. Med., *20*:233–242, 1969.

89. Passer, J.: Incomplete distal renal tubular acidosis in hypomagnesemia-dependent hypocalcemia. Arch. Intern. Med., *136*:462–466, 1976.

90. Balint, J. A., and Hirschowitz, B. I.: Hypomagnesemia with tetany in nontropical sprue. N. Engl. J. Med., *265*:631–633, 1961.

91. Goldman, A. S., VanFossan, D. D., and Baird, E. E.: Magnesium deficiency in celiac disease. Pediatrics, *29*:948–952, 1962.

92. Fletcher, R. F., Henly, A. A., Sammons, H. G., and Squire, J. R.: A case of magnesium deficiency following massive intestinal resection. Lancet, *1*:522–525, 1960.

93. Opie, L. H., Hunt, B. G., and Finlay, J. M.: Massive small bowel resection with malabsorption and negative magnesium balance. Gastroenterology, *47*:415–420, 1964.

94. Fishman, R. A.: Neurological aspects of magnesium metabolism. Arch. Neurol., *12*:562–569, 1965.

95. Kellaway, G., and Ewen, K.: Magnesium deficiency complicating prolonged gastric suction. N.Z. Med. J., *61*:137–142, 1962.

96. Edmondson, H. A. Berne, C. J., Hamann, R. E., Jr., and Westman, M.: Calcium, potassium, magnesium, amylase disturbances in acute pancreatitis. Am. J. Med., *12*:34–42, 1952.

97. Sullivan, J. F., Lankford, H. G., Swartz, M. J., and Farrell, C.: Magnesium metabolism in alcoholism. Am. J. Clin. Nutr., *13*:297–303, 1963.

98. Agna, J. W., and Goldsmith, R. E.: Primary hyperparathyroidism associated with hypomagnesemia. N. Engl. J. Med., *258*:222–225, 1958.

99. Hanna, S., North, K. A. K., MacIntyre, I., and Fraser, R.: Magnesium metabolism in parathyroid disease. Br. Med. J., *2*:2153–2156, 1961.

100. Jones, K. H., and Fourman, P.: Effects of infusions of magnesium and of calcium in parathyroid insufficiency. Clin. Sci., *30*:139–150, 1966.

101. Horton, R., and Biglieri, E. G.: Effect of aldosterone on the metabolism of magnesium. J. Clin. Endocrinol. Metab., *22*:1187–1192, 1962.

102. Wacker, W. E. C., and Vallec, B. L.: Magnesium metabolism. N. Engl. J. Med., *259*:431–438, 475–482, 1958.

103. Smith, W. O., Kyriakopoulos, A. A., and Hammarstein, J. F.: Magnesium depletion induced by various diuretics. J. Okla. State Med. Assoc., *55*:258–260, 1962.

104. Wacker, W. E. C.: Effect of hydrochlorothiazide on magnesium excretion. J. Clin. Invest., *40*:1086, 1961.

105. George, W. K., George, W. D., Haan, C. L., and Fisher, R. G.: Vitamin D and magnesium. Lancet, *1*:1300–1301, 1962.

106. Flink, E. B.: Therapy of magnesium deficiency. Ann. N.Y. Acad. Sci., *162*:901–905, 1969.

107. Somjen, G., Hilmy, M., and Stephen, C. R.: Failure to anesthetize human subjects by intravenous administration of magnesium sulfate. J. Pharmacol. Exp. Ther., *154*:652–659, 1966.

108. Randall, R. E., Jr., Cohen, M. D., Spray, C. C., Jr.,

and Rossmeisl, E. C.: Hypermagnesemia in renal failure. Etiology and toxic manifestations. Ann. Intern. Med., *61*:73–88. 1964.

109. Abbott, W. M., Abel, R. M., and Fischer, J. E.: The effects of total parenteral nutrition upon serum lipid levels. Surg. Gynecol. Obstet., *142*:565–568, 1976.

110. DenBesten, L., Reyna, R. H., Connor, W. E., and Steglink, L. D.: The different effects on the serum lipids and fecal steroids of high carbohydrate diets given orally or intravenously. J. Clin. Invest., *52*:1384–1393, 1973.

111. Torsvik, H., Fischer, J. E., Feldman, H. A., and Lees, R. S.: Effects of intravenous hyperalimentation on plasma-lipoproteins in severe familial hypercholesterolemia. Lancet, *1*:601–603, 1975.

112. Burr, G. O., and Burr, M. M.: A new deficiency disease produced by the rigid exclusion of fat from the diet. J. Biol. Chem. *82*:345–367, 1929.

113. Richardson, T. J., and Sgoutas, D.: Essential fatty acid deficiency in four adult patients during total parenteral nutrition. Am. J. Clin. Nutr., *28*:258–263, 1975.

114. Tashiro, T., Ogata, H., Yokoyama, H., Mashima, Y., and Iwasaki, I.: The effects of fat emulsion on essential fatty acid deficiency during intravenous hyperalimentation in pediatric patients. J. Pediatr. Surg., *10*:203–213, 1975.

115. Riela, M. D., Broviac, J. W., Wells, M., and Scribner, B. H.: Essential fatty acid deficiency in human adults during total parenteral nutrition. Ann. Intern. Med., *83*:786–789, 1975.

116. Holman, R. T.: The ratio of trienoic:tetraenoic acids in tissue lipids as a measure of essential fatty acid requirement. J. Nutr., *70*:405–410, 1960.

117. Hansen, A. E., Haggard, M. E., Boelsche, A. N., Adams, D. J. D., and Wiese, H. F.: Essential fatty acids in infant nutrition. III. Clinical manifestations of linoleic acid deficiency. J. Nutr., *66*:565–576, 1958.

118. Caldwell, M. D., Jonsson, H. T., and Othersen, H. B., Jr.: Essential fatty acid deficiency in an infant receiving prolonged parenteral alimentation. J. Pediatr., *81*:894–898, 1972.

119. Collins, F. D., Sinclair, A. J., Royle, J. P., Coats, D. A., Maynard, A. T., and Leonard, R. F.: Plasma lipids in human linoleic acid deficiency. Nutr. Metab., *13*:150–167, 1971.

120. Jeejeebhoy, K. N., Zohrab, W. J., Langer, B., Phillips, M. J., Kuksis, A., and Anderson, G. H.: Total parenteral nutrition at home for 23 months without complication, and with good rehabilitation. A study of technical and metabolic features. Gastroenterology, *65*:811–820, 1973.

121. Press, M., Hartop, P. J., and Prottey, C.: Correction of essential fatty acid deficiency in man by the cutaneous application of sunflowerseed oil. Lancet, *1*:597–599, 1974.

122. Skolnik, P., Eaglstein, W. H., and Ziboh, V. A.: Human essential fatty acid deficiency. Treatment by topical application of linoleic acid. Arch. Dermatol. *113*:939–941, 1977.

123. Sinclair, H. M.: Effects of deficiency of essential fatty acids: Deficiency of essential fatty acids in lower animals. In Sinclair, H. M. (ed.): Essential Fatty Acids. Fourth International Conference on Biochemical Problems of Lipids. London, Butterworth & Co. (Publishers), 1958, Chapter 36.

124. Lehninger, A. L.: The enzymatic and morphologic organization of the mitochondria. Pediatrics., 26:466–475, 1960.

125. Soderhjelm, L., Wiese, H. F., and Holman, R. T.: The role of polyunsaturated acids in human nutrition and metabolism. Prog. Chem. Fats Other Lipids, 9:555–585, 1970.

126. Klein, P. D., and Johnson, R. M.: Phosphorus metabolism in unsaturated fatty acid deficient rats. J. Biol. Chem., 211:103–110, 1954.

127. Heird, W. C., and Winters, R. W.: Total parenteral nutrition: The state of the art. J. Pediatr., 86:2–16, 1975.

128. Holman, R. T.: Essential fatty acid deficiency, Prog. Chem. Fats Other Lipids, 9:275–348, 1971.

129. Paulsrud, J. R., Pensler, L., Whitten, C. F., Stewart, S., and Holman, R. T.: Essential fatty acid deficiency in infants induced by fat-free intravenous feeding. Am. J. Clin. Nutr., 25:897–904, 1972.

130. O'Neill, J. A., Jr., Caldwell, M. D., and Meng, H. C.: Essential fatty acid deficiency in surgical patients. Ann. Surg., 185:535–542, 1977.

131. Holman, R. T.: Essential fatty acid deficiency. Prog. Chem. Fats Other Lipids, 9:329–331, 1971.

132. Hansen, A. E., Stewart, R. A., Hughes, G., and Soderhjelm, L.: The relation of linoleic acid to infant feeding. Acta Paediatr. Scand., 51(Suppl. 137):1–41, 1962.

133. Mohrhauer, H., and Holman, R. T.: The effect of dose level of essential fatty acids upon fatty acid composition of the rat liver. J. Lipid Res., 4:151–159, 1963.

134. Wesson, L. G., and Burr, G. O.: The metabolic rate and respiratory quotients of rats on a fat-deficient diet. J. Biol. Chem., 91:525–539, 1931.

135. Hansen, A. E., Adam, D. J. D., Wiese, H. F., Boelsche, A. N., and Haggard, M. E.: Essential fatty acid deficiency in infants. In Sinclair, H. M. (ed.): Essential Fatty Acids. Fourth International Conference on Biochemical Problems of Lipids. London, Butterworth & Co. (Publishers) 1958, Chapter 32.

136. Bohles, H., Bieber, M. A., and Heird, W. C.: Reversal of experimental essential fatty acid deficiency by cutaneous administration of safflower oil. Am. J. Clin. Nutr., 29:398–401, 1976.

137. Hansen, L. M., Hardie, W. R., and Hidalgo, J.: Fat emulsion for intravenous administration: Clinical experience with Intralipid 10%. Ann. Surg., 184:80–88, 1976.

138. Wene, J. D., Connor, W. E., and DenBesten, L.: The development of essential fatty acid deficiency in healthy men fed fat-free diets intra-venously and orally. J. Clin. Invest., 56:127–134, 1975.

139. Rothschild, M. A., Oratz, M., and Schreiber, S. S.: Albumin synthesis. N. Engl. J. Med., 286:748–757, 816–821, 1972.

140. Rothschild, M. A., Bauman, A., Yalow, R. S., and Bernson, S. A.: Tissue distribution of I-131 labeled human albumin following intravenous administration. J. Clin. Invest., 34:1354–1358, 1955.

141. Rothschild, M. A., Oratz, M., and Schreiber, S. S.: Albumin Synthesis. N. Engl. J. Med., 286:748–757, 816–821, 1972.

142. Bernson, S. A., and Yalow, R. S.: The distribution of I-131 labeled human serum albumin introduced into ascitic fluid: Analysis of the kinetics of a three compartment catenary transfer system in man and speculations on possible sites of degradation. J. Clin. Invest., 33:377–387, 1954.

143. Waterlow, J. C.: Observations on the mechanism of adaptation to low protein intakes. Lancet, 2:1091–1097, 1968.

144. Cohen, S., and Hansen, D. L.: Metabolism of albumin and gamma-globulin in kwashiorkor. Clin. Sci., 23:351–359, 1962.

145. Hoffenberg, R., Black, E., and Brock, J. F.: Albumin and gamma-globulin tracer studies in protein depletion states. J. Clin. Invest., 45:143–152, 1966.

146. Freeman, T., and Gordan, A. H.: Metabolism of albumin and gamma-globulin in protein deficient rats. Clin. Sci., 26:17–26, 1964.

147. Eckart, J., Tempel, G., Schreiber, V., Schaaf, H., Oeff, K., and Schurubrand, P.: The turnover of I-125-labeled serum albumin after surgery and injury. In Wilkinson, A. W. (ed.): Parenteral Nutrition. Edinburgh, Churchill Livingstone, 1972, pp. 288–298.

148. Davis, M. M., and Richmond, J. E.: Effect of dietary protein on serum proteins. Am. J. Physiol., 215:366–369, 1968.

149. Elman, R., Brown, F. A., Jr., and Wolf, H.: Studies on hypoalbuminemia produced by protein-deficient diets. II. Rapid correction of hypoalbuminemia with an ad libitum meat diet. J. Exp. Med., 75:461–464, 1942.

150. Steiger, E., Daly, J. M., Allen, T. R., Dudrick, S. J., and Vars, H. M.: Postoperative intravenous nutrition: Effects on body weight, protein regeneration, wound healing, and liver morphology. Surgery, 73:686–691, 1973.

151. Moss, G. K., and Koblenz, G.: Postoperative positive nitrogen balance: Effects upon wound and plasma protein synthesis. Surg. Forum, 21:71–73, 1970.

152. Skillman, J. J., Rosenoer, V. M., Smith, P. C., and Fang, M. S.: Improved albumin synthesis in postoperative patients by amino acid infusion. N. Engl. J. Med., 295:1037–1040, 1976.

153. Caldwell, M. D., O'Neill, J. A., Meng, H. C., and Stahlman, M. H.: Evaluation of a new amino acid source for use in parenteral nutrition. Ann. Surg., 185:153–161, 1977.

154. Olson, R. E.: Protein-Calorie Malnutrition. New York, Academic Press, Inc., 1975, p. 275.

155. Elman, R.: Parenteral Alimentation in Surgery. New York, Hoeber Medical Books (Harper & Row, Publishers, Inc.) 1947.

156. Garrow, J. S.: Protein nutrition and wound healing. Proc. Nutr. Soc., 28:242–248, 1969.

157. Alexander, H. C., and Prudden, J. F.: The causes of abdominal wound disruption. Surg. Gynecol. Obstet., 122:1223–1229, 1966.

158. Daly, J. M.,Vars, H. M., and Dudrick, S. J.: Correlation of protein depletion with colonic anastomotic strength in rats. Surg. Forum, 21:77–78, 1970.

159. Daly, J. M., Vars, H. M., and Dudrick, S. J.: Effects of protein depletion on strength of colonic anastomoses. Surg. Gynecol. Obstet., 134:15–21, 1972.

160. Irvin, T. T., and Goligher, J. C.: Aetiology of disruption of intestinal anastomoses. Br. J. Surg., 60:461–464, 1973.

161. Rhoads, J. E., and Kasinskas, W.: The influence of hypoproteinemia on the formation of callus in experimental fracture. Surgery, 11:38–44, 1942.

162. Law, D. K., Dudrick, S. J., and Abdou, H. I.: Immunocompetence of patients with protein-calorie malnutrition: The side effects of nutritional repletion. Ann. Intern. Med., 79:545–550, 1973.

163. Cannon, P. R.: The importance of proteins in resistance to infection. J.A.M.A., 128:360–363, 1945.

164. Rhoads, J. E., and Alexander, C. E.: Nutritional problems of surgical patients. Ann. N.Y. Acad. Sci., 63:268–275, 1955.

165. Mecray, P. M., Jr., Barden, R. P., and Ravdin, I. S.: Nutritional edema: Its effect on gastric emptying time before and after gastric operations. Surgery, 1:53–64, 1927.

166 Barden, R. P., Thompson, W. D., Ravdin, I. S., and Frank, I. L.: The influence of serum protein on motility of the small intestine. Surg. Gynecol. Obstet., 66:819–821, 1938.

167. Moss, G.: Plasma albumin and postoperative ileus. Surg. Forum, 18:333–334, 1967.

168. Moss, G.: Postoperative metabolism. The role of plasma albumin in the absorption of water and electrolytes. Pacific Medicine and Surgery, 75:355–358, 1967.

169. Howland, W. S., Schweizer, O., Ragasa, J., and Jascott, D.: Colloid oncotic pressure and levels of albumin and total protein during major surgical procedures. Surg. Gynecol. Obstet., 143:592–596, 1976.

170. Holcroft, J. W., and Trunkey, D. D.: Pulmonary extravasation of albumin during and after hemorrhagic shock in baboons. J. Surg. Res., 18:91–97, 1975.

171. Johnson, J. D., Albritton, W. L., and Sunshine, P.: Hyperammonemia accompanying parenteral nutrition in newborn infants. J. Pediatr., 81:154–161, 1972.

172. Walker, F. A.: Ammonia in fibrin hydrolysates. N. Engl. J. Med., 285:1324–1325, 1971.

173. Ghadimi, H., and Kumar, S.: High ammonia content of protein hydrolysates. Biochem. Med., 5:548–551, 1971.

174. Heird, W. C., Nicholson, J. F., Driscoll, J. M., Jr., Schullinger, J. N., and Winters, R. W.: Hyperammonemia resulting from intravenous alimentation using a mixture of synthetic L-amino acids: A preliminary report. J. Pediatr., 81:162–165, 1972.

175. Fortner, C. L., Foley, T., and Cradock, J. C.: Reduction in serum $CO_2$ content during hyperalimentation therapy. Am. J. Hosp. Pharm., 28:121–122, 1971.

176. Chan, J. C. M., Asch, M. J., Lin, S., and Hays, D. M.: Hyperalimentation with amino acid and casein hydrolysate solutions. Mechanism of acidosis. J.A.M.A., 220:1700–1705, 1972.

177. Hull, R. L.: Physiochemical considerations in intravenous hyperalimentation. Am. J. Hosp. Pharm., 31:236–243, 1974.

178. Heird, W. C., Dell, R. B., Driscoll, J. M., Jr., Grebin, B., and Winters, R. W.: Metabolic acidosis resulting from intravenous alimentation mixtures containing synthetic amino acids. N. Engl. J. Med., 287:943–948, 1972.

179. Guyton, A. C.: Textbook of Medical Physiology, 4th Edition. Philadelphia, W. B. Saunders Company, 1971, p. 437.

180. Rector, F. C., Jr.: Acidification of the urine. In Orloff, J., Berline, R. W., and Geiger, S. R. (eds.): Handbook of Physiology. Washington, D. C., American Physiological Society, 1973, p. 447.

181. Pitts, R. F.: Physiology of the Kidney and Body fluids, 2nd Edition. Chicago, Year Book Medical Publishers, Inc., 1972, p. 188.

182. Grant, J. P., Cox, C. E., Kleinman, L. M., Maher, M. M., Pittman, M. A., Tangrea, J. A., Brown, J. H., Gross, E., Beazley, R. M., and Jones, R. S.: Serum hepatic enzyme and bilirubin elevations during parenteral nutrition. Surg. Gynecol. Obstet., 145:573–580, 1977.

183. Ghadimi, H., Abaci, F., Kumar, S., and Rathi, M.: Biochemical aspects of intravenous alimentation. Pediatrics, 48:955–965, 1971.

184. Wigger, J. H.: Hepatic Changes in Premature Infants Receiving Intravenous Alimentation. Toronto, Pediatric Pathology Club, 1971. (abstract)

185. Shils, M.: Guidelines for parenteral nutrition. J.A.M.A., 220:1721–1729, 1972.

186. Parsa, M. H., Ferrer, J. M., Habif, D. V., Forde, K. A., Sampath, A., and Lipton, R.: Experiences with central venous nutrition: Problems and their prevention. A scientific exhibit, 57th Annual Clinical Congress, American College of Surgeons, Atlantic City, N.J., Oct., 1971.

187. Parsa, M. H., Habif, D. V., Ferrer, J. M., Lipton, R., and Yoshimura, N. N.: Intravenous hyperalimentation: Indications, technique and complications. Bull. N.Y. Acad. Med., 48:920–942, 1972.

188. Host, W. R., Serlin, O., and Rush, B. F., Jr.: Hyperalimentation in cirrhotic patients. Am. J. Surg., 123:57–62, 1971.

189. Sheldon, G. F., Peterson, S. R., and Sanders, R.: Hepatic dysfunction during hyperalimentation. Arch. Surg., 113:504–508, 1978.

190. Touloukian, R. J., and Downing, S. E.: Cholestasis

associated with long term parenteral hyperalimentation. Arch. Surg., *106*:56–62, 1973.

191. Peden, V. H., Witzleben, C. L., and Skelton, M. A.: Total parenteral nutrition. J. Pediatr., *78*:180, 1971.

192. Heird, W. C., Driscoll, J. M., Jr., Schullinger, J. N., Grebin, B., and Winters, R. W.: Intravenous alimentation in pediatric patients. J. Pediatr., *80*:351–372, 1972.

193. Popper, H.: Cholestasis. Am. Rev. Med., *19*:39–56, 1968.

194. Silvis, S. E., and Badertscher, V.: Treatment of severe liver failure with hyperalimentation. Am. J. Gastroenterol., *59*:416–422, 1973.

195. Kleinman, L. M., Tangrea, J. A., Galleli, J. F., Brown, J. H., and Gross, E.: Stability of solutions of essential amino acids. Am. J. Hosp. Pharm., *30*:1054–1057, 1973.

196. Wilmore, D. W., Moylan, J. A., Bristow, B. F., Mason, A. D., Jr., and Pruitt, B. A., Jr.: Anabolic effects of human growth hormone and high caloric feedings following thermal injury. Surg. Gynecol. Obstet., *138*:875–884, 1974.

197. Hinton, P., Littlejohn, S., Allison, S. P., and Lloyd, J.: Insulin and glucose catabolic response to injury in burned patients. Lancet, *1*:767–769, 1971.

198. Wilmore, D. W., Long, J. M., Mason, A. D., Jr., Skreen, R. W., and Pruitt, B. A., Jr.: Catecholamines: Mediator of the hypermetabolic response following thermal injury. Ann. Surg., *180*:653–669, 1974.

199. Bozzetti, F.: Parenteral nutrition in surgical patients. Surg. Gynecol. Obstet., *142*:16–20, 1976.

200. Flack, H. L., Gans, J. A., Serlick, S. E., and Dudrick, S. J.: The current status of parenteral hyperalimentation. Am. J. Hosp. Pharm., *28*:326–335, 1971.

201. Barac-Nieto, M., Spurr, G. B., Lotero, H., and Maksud, M. G.: Body composition in chronic undernutrition. Am. J. Clin. Nutr., *31*:23–40, 1978.

202. Sanders, R., Sheldon, G. F., Garcia, J., Schooley, J., and Fuchs, R.: Erythropoietin synthesis in rats during total parenteral nutrition. J. Surg. Res., *22*(6):649–653, 1977.

203. Klingman, A. M.: Pathologic dynamics of human hair loss. Arch. Dermatol., *83*:175–198, 1961.

# Chapter 10

# TRACE ELEMENT REQUIREMENTS AND DEFICIENCY SYNDROMES

The nutritional requirement for elements present only in trace amounts within the human body has been under intensive study during the past 10 years. Prior to 1957, only 7 trace elements were recognized as essential in the mammalian diet. Now at least 15 are thought to be essential (Table 10–1). Deficiency syndromes of trace elements have been only partially defined because of the difficulty of establishing a completely trace-element–free environment and highly purified diets. With the development of parenteral nutrition solutions containing highly purified constituents, it has been possible to design experiments using diets deficient in trace elements. In addition, more sensitive techniques for detecting trace elements have led to the definition of some deficiency states in humans that can be correlated with experimental findings in laboratory animals.

In this chapter, proposed metabolic function, symptomatology of deficiency states, and estimated daily requirements for trace elements will be reviewed. As interest in trace elements increases, greater knowledge of human requirements will be acquired. Eventually, commercial trace element solutions might well be available. Until then, administration of trace elements should be limited to centers that can confirm deficiency states, formulate sterile, non-pyrogenic trace element solutions, and document clinical results.

*Cadmium.* The biologic half-life of cadmium has been estimated at 16 to 33 years. Interest in cadmium has therefore focused mostly on undesirable effects of accumulation in the body. Following dietary absorption, cadmium is bound to a low molecular weight protein called metallothionein. This protein is involved in both transportation of cadmium in the serum and its selective storage. Metallothionein and cadmium are found in large amounts in the renal cortex, liver, and gastrointestinal mucosa. Renal damage may occur if the concentration of cadmium exceeds 20 mg/kg wet weight.[1]

Much of the importance of cadmium appears to be in its interactions with other trace elements. It may compete directly with zinc for certain intracellular ligands. Research has shown that zinc infusion counteracts some of the adverse effects of excess cadmium, including cadmium-induced hypertension. A low or marginal body copper content appears to decrease tolerance to cadmium, and cadmium has been demonstrated to interfere with the intestinal uptake of copper. Finally, selenium apparently protects against cadmium toxicity in experimental animals. Deficiency states of cadmium in the human have yet to be described, and daily requirements are unknown. Because of its long metabolic half-life, supplementation during parenteral nutrition is unnecessary.

*Chromium.* Chromium concentration in human plasma averages between 0.3 and 0.72 micrograms per 100 ml.[2] Wide variations are found, however, because of geo-

**Table 10-1**   TRACE ELEMENT INFUSION IN 70 Kg MAN

| ELEMENT | RDA* | NORMAL CONC. PER 100 ml† | AUTHOR | | | | | CONC. IN TPN SOL./LITER‡ |
|---|---|---|---|---|---|---|---|---|
| | | | Shils[118] | Hull[122] | Wretlind[119] | Jeejeebhoy[13,120] | Blackburn[123] | |
| Cadmium | | ? | – | – | – | – | – | – |
| Chromium | [52-78 µg] | P 0.31-0.72 µg<br>B 0.49-0.95 µg | 15 µg | – | – | 2-20 µg | 200 µg | 0.8-24 µg |
| Cobalt | ? | P 29 ng<br>B 35 ng | – | 70 µg | – | – | 50 µg | – |
| Copper | 0.63-1.78 mg | P 0.07-0.15 mg<br>B 0.07-0.11 mg | 1 mg | 0.11 mg | 1.1 mg | 1.6 mg | 2 mg | 0.008-1.04 mg |
| Fluorine | (1-2 mg) | P 14-19 µg<br>B 4-36 µg | 1-2 mg | – | 3.4 mg | – | – | – |
| Iron | 0.5-2 mg | P 0.058-0.21 mg<br>B 0.04-0.056 mg | 1 mg | – | 6.7 mg | 1.8 mg | 1 mg | 0.025-1.39 mg |
| Manganese | [0.7-22 mg] | P 0.18-0.31 mg<br>B 0.3-1.38 mg | 1-12 mg | 0.2 mg | 3.3 mg | 2 mg | 5 mg | 0.04-0.28 mg |
| Molybdenum | [0.045-0.5 mg] | 4 µg | – | – | – | – | – | – |
| Nickel | [0.3-0.6 mg] | P 0.12-0.42 µg | – | – | – | – | – | – |
| Selenium | ? | B 2-22 µg | – | – | – | 120 µg | – | – |
| Silicon | ? | P ~1 mg | – | – | – | – | – | – |
| Tin | [3.5-17 mg] | ? | – | – | – | – | – | – |
| Vanadium | [1-3 mg] | ? | – | – | – | – | – | – |
| Zinc | 1-2.2 mg | P 0.1-0.3 mg<br>B 0.88-1.6 mg | 2-4 mg | 0.2 mg | 3.9 mg | 3 mg | 10 mg | 0.026-4.04 mg |
| Iodide | 0.05-0.075 µg | P 3.6-6 µg | 0.07-0.14 mg | 0.075 mg | 0.3 mg | 0.12 mg | 0.5 mg | – |

*Estimated amount of element absorbed from daily oral diet containing recommended dietary allowance; ( )-recommended dietary allowance; [ ]-estimated dietary intake – requirements unknown; ?-dietary information unavailable.
†Range of means for plasma (P) and blood (B). See references 1, 2, 13, 23, 36, 39, 47, 120, 128–134.
‡See references 30, 124–126, 129.

graphical differences in dietary intake. Hair chromium levels may better reflect body chromium stores, with 350 to 450 ppb being normal.[3]

Of ingested chromium, only about 0.5 per cent is absorbed through the gastrointestinal tract, and most of this is the hexavalent form, which is more easily absorbed than the trivalent form.[4, 5] Chromium localizes in skin, muscle, fat, testes, bone, liver, and spleen, and low concentrations are found in brain. It is excreted almost exclusively via the urine (7 to 10 micrograms per day) except for small amounts lost through the gastrointestinal tract.[6]

Chromium may act to stabilize the tertiary structures of proteins and nucleic acids, where it is found in high concentrations, and it apparently stimulates hepatic synthesis of fatty acids and cholesterol from acetate.[7] Normal glucose utilization in humans requires chromium,[8] which affects the sensitivity of peripheral tissues to insulin.[7]

Increasingly, chromium deficiency is being recognized in humans. Schroeder et al.[9] found progressively declining levels of tissue chromium with increasing age. The reasons for the decline are not known. Patients on high-carbohydrate diets tend to develop chromium deficiency as a result of increased urinary chromium excretion.[6] Further, insulin administration increases urinary losses of chromium and may be associated with total body chromium depletion. Chromium deficiency can best be detected by measurement of tissue concentrations, particularly in the hair.[3] It has also been suggested that the absence of increased chromium excretion following a glucose load may be a reliable indicator of chromium deficiency.[10]

Experimentally, deficiency states have led to retarded growth, decreased glycogen reserves, increased incidence of aortic lesions, and impaired amino acid utilization in protein synthesis. A diabetes-like syndrome has been observed in chromium-deficient rats raised in a controlled environment[11] and also in man.[8, 12, 13] It is postulated that trivalent chromium ion is an essential part of a complex substance called glucose tolerance factor.[10, 14, 15] This factor facilitates the reaction of insulin with receptor sites of sensitive tissues.[7] Administration of 150 to 250 micrograms of chromium per day as chromic chloride has improved glucose tolerance in adult and elderly patients.[8, 16] Hopkins et al.[12] demonstrated improved removal rates of intravenously infused glucose in children with kwashiorkor malnutrition following single doses of 250 micrograms of chromium III. Jeejeebhoy[13] described a case of chromium deficiency in a patient receiving home parenteral nutrition for three years. Symptoms included weight loss, abnormal glucose tolerance, and diabetic neuropathy. Laboratory studies demonstrated marginal nitrogen balance, a respiratory quotient consistent with mainly fat metabolism, and markedly depressed chromium content in blood and hair. Administration of 250 micrograms of chromium daily for two weeks reversed all clinical and laboratory findings.

The minimum daily oral requirement for chromium has not been defined, but it is estimated that the typical daily diet contains 52 to 78 micrograms.[8, 9] Based on the few studies during parenteral nutrition, an intravenous intake of 20 micrograms chromium per day appears sufficient.

*Cobalt.* The only known human requirement for cobalt is that amount necessary for the structure of vitamin $B_{12}$. Approximately 2 micrograms of cyanocobalamine are necessary in the daily human diet. There is some suggestion that cobalt interferes with iodine metabolism in rats[17] and may induce goiters when in excess. No minimal daily requirement for cobalt has been established.

*Copper.* The adult body contains 75 to 150 mg of copper, which is located mainly in brain, liver, heart, spleen, kidneys, and blood.[18] Serum copper ranges from 75 to 150 micrograms per 100 ml, of which approximately 95 per cent is bound to a circulating alpha$_2$-globulin, ceruloplasmin. The major excretory route is the biliary system, with $25 \pm 13$ micrograms/kg/day being lost.[19, 20]

Copper belongs to the same group of transition elements in the periodic table as iron and has many biologically similar functions, including formation of hemoglobin and red cells. Also, it is apparently involved in the activity of cytochrome oxidase, the terminal oxidase in the electron transport mechanism, from which high-energy phosphate bonds are derived.[21] Copper plays an essential role in connective-tissue integrity. It is necessary for maintenance of normal amine oxidase activity, which converts lysine to desmosine and isodesmosine, the amino acids required for cross-linkage of elastin.[22] Lysyl oxidase, another enzyme required for collagen cross-linkage, is also copper-dependent. Deficiencies of copper have resulted in delayed wound healing and aortic aneurysms in animals. Copper is apparently a functional part of the enzyme tyrosinase, which is essential for conversion of tyrosine to melanin. In animals, copper deficiency has resulted in loss of hair color.[23] Finally, copper-containing proteins from the brain (cerebrocuprein) and from the liver (hepatocuprein and mitochondrocuprein) have been isolated. The function of these proteins is unknown.

Until recently, copper deficiency was rare in human beings, occurring mainly in infants with abnormal losses of ceruloplasmin and impaired copper retention.[24, 25] More recently, copper deficiency in adults and infants has been reported during copper-deficient intravenous feeding,[25-27] when serum copper concentration may fall as much as 11 micrograms/100 ml per week.[28] In the human being, copper deficiency has produced variable combinations of anemia, leukopenia, hypoproteinemia with periorbital or pretibial edema, and bony changes.[25, 26] The leukopenia, which is characterized by neutropenia, occurs early and corrects rapidly with copper replacement.

We have observed two cases of acute copper deficiency characterized by leukopenia, both in young women. Both clinical courses were similar, and only one will be reviewed here. An 18-year-old female patient had been repeatedly hospitalized over a three-year period for a combination of anorexia nervosa and intestinal pseudo-obstruction. She had lost 20 kg over that period as a result of nausea, vomiting, bloating, and poor dietary habits. When first examined by the Nutritional Support Service, she exhibited malaise, weakness, and severe protein–calorie malnutrition of the marasmic-kwashiorkor type. Parenteral nutrition was begun on March 20, 1978, at which time she weighed 24.5 kg, and was continued for the next five months, during which time she gained 16 kg. Her oral intake remained between 300 and 600 kcal/day until the last two weeks, when it improved to greater than 1800 kcal/day. Laboratory data are presented in Table 10–2.

She was given 2 to 2.4 liters a day of a nutritional solution providing 600 grams of carbohydrate, 13.5 grams of nitrogen, and added electrolytes, minerals, and vitamins. No trace elements were given, but essential fatty acid requirements were met with infusion of 1500 ml a week of Intralipid 10%. After ten weeks of nutritional support the patient exhibited a sharp decline in the white blood count, with a marked decrease in polymorphonuclear cells (from 56 per cent to 9 per cent). No change was seen in either the red blood cell or platelet populations. Serum copper concentration, which was initially 46 micrograms/100 ml, had fallen to only 12 micrograms/100 ml. The patient was given intravenous copper sulfate supplementation, which added 900 micrograms of copper per day to her nutrition solution. The serum copper concentration returned to normal over the next three weeks, and there was a rapid increase in both the total white blood count and percentage of polymorphonuclear cells.

The anemia associated with copper deficiency is often hypochromic normocytic with a depressed reticulocyte count. It is due in part to a reduced rate of red cell synthesis, decreased red blood cell survival, and an impairment in the formation of transferrin from ferrous iron because of low levels of ceruloplasmin, a feroxidase enzyme.[25, 29] Impaired hematopoiesis is usually seen when serum copper concentra-

**Table 10-2  HEMATOLOGICAL CHANGES IN ACUTE COPPER DEFICIENCY**

| | DAYS OF TOTAL PARENTERAL NUTRITION | | | | | | | | | | | | |
|---|---|---|---|---|---|---|---|---|---|---|---|---|---|
| | 0 | 26 | 31 | 45 | 46 | 47 | 48 | 50 | 56 | 59 | 68 | 73 | 83 |
| Weight | 24.5 | 33 | | 35.9 | | | | 36.8 | | | 38.9 | | 40.7 |
| WBC | 8.2 | 4.6 | 6.6 | 2.2 | 2.6 | 1.8 | 2.6 | 2.8 | 2.8 | 4.5 | 5.1 | 5.4 | 4.9 |
| Per Cent PMN | 67 | 56 | 58 | 21 | 9 | 15 | 13 | 18 | 26 | 39 | 65 | 58 | 55 |
| Hct | 28 | 30 | 30 | 30 | 28 | 29 | 29 | 32 | | 35 | | 34 | 34 |
| Copper | 46 | | | | | | 12 | 29 | 57 | | 98 | | |
| Folate | 9.1 | | | | | | 8.9 | | | | | | |
| Vitamin $B_{12}$ | 472 | | | | | | 756 | | | | | | |
| Copper supplementation | | | | | | | | 900 micrograms/day →→→→→→ | | | | | |

Weight in kilograms
WBC: white blood count × 1000
Per cent PMN: per cent polymorphonuclear cells
Hct: hematocrit in per cent
Copper in micrograms per 100 milliliters (normal 80 to 120)
Folate in nanograms per milliliter (normal 3 to 15)
Vitamin $B_{12}$ in picograms per milliliter (normal 300 to 1000)

tions fall below 20 micrograms per 100 ml.[25, 27, 30] The bone marrow is hypochromic with erythroid hypoplasia. In addition, there is a tendency for the myeloid elements to be immature. Scorbutic-type bony changes, including retarded bone age, "ground glass" appearance of osteoporosis, metaphyseal irregularities and spurring, and a radiolucent zone in the metaphyses, are probably due to decreased activity of ascorbate oxidase, a cuproenzyme.[26]

All symptoms of copper deficiency can be reversed with administration of copper. The neutropenia and leukopenia respond rapidly, while the anemia, and especially the bony changes, respond more slowly. Daily oral requirements have been estimated at 30 micrograms per kilogram, of which 30 to 80 per cent is thought to be absorbed, mainly in the stomach and proximal duodenum.[18, 25] Intravenous requirements for copper remain to be established. Dudrick and Rhoads[31] recommend approximately 22 microgram/kg/day, an amount found adequate by Vilter et al.[27] to replace copper in one of their patients.

Acute copper toxicity, such as that following the ingestion of more than 15 mg of elemental copper, has been associated with nausea, vomiting, diarrhea, and intestinal cramps. Intravascular hemolysis has occurred with larger ingestions. The hemolysis is due to an inhibition of glucose-6-phosphate dehydrogenase activity, inhibition of erythrocyte glycolysis, denaturation of hemoglobin, and oxidation of glutathione.[32] In India, where ingestion of copper sulfate is a relatively common way of committing suicide, autopsies have demonstrated jaundice, dilation of the central veins of the liver, and varying degrees of acute hepatic necrosis, as well as tubular swelling, glomerular congestion, and hemoglobin casts in the kidneys.[33]

*Fluorine.* It has been suggested that fluorine plays an important role in fertility, growth, and the maintenance of a normal hematocrit.[34, 35] Fluorine is beneficial in the maintenance of teeth and of a normal skeleton in the adult.[36] A deficiency syndrome in man and daily requirements remain to be determined. The average daily diet provides from 0.25 to 0.35 mg of fluoride, which is supplemented by an average adult ingestion of 1.0 to 1.5 mg from drinking and cooking water.[37]

*Iodine.* Iodine is an integral part of the thyroid hormones thyroxine and triiodothyronine and is, therefore, essential for regulation of body metabolism. Deficiencies of iodine lead to thyroid enlargement with an increase in size and number of epithelial cells. The daily iodine requirement to prevent goiter development in adults is approximately 1.0 microgram per kilogram.[38]

*Iron.* The adult body contains 3 to 5 grams of iron. Slightly more than half is present in hemoglobin, 30 to 35 per cent is in storage forms, and the remainder is in various tissue components and enzymes.[39] It is estimated that daily losses of iron include less than 0.1 mg in the urine, 0.3 to 0.5 mg in the feces, and a variable amount in sweat and desquamated skin. Total daily losses are approximately 0.5 to 1.0 milligram per day. Recommended daily intake for adult males and post-menopausal females is 0.5 to 1.0 mg; for menstruating females, 1 to 2 mg; for pregnant females, 1.5 to 2.5 mg; and for children, on the average, 1 mg.[40]

The average daily diet contains 16 to 18 mg iron, of which only 5 to 10 per cent is absorbed, mostly in the upper small intestine. Iron apparently enters the mucosal cells, either in an ionic form or bound to a non-protein substance of low molecular weight by a process that does not require energy. The iron complex diffuses directly to the vascular border, where it is transferred across the membrane into the plasma by a process requiring oxidative energy. This latter process appears to be the rate-limiting step.[41] In the plasma, iron is transported bound to a protein called transferrin, or siderophilin, which is formed in the liver. It is cleared from the plasma with a half-time of approximately 60 to 120 minutes and is either taken up by erythroid precursors of the bone marrow or deposited in storage complexes.

Biochemically, iron is necessary for production of hemoglobin and myoglobin and for the functioning of some essential metabolic enzymes. Deficiency states are characterized by a hypochromic macrocytic anemia, lowered serum iron concentration, and frequently an elevated total iron-binding capacity. In addition, iron deficiency may increase susceptibility to helminth infections, depress cellular immunity,[42] and decrease bactericidal activity of leukocytes.[43, 44] On the other hand, decreased serum iron results in less available iron for iron-dependent microbes and an apparent increase in host resistance to some infections.[45] To calculate iron needed for restoration of hemoglobin and replenishment of iron stores, the following formula may be used:

$$Fe = 0.3 \text{ (weight in lbs)} \times$$
$$(100 - \frac{Hgb \times 100}{14.8}) = \text{mg iron needed}$$

The iron is given intravenously on a daily or monthly basis as iron dextran.[46]

*Manganese.* A 70 kg adult human body contains 12 to 20 mg of manganese.[47] Daily oral intake varies greatly, depending on the locality and diet, but has been estimated to be between 0.7 and 22 mg per day.[48] Manganese is poorly absorbed from the gastrointestinal tract, and only about 12 per cent is retained. The mechanism of absorption remains to be determined. Absorbed manganese is distributed throughout the body, with highest concentrations in the brain, kidney, pancreas, liver, and bones. It is bound in serum by a specific protein designated transmanganin.[49] Normal serum concentrations are low, averaging 8.44 ± 2.73 micrograms/liter. However, reports vary widely, and the true normal serum concentration remains to be determined.[50] Manganese is excreted almost exclusively through the gastrointestinal tract, with bile and pancreatic juices contributing large amounts. Some reabsorption from the duodenum, jejunum, and ileum occurs. Almost no manganese is excreted in the urine.[50, 51]

Manganese is known to activate many enzyme systems.[52] One system in which a clinical effect of manganese deficiency has been demonstrated is chondroitin sulfate synthesis.[53] Other studies have shown the important role manganese plays in initiating protein synthesis by stimulating RNA and DNA polymerase activity.[54]

The first case of human manganese deficiency was reported by Doisy in 1972.[55] Symptoms included weight loss, transient dermatitis, occasional nausea and vomiting, slow growth, and changes in hair and beard color. Protein synthesis appeared unaltered. Marked hypocholesterolemia was noted. In addition, experimentally induced manganese deficiency has been reported in many domestic animals. Symptoms include slow growth, decreased testicular and ovarian function, and accumulation of fat. Skeletal abnormalities such as shortening and bowing of the forelegs and chondrodystrophy have also been documented (see review in reference 50).

The role of manganese in glucose utilization is of particular interest in parenteral nutrition. A diabetes-like glucose tolerance curve found in manganese-deficient guinea pigs was corrected by manganese supplementation.[56] A potential relationship between insulin and manganese is also suggested by the decreased concentrations of manganese found in blood and tissues of pancreatectomized dogs and patients with untreated diabetes mellitus.[47]

Manganese appears to be the least toxic of trace metals.[50] Toxic symptoms, however, have been reported in Chilean miners after 7 months to 20 years of exposure in manganese mines.[57] There is permanent damage to the extrapyramidal system, with symptoms similar to Parkinson's disease. Curiously, levodopa, with known benefit in the treatment of Parkinsonism, is sometimes successful in alleviating symptoms of manganese toxicity.[58] Metabolic balance studies have indicated that intravenous administration of approximately 2 to 3 mg manganese per day (0.006 mEq/kg/day) is adequate to prevent deficiencies.

*Molybdenum.* There are no defined symptoms of molybdenum deficiency in man. Animal experiments, however, suggest that molybdenum deficiency adversely affects growth and may contribute to dental caries. The metal is an essential component of the enzyme xanthine oxidase.[59] The average daily diet contains 45 to 500 micrograms of molybdenum.[3] Studies have indicated that molybdenum equilibrium or a slight positive balance can be maintained in man if the diet provides 2 micrograms per kilogram body weight.

*Nickel.* Only recently has nickel been demonstrated to be essential in the mammalian diet.[60, 61] Symptoms of nickel deficiency in animals include impaired reproduction, a sparse, rough hair coat, and decreased oxygen uptake by liver homogenates. Histologically, hepatocytes show dilated cisterns of the rough endoplasmic reticulum and swelling of the mitochondria. Patients likely to develop nickel deficiency include those with cirrhosis of the liver, chronic uremia, or malabsorption, those under extreme physiologic stress,[62] and those with large losses of sweat, which contains up to 49 micrograms of nickel per liter.[63] Daily requirements for nickel have yet to be determined in man, although it has been suggested that 50 to 80 ng of nickel per gram of diet are necessary for the rat and chick.

*Selenium.* The need for selenium by a variety of laboratory and farm animals is well documented.[64, 65] In lambs and calves a muscle degeneration termed "white muscle disease" has been attributed to selenium deficiency. This disease is characterized by a classic Zenker's degeneration and a progressive calcification of skeletal muscle. Selenium deficiency in experimental animals has also resulted in mild growth retardation, reproductive failure, eye changes, and fibrotic degeneration of the pancreas. Selenium is a component of the glutathione peroxidase system and is required for efficient oxidation of sulphydryl groups. A deficiency syndrome in man has yet to be observed, and minimal daily requirements are unknown.

*Silicon.* The first clear evidence that silicon was an essential element was reported in 1972 when a depressed growth rate and pallor of the skin and mucous membrane were observed in experimental chickens fed a silicon-free diet.[66] Silicon appears to be involved in bone calcification and the structure of cartilage matrix. It may also play a role in mucopolysaccharide metabolism and function as a biologic cross-linking agent contributing to the structure and resiliency of connective tissue. Deficiency states in the human have yet to be reported, and minimal daily requirements are unknown. An excellent source for silicon, if oral liquids are tolerated, is beer, which contains up to 1.2 mg per gram of fluid.[61]

*Tin.* A 1970 report found tin to be essential for the growth of rats maintained on purified amino acid diets in a trace-element–controlled environment.[67] The ability of tin to form complexes with four to six, and possibly eight, ligands has led to speculation that it may contribute to the tertiary structure of proteins or other components of biologic importance. A deficiency state in humans has yet to be defined, and daily requirements are unknown.

*Vanadium.* The requirement for vanadium in the mammalian diet was first reported in 1971.[68] Symptoms observed in rats and chickens have included reduced body growth,[69] increased packed red blood cell volume, increased plasma triglyceride levels, impaired reproductive performance,[70] and a shortened, thickened leg structure secondary to impaired bony development. Deficiency syndromes in man have yet to be reported, and minimal daily requirements are unknown.

*Zinc.* Total body zinc ranges from 1.4 to 2.3 grams. Normal plasma concentrations are greater than 80 micrograms per 100 ml,[71, 72] with hair concentrations of 103.3 ± 4.4 ppm.[73] An average oral diet contains 10 to 15 mg zinc, of which 1 to 2 mg are absorbed, primarily from the upper small intestine. Zinc absorption is thought to be regulated, in part, by the amount of zinc intake, the intake of other elements and dietary components, and mucosal cell zinc concentrations.[74] The major excretory route for zinc is via the feces by a poorly understood mechanism.[75] Pancreatic secretions appear to have high concentrations of zinc.[76] Sweat contains around 1 mg zinc per liter.[47] Normal urinary zinc ranges from 300 to 700 micrograms per 24 hours.[71] During stress up to 8000 micrograms zinc may be lost per day in the urine, primarily because of catabolism of skeletal muscle, which contains relatively high concentrations of zinc.[77, 78] Urinary zinc excretion has been proposed as an indicator of an anabolic status.[72]

Zinc was first shown to be essential in the mammalian diet by Todd et al. in 1934.[79] In 1956 Vallee suggested that zinc was essential in man as summarized in reference 80. Prasad et al.[81-83] described a syndrome of iron-deficiency anemia, hepatosplenomegaly, geophagia, hypogonadism, and dwarfism in Iranian and Egyptian males with chronic zinc deficiency. Following zinc replacement, an increase in growth rate and sexual development was observed.[84] Although other studies have cast some doubt on these effects,[85, 86] Hambidge et al.[87] found poor growth in American children with low hair zinc concentrations. Although the actual role of zinc remains to be determined, preliminary evidence indicates that sexual maturation, growth, and development depend on adequate dietary zinc. Biochemically, zinc is essential for mobilization of vitamin A from the liver[88] and functions as an integral component of more than 70 known metaloenzymes[89, 90] through its involvement in protein, DNA, and RNA synthesis.[91] More than 90 per cent of enzymatic zinc is present in the erythrocyte as carbonic anhydrase.[92]

A syndrome of acute zinc deficiency in adult human beings was first outlined by Kay et al. in 1975 and 1976.[93, 94] They observed diarrhea, mental depression, alopecia, and paranasal, periorbital, and perioral dermatitis in patients given intravenous nutrition with zinc-free solutions. The diarrhea invariably preceded other symptoms, was at times quite severe, and occasionally occurred with only minimally depressed plasma zinc concentrations. The diarrhea resolved within 24 to 48 hours of zinc administration. Apathy and depression occurred fairly early as well, while the dermatitis appeared only after plasma zinc concentrations fell below 20 micrograms per 100 ml. The dermatitis, which resem-

bles the parakeratosis of fungal infections, rapidly spread to other areas of the body, especially the face and scrotum. It did not respond to antifungal agents. Alopecia appeared 7 to 14 days after the dermatitis and responded slowly to zinc infusion (the presence of telogen effluvium was not considered in their report, and the etiology of the hair loss remains uncertain). Okada et al.[95] and Tucker et al.[96] reported a similar clinical syndrome in adults, and Arakawa et al.[97] reported the syndrome in infants. We have observed one case of probable zinc deficiency in a chronically ill patient after 17 days of zinc-free parenteral nutrition. It was characterized by a marked dermatitis about the mouth and eyes and over the nose and chin (Fig. 10–1). The patient also reported a change in both taste and smell acuity. She was placed on 300 micrograms of zinc per kg (10 mg per day) given as zinc sulfate with the parenteral nutrition solution. Clearing of the skin lesions and improvement in both taste and smell occurred over the next 6 days, and zinc infusion was discontinued after 16 days. Two months later the rash recurred in the same areas, and zinc infusion was reinstituted. The rash again cleared over 5 days, and the patient was maintained on 10 mg zinc for the next 30 days, during which time her appetite improved and an oral diet was resumed.

The beneficial effect of zinc on healing of surgical wounds was suggested by Pories et al.[98, 99] Others have since demonstrated that zinc deficiency is associated with decreased synthesis of protein and collagen in surgical wounds.[99-103] Yet, not all studies have demonstrated clear benefits of zinc administration on wound healing, as reviewed by Lee et al.[104] and Chvapil et al.[105] Most data suggest that zinc supplementation in patients with normal zinc stores is of little value in wound healing, but that administration of zinc to patients with zinc deficiency significantly improves wound healing.

Henkin et al.[106, 107] have described decreased taste and olfactory acuity, occasionally associated with perverted taste and smell, in zinc-deficient patients. The pa-

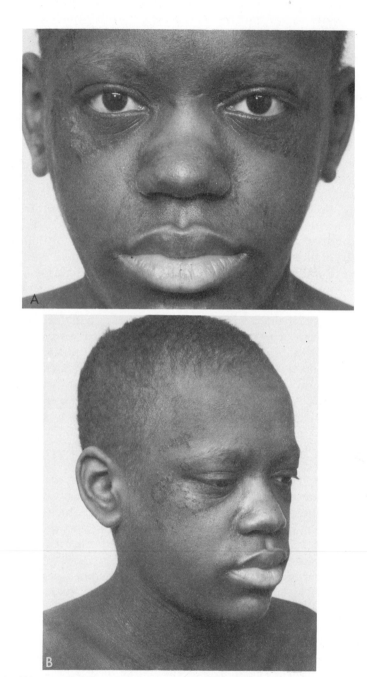

**Figure 10–1**  Skin manifestations of acute zinc deficiency during parenteral nutrition. Non-pruritic dermatitis about mouth and eyes and over nose and chin is evident.

tients often developed anorexia, weight loss, and psychological difficulties. All symptoms were reversed with the administration of zinc.

Finally, although not documented in humans, zinc deficiency has been associated with congenital anomalies, decreased fertility, and *in utero* fetal reabsorption in animals (see review in reference 47).

Certain patients are prone to develop zinc deficiency. They include patients with cirrhosis,[71, 108, 109] those who are receiving long-term corticosteroid therapy or who have undergone bilateral adrenalectomy,[110] major-surgical patients or ones with significant trauma,[111] and those on zinc-deficient diets or with malabsorption syndromes.[71] The recommended daily oral intake for zinc is 15 mg of which 1 to 2 mg are absorbed.[37, 112] The intravenous dose suggested to reverse clinical features of acute zinc deficiency is 16 to 32 mg zinc per day given as zinc sulfate.[93] The intravenous maintenance dose during prolonged parenteral nutrition remains to be determined, although 2 to 10 mg per day has been suggested (see Table 10–1). Recently, Jeejeebhoy et al.[113] have suggested giving 2 mg zinc, plus 17.1 mg per kilogram of stool or ileostomy output, or 12.2 mg per kilogram of gastric, duodenal, or jejunal fluid loss per day.

Paradoxically, replacement of zinc deficiency by oral zinc sulfate has been observed to decrease serum zinc concentrations initially.[114] This decline may represent a shift of zinc into intracellular spaces or perhaps increased excretion by the pancreas. Zinc sulfate is a relatively non-toxic compound.[115, 116] Excessive ingestion has, however, resulted in fever, nausea, vomiting, and diarrhea. Chronic ingestion of large amounts of zinc by animals has led to poor growth and anemia.[89]

## DISCUSSION

The above review presents data accumulated, for the most part, from study of animals, or man under normal conditions. If these data appear inadequate, no apology need be made, as interest in trace elements has only recently been awakened. Furthermore, the analytical procedures are complex, require special instrumentation, and are not routinely available. Changes in trace element metabolism during stress, prolonged malnutrition, and abnormal body fluid losses compound the problem.

As in many other aspects of medicine, appreciation of the need for trace elements during parenteral nutrition has preceded basic scientific knowledge. Early investigators proposed that the suspected requirements for trace elements be met by weekly administration of fresh-frozen plasma.[117] This concept is still supported by some. Yet, Table 10–1, summarizing the serum concentrations of the various trace elements and the estimated daily requirements for each, points out the obvious inadequacy of plasma infusion. The tangible risk of serum hepatitis raises further caution about its use.

More recently, several investigators have suggested the infusion of trace element solutions with parenteral nutrition to avoid possible deficiencies[13, 118-120, 122, 123] (see Table 10–1). The value of the various formulas is questionable, as suggested by the wide range of proposals for trace element supplementation. Further, special care must be taken to avoid toxic complications. The intestinal mucosa functions as a protective barrier against absorption of excessive amounts of some trace elements, especially those poorly excreted by the kidneys. Administration of trace elements intravenously bypasses this protective effect. In addition, decisions on trace element administration must take into account those elements already present in parenteral nutrition solutions, some of which are quite common (Table 10–1).

More appropriate trace-element formulas must await further research on trace element requirements and metabolism. A contribution in this area has been made by Hankins et al.,[121] who studied the effects of long-term parenteral nutrition on trace element concentrations in blood. They demonstrated a significant increase in manganese, which reflected the relatively high manganese content of the solution used. Bromine and rubidium were consistently low and antimony was elevated, while blood concentrations of chromium, iron, zinc, cobalt, and selenium were unaltered. Fleming et al.[30] and Lowry et al.[127] found serum zinc and copper levels to decline progressively during parenteral nutrition. With further studies of human requirements and the development of improved laboratory techniques for trace element measurements, currently unsuspected effects of trace element deficiencies or excesses might be avoided. For the present, deficiency syndromes should be carefully sought and vigorously treated by oral or intravenous supplementation of appropriate trace elements. The safety of routine trace element infusion remains to be proven, as does the effect of trace elements already present in parenteral nutrition solutions.

## REFERENCES

1. Trace Elements in Human Nutrition. W.H.O. Tech. Rep. Ser., *532*:41–43, 1973.
2. Hambidge, K. M.: Chromium nutrition in man. Am. J. Clin. Nutr., *27*:505–514, 1974.
3. Dietary Allowances Committee and Food and Nutrition Board: Recommended Dietary Allowances, 8th Edition. Washington, D.C., National Academy of Science, 1974.
4. Donaldson, R. M., and Barreras, R. F.: Intestinal absorption of trace quantities of chromium. J. Lab. Clin. Med., *68*:484–493, 1963.
5. Mertz, W., Roginski, E. E., and Reba, R. C.: Biological activity and fate of intravenous chromium (3) in the rat. Am. J. Physiol., *209*:489–494, 1965.
6. Schroeder, H. A.: The role of chromium in mammalian nutrition. Am. J. Clin. Nutr., *21*:230–244, 1968.
7. Mertz, W.: Chromium occurrence and function in biological systems. Physiol. Rev., *49*:163–239, 1969.
8. Levine, R. A., Streeten, D. H. P., and Doisy, R. J.: Effects of oral chromium supplementation on the glucose tolerance of elderly human subjects. Metabolism, *17*:114–125, 1968.
9. Schroeder, H. A., Balassa, J. J., and Tipton, I. H.: Abnormal trace metals in man: Chromium. J. Chronic Dis., *15*:941–964, 1962.
10. Mertz, W.: Effects and metabolism of glucose tolerance factor. Nutr. Rev., *33*:129–135, 1975.
11. Mertz, W., Roginski, E. E., and Schroeder, H. A.: Some aspects of glucose metabolism of chromium-deficient rats raised in a strictly controlled environment. J. Nutr., *86*:107–112, 1965.
12. Hopkins, L. L., Jr., Ransome-Kuti, O., and Majaj, A. S.: Improvement of impaired carbohydrate metabolism by chromium (III) in malnourished infants. Am. J. Clin. Nutr., *21*:203–211, 1968.
13. Jeejeebhoy, K. N., Chu, R. C., Marliss, E. B., Greenberg, G. R., and Bruce-Robertson, A.: Chromium deficiency, glucose intolerance, and neuropathy reversed by chromium supplementation, in a patient receiving long-term total parenteral nutrition. Am. J. Clin. Nutr., *30*:531–538, 1977.
14. Schwarz, K., and Mertz, W.: A glucose tolerance factor and its differentiation from Factor 3. Arch. Biochem. Biophys., *72*:515–518, 1957.
15. Schwarz, K., and Mertz, W.: Chromium (III) and the glucose tolerance factor. Arch. Biochem. Biophys., *85*:292–295, 1959.
16. Glinsmann, W. H., and Mertz, W.: Effect of trivalent chromium on glucose tolerance. Metabolism, *15*:510–520, 1966.
17. Novikova, E. P.: Effect of different amounts of dietary cobalt on iodine content of rat thyroid gland. Fed. Proc., *23*:459–460, 1964.
18. Cartwright, G. E., and Wintrobe, M. M.: Copper metabolism in normal subjects. Am. J. Clin. Nutr., *14*:224–232, 1964.
19. Evans, G. W.: Copper homeostasis in the mammalian system. Physiol. Rev., *53*:535–570, 1973.
20. van Berge Henegouwen, G. P., Tangedahl, T. N., Hofmann, A. F., Northfield, T. C., LaRusso, N. F., and McCall, J. T.: Biliary secretion of copper in healthy man. Gastroenterology, *72*:1228–1231, 1977.
21. Linder, M. C., and Munro, H. N.: Iron and copper metabolism during development. Enzyme, *15*:111–138, 1973.
22. Kim, C. S., and Hill, C. H.: The interrelationship of dietary copper and amine oxidase in the formation of elastin. Biochem. Biophys. Res. Commun., *24*:395–400, 1966.
23. Maynard, L. A., and Loosli, J. K.: Animal Nutrition. New York, McGraw-Hill Book Company, 1962, p. 154.
24. Schubert, W. K., and Lahey, M. E.: Copper and protein depletion complicating hypoferric anemia of infancy. Pediatrics, *24*:710–733, 1959.
25. Dunlap, W. M., James, G. W., III, and Hume, D. M.: Anemia and neutropenia caused by copper deficiency. Ann. Intern. Med., *80*:470–476, 1974.
26. Karpel, J. T., and Peden, V. H.: Copper deficiency in long-term parenteral nutrition. J. Pediatr., *80*:32–36, 1972.
27. Vilter, R. W., Bozian, R. C., Hess, E. V., Zellner, D. C., and Petering, H. G.: Manifestations of copper deficiency in a patient with systemic sclerosis on intravenous hyperalimentation. N. Engl. J. Med., *291*:188–191, 1974.
28. Solomons, N. W., Layden, T. J., Rosenberg, I. H., Vo-Khactu, K., and Sandstead, H. H.: Plasma trace metals during total parenteral alimentation. Gastroenterology, *70*:1022–1025, 1976.

29. Roeser, H. P., Nacht, L. S., and Cartwright, G. E.: The role of ceruloplasmin in iron metabolism. J. Clin. Invest., *49*:2408–2417, 1970.

30. Fleming, C. R., Hodges, R. E., and Hurley, L. S.: A prospective study of serum copper and zinc levels in patients receiving total parenteral nutrition. Am. J. Clin. Nutr., *29*:70–77, 1976.

31. Dudrick, S. J., and Rhoads, J. E.: New horizons for intravenous feeding. J.A.M.A., *215*:939–949, 1971.

32. Fairbanks, V. F.: Copper sulfate-induced hemolytic anemia. Arch. Intern. Med., *120*:428–432, 1967.

33. Chuttani, H. K., Gupta, P. S., Gulati, S., and Gupta, D. N.: Acute copper sulfate poisoning. Am. J. Med., *39*:849–854, 1965.

34. Messer, H. H., Wong, K., Wegner, M., Singer, I., and Armstrong, W. D.: Effect of reduced fluoride intake by mice on haematocrit values. Nature (New Biol.), *240*:218–219, 1972.

35. Schwartz, K., and Milne, D. B.: Fluorine requirement for growth in the rat. Bioinorg. Chem., *1*:331, 1972.

36. Underwood, E. J.: Trace Elements in Human and Animal Nutrition, 3rd Edition. New York, Academic Press, Inc., 1971, p. 369.

37. Passmore, R., Nicol, B. M., Rao, M. N., et al.: Handbook on Human Nutritional Requirements. F.A.O. Nutr. Stud., *28*:1–66, 1974. [Also W.H.O. Monogr. Ser., *0*(61):1–64, 1974.]

38. Food and Nutrition Board: Iodine Nutriture in the United States. Washington, D.C., National Academy of Science, 1970.

39. Peden, J. C., Jr.: Present knowledge of iron and copper. Nutr. Rev., *25*:321–324, 1967.

40. Moore, C. V.: Iron nutrition. *In* Gross, F. (ed.): Iron Metabolism. Berlin, Springer Verlag, 1964, p. 251.

41. Dowdle, E. B., Schachter, D., and Schenker, H.: Active transport of Fe-59 by everted segments of rat duodenum. Am. J. Physiol., *198*:609–613, 1960.

42. Joynson, D.H.M., Walker, D.M., Jacobs, A., and Dolby, A. E.: Defect of cell-mediated immunity in patients with iron-deficiency anaemia. Lancet, *2*:1058–1059, 1972.

43. Arbeter, A., Echeverri, L., Franco, D., Munson, D., Velez, H., and Vitale, J. J.: Nutrition and infection. Fed. Proc., *30*:1421–1428, 1971.

44. Chandra, R. K.: Reduced bactericidal capacity of polymorphs in iron deficiency. Arch. Dis. Child., *48*:864–866, 1973.

45. Weinberg, E. D.: Iron and susceptibility to infectious disease. Science, *184*:952–956, 1974.

46. Mays, T., and Mays, T.: Intravenous iron-dextran therapy in the treatment of anemia occurring in surgical, gynecologic, and obstetric patients. Surg. Gynecol. Obstet., *143*:381–384, 1976.

47. Burch, R. E., Hahn, H. K. J., and Sullivan, J. F.: Newer aspects of the roles of zinc, manganese, and copper in human nutrition. Clin. Chem., *21*:501–520, 1975.

48. McLeod, B. E., and Robinson, M. F.: Metabolic balance of manganese in young women. Br. J. Nutr., *27*:221–227, 1972.

49. Cotzias, G. C., and Bertinchamps, A. J.: Transmanganin, the specific manganese-carrying protein in human plasma. J. Clin. Invest., *39*:979, 1960. (abstract)

50. Underwood, E. J.: Trace Elements in Human and Animal Nutrition, 3rd Edition. New York, Academic Press, Inc., 1971, p. 177.

51. Bertinchamps, A. J., Miller, S. T., and Cotzias, G. C.: Interdependence of routes excreting manganese. Am. J. Physiol., *211*:217–224, 1966.

52. O'Dell, B. L., and Campbell, B. J.: Trace elements: Metabolism and metabolic function. *In* Florkin, M., and Stotz, E. (eds.): Comprehensive Biochemistry. New York, Elsevier North-Holland, Inc., 1971, p. 223.

53. Leach, R. M., Jr., Muenster, A. M., and Wien, E. M.: Studies on the role of manganese in bone formation. II. Effect upon chondroitin sulfate synthesis in chick epiphyseal cartilage. Arch. Biochem. Biophys., *133*:22–28, 1969.

54. Luck, G., and Zimmer, C.: Conformational aspects and reactivities of DNA: Effects of manganese and magnesium ions on interaction with DNA. Eur. J. Biochem., *29*:528–536, 1972.

55. Doisy, E. A., Jr.: Micronutrient control on biosynthesis of clotting proteins and cholesterol. *In* Hemphill, D. D. (ed.): Proceedings of the University of Missouri's 6th Annual Conference on Trace Substances in Environmental Health. Columbia, Mo., University of Missouri Press, 1973, p. 193.

56. Everson, G. J., and Shrader, R. E.: Abnormal glucose tolerance in manganese-deficient guinea pigs. J. Nutr., *94*:89–94, 1968.

57. Mena, I., Marin, O., Fuenzalida, S., and Cotzias, G. C.: Chronic manganese poisoning: Clinical picture and manganese turnover. Neurology, *17*:128–136, 1967.

58. Cotzias, G. C., Papavasilion, P. S., Ginos, J., Steck, A., and Duby, S.: Metabolic modification of Parkinson's disease and chronic manganese poisoning. Annu. Rev. Med., *22*:305–326, 1971.

59. Richert, D. A., and Westerfeld, W. W.: Isolation and identification of the xanthine oxidase factor as molybdenum. J. Biol. Chem., *203*:915–923, 1953.

60. Nielsen, F. H., and Ollerich, D. A.: Nickel: A new essential trace element. Fed. Proc., *33*:1767–1772, 1974.

61. Nielson, F. H., and Sandstead, H. H.: Are nickel, vanadium, silicon, fluorine and tin essential for man? A review. Am. J. Clin. Nutr., *27*:515–520, 1974.

62. McNeely, M. D., Sunderman, F. W., Jr., Nechay, M. W., and Levine, H.: Abnormal concentrations of nickel in serum in cases of myocardial infarction, stroke, burns, hepatic cirrhosis, and uremia. Clin. Chem., *17*:1123–1128, 1971.

63. Horak, E., and Sunderman, F. W., Jr.: Fecal nickel excretion by healthy adults. Clin. Chem., *19*:429–430, 1973.

64. McLean, J. W., Thomson, G. G., and Claxton, J. H.: Growth responses to selenium in lambs. Nature, *184*:251–252, 1959.

65. Muth, O. H.: White muscle disease, a selenium-responsive myopathy. J. Am. Vet. Med. Assoc., *142*:272–277, 1963.

66. Carlisle, E. M.: Silicon: An essential element for the chick. Science, *178*:619–621, 1972.

67. Schwarz, K., Milne, D. B., and Vinyard, E.: Growth effects of tin compounds on rats maintained in a trace element controlled environment. Biochem. Biophys. Res. Commun., *40*:22–29, 1970.

68. Hopkins, L. L., Jr., and Mohr, H. E.: The biological essentiality of vanadium. *In* Mertz, W., and Cornatzer, W. W. (eds.): Newer Trace Elements in Nutrition. New York, Marcel Dekker, Inc., 1971, p. 195.

69. Schwarz, K., and Milne, D. B.: Growth effects of vanadium in the rat. Science, *174*:426–428, 1971.

70. Hopkins, L. L., Jr., and Mohr, H. E.: Vanadium as an essential element. Fed. Proc., *33*:1773–1775, 1974.

71. Walker, B. E., Dawson, J. B., Kelleher, J., and Lasowsky, M. S.: Plasma and urinary zinc in patients with malabsorption syndromes or hepatic cirrhosis. Gut, *14*:943–948, 1973.

72. Fell, G. S., Cuthbertson, D. P., Morrison, C., Fleck, A., Queen, K., Bessent, R. G., and Husain, S. L.: Urinary zinc levels as an indication of muscle catabolism. Lancet, *1*:280–282, 1973.

73. Strain, W. H., Steadman, L. T., Lankau, C. A., Jr., Berliner, W. P., and Pories, W. J.: Analysis of zinc levels in hair for the diagnosis of zinc deficiency in man. J. Lab. Clin. Med., *68*:244–249, 1966.

74. Evans, G. W., Grace, C. I., and Hahn, C.: Homeostatic regulation of zinc absorption in the rat. Proc. Soc. Exp. Biol. Med., *143*:723–725, 1973.

75. Cotzias, G. C., Borg, D. C., and Selleck, B.: Specificity of zinc pathway through the body: Turnover of Zn-65 in the mouse. Am. J. Physiol., *202*:359–363, 1962.

76. Sullivan, J. F., O'Grady, J., and Lankford, H. G.: The zinc content of pancreatic secretion. Gastroenterology, *48*:438–443, 1965.

77. Lindeman, R. D., Bottomley, R. G., Cornelison, R. L., Jr., and Jacobs, L. A.: Influence of acute tissue injury on zinc metabolism in man. J. Lab. Clin. Med., *79*:452–460, 1972.

78. Cuthbertson, D. P., Fell, G. S., Smith, C. M., and Tilstone, W. J.: Metabolism after injury. I. Effects of severity, nutrition, and environmental temperature on protein, potassium, zinc, and creatine. Br. J. Surg., *59*:925–931, 1972.

79. Todd, W. R., Elvehjem, C. A., and Hart, E. B.: Zinc in the nutrition of the rat. Am. J. Physiol., *107*:146–156, 1934.

80. Vallee, B. L.: Biochemistry, physiology and pathology of zinc. Physiol. Rev., *39*:443–490, 1959.

81. Prasad, A. S., Halsted, J. A., and Nadimi, M.: Syndrome of iron deficiency anemia, hepatosplenomegaly, hypogonadism, dwarfism, and geophagia. Am. J. Med., *31*:532–546, 1961.

82. Prasad, A. S., Miale, A., Jr., Farid, Z., Sandstead, H. H., and Schulert, A. R.: Zinc metabolism in patients with the syndrome of iron deficiency anemia, hepatosplenomegaly, dwarfism, and hypogonadism. J. Lab. Clin. Med., *61*:537–549, 1963.

83. Prasad, A. S., Miale, A., Jr., Farid, Z., Sandstead, H. H., Schulert, A. R., and Darby, W. J.: Biochemical studies on dwarfism, hypogonadism, and anemia. Arch. Intern. Med., *111*:407–428, 1963.

84. Sandstead, H. H., Prasad, A. S., Schulert, A. R., Farid, Z., Miale, A., Jr., Bassilly, S., and Darby, W. J.: Human zinc deficiency, endocrine manifestations and response to treatment. Am. J. Clin. Nutr., *20*:422–442, 1967.

85. Coble, Y. D., VanReen, R., Schulert, A. R., Koshakji, R. P., Farid, Z., and Davis, J. T.: Zinc levels and blood enzyme activities in Egyptian male subjects with retarded growth and sexual development. Am. J. Clin. Nutr., *19*:415–421, 1966.

86. Coble, Y. D., Schulert, A. R., and Farid, Z.: Growth and sexual development of male subjects in an Egyptian oasis. Am. J. Clin. Nutr., *18*:421–425, 1966.

87. Hambidge, K. M., Hambidge, C., Jacobs, M., and Baum, J. D.: Low levels of zinc in hair, anorexia, poor growth, and hypogeusia in children. Pediatr. Res., *6*:868–874, 1972.

88. Smith, J. C., Jr., McDaniel, E. G., Fan, F. F., and Halsted, J. A.: Zinc: A trace element essential in vitamin A metabolism. Science, *181*:954–955, 1973.

89. Mikac-Devic, D.: Methodology of zinc determinations and the role of zinc in the biochemical processes. Adv. Clin. Chem., *13*:271–333, 1970.

90. Parisi, A. F., and Vallee, B. L.: Zinc metalloenzymes: Characteristics and significance in biology and medicine. Am. J. Clin. Nutr., *22*:1222–1239, 1969.

91. Zinc in relation to DNA and RNA synthesis in regenerating rat liver. Nutr. Rev., *27*:211–213, 1969.

92. Widdowson, R. M.: Trace elements in foetal and early postnatal development. Nutr. Soc. Proc., *33*:275–284, 1974.

93. Kay, R. G., Tasman-Jones, C., Pybus, J., Whiting, R., and Black, H.: A syndrome of acute zinc deficiency during total parenteral alimentation in man. Ann. Surg., *183*:331–340, 1976.

94. Kay, R. G., and Tasman-Jones, C.: Acute zinc deficiency in man during intravenous alimentation. Aust. N.Z. J. Surg., *45*(4):325–330, 1975.

95. Okada, A., Takagi, Y., Itakura, T., Satani, M., Manabe, H., Iida, Y., Tanigaki, T., Iwasaki,

M., and Kasahara, N.: Skin lesions during intravenous hyperalimentation: Zinc deficiency. Surgery, *80*:629–635, 1976.

96. Tucker, S. B., Schroeter, A. L., Brown, P. W., Jr., and McCall, J. T.: Acquired zinc deficiency: Cutaneous manifestations typical of acrodermatitis enteropathica. J.A.M.A., *235*:2399–2402, 1976.

97. Arakawa, T., Tamura, T., Igarashi, Y., Suzuki, H., and Sandstead, H. H.: Zinc deficiency in two infants during total parenteral alimentation for diarrhea. Am. J. Clin. Nutr., *29*:197–204, 1976.

98. Pories, W. J., and Strain, W. H.: Zinc and wound healing. *In* Prasad, A. S. (ed.): Zinc Metabolism. Springfield, Ill., Charles C Thomas, Publisher, 1966, p. 378.

99. Pories, W. J., Henzel, J. H., Rob, C. G., and Strain, W. H.: Acceleration of healing with zinc sulfate. Ann. Surg., *165*:432–436, 1967.

100. Sandstead, H. H., and Shepard, G. H.: The effect of zinc deficiency on the tensile strength of healing surgical incisions in the integument of the rat. Proc. Soc. Exp. Biol. Med., *128*:687–689, 1968.

101. Oberleas, D., Seymour, J. K., Lenaghan, R., Hovanesian, J., Wilson, R. F., and Prasad, A. S.: Effect of zinc deficiency on wound healing in rats. Am. J. Surg., *121*:566–568, 1971.

102. Hsu, J. M., and Anthony, W. L.: Zinc deficiency and collagen synthesis in rat skin. *In* Hemphill, D. D. (ed.): Proceedings of the University of Missouri's 6th Annual Conference on Trace Substances in Environmental Health. Columbia, Mo., University of Missouri Press, 1973, p. 137.

103. Savlov, E. D., Strain, W. H., and Huegin, F.: Radiozinc studies in experimental wound healing. J. Surg. Res., *2*:209–212, 1962.

104. Lee, P. W. R., Green, M. A., Long, W. B., III, and Gill, W.: Zinc and wound healing. Surg. Gynecol. Obstet., *143*:549–554, 1976.

105. Chvapil, M., Elias, S. L., Ryan, J. N., and Zukoski, C. F.: Pathophysiology of zinc. *In* Pfeiffer, C. C. (ed.): Neurobiology of the Trace Metals Zinc and Copper. New York, Academic Press, Inc., 1972, p. 105.

106. Henkin, R. I.: Newer aspects of copper and zinc metabolism. *In* Mertz, W., and Cornatzer, W. E. (eds.): Newer Trace Elements in Nutrition. New York, Marcel Dekker, Inc., 1971, p. 255.

107. Henkin, R. I., Schechter, P. J., Hoye, R., and Matten, C. F. T.: Idiopathic hypogeusia with dysgeusia, hyposmia and dysosmia. A new syndrome. J.A.M.A., *217*:434–440, 1971.

108. Vallee, B. L., Wacker, W. E. C., Bartholomay, A. F., and Robin, E. D.: Zinc metabolism in hepatic dysfunction. I. Serum zinc concentrations in Laennec's cirrhosis and their validation by sequential analysis. N. Engl. J. Med., *255*:403–408, 1956.

109. Vallee, B. L., Wacker, W. E., Bartholomay, A. F., and Hock, F. L.: Zinc metabolism in hepatic dysfunction. II. Correlation of metabolic patterns with biochemical findings. N. Engl. J. Med., *257*:1055–1065, 1957.

110. Flynn, A., Strain, W. H., Pories, W. J., and Hill, O. A.: Zinc deficiency with altered adrenocortical function and its relation to delayed healing. Lancet, *1*:789–791, 1973.

111. Henzel, J. H., DeWeese, M. S., and Pories, W. J.: Significance of magnesium and zinc metabolism in the surgical patient. Arch. Surg., *95*:991–999, 1967.

112. Dietary Allowances Committee and Food and Nutrition Board: Recommended Dietary Allowances. 8th Edition. Washington, D.C., National Academy of Science, 1974.

113. Wolman, S. L., Anderson, G. H., Marliss, E. B., and Jeejeebhoy, K. N.: Zinc in total parenteral nutrition: Requirements and metabolic effects. Gastroenterology, *76*:458–467, 1979.

114. Spencer, H., Olsis, P., Kramer, L., and Weatrowski, E.: Studies of zinc metabolism in normal man and in patients with neoplasia. *In* Pories, W. J., Strain, W. H., Hsu, J. M., and Woosley, R. L. (eds.): Clinical Applications of Zinc Metabolism. Springfield, Ill., Charles C Thomas, Publisher, 1974, Chapter 8.

115. Brocks, A., Reid, H., and Glazer, G.: Acute intravenous zinc poisoning. Br. Med. J., *1*:1390–1391, 1977.

116. Murphy, J. V.: Intoxication following ingestion of elemental zinc. J.A.M.A., *212*:2119–2120, 1970.

117. Dudrick, S. J., Wilmore, D. W., Vars, H. M., and Rhoads, J. E.: Can intravenous feeding as the sole means of nutrition support growth in the child and restore weight loss in the adult? Ann. Surg.. *169*:974–984, 1969.

118. Shils, M. E.: Minerals in total parenteral nutrition. Drug Intelligence and Clinical Pharmacy, *6*:385–391, 1972.

119. Wretlind, A.: Complete intravenous nutrition: Theoretical and experimental background. Nutr. Metab., *14*(Suppl.):1–57, 1972.

120. Jeejeebhoy, K. N., Langer, B., Tsallas, G., Chu, R. C., Kuksis, A., and Anderson, G. H.: Total parenteral nutrition at home: Studies in patients surviving 4 months to 5 years. Gastroenterology, *71*:943–953, 1976.

121. Hankins, D. A., Riella, M. C., Scribner, B. H., and Babb, A. L.: Whole blood trace element concentrations during total parenteral nutrition. Surgery, *79*:674–677, 1976.

122. Hull, R. L.: Use of trace elements in intravenous hyperalimentation solutions. Am. J. Hosp. Pharm., *31*:759–761, 1974.

123. Blackburn, G. L., and Bistrian, B. R.: Nutritional care of the injured and/or septic patient. Surg. Clin. North Am., *56*:1195–1224, 1976.

124. Hoffman, R. P., and Ashby, D. M.: Trace element concentrations in commercially available solutions. Drug Intelligence and Clinical Pharmacy, *10*:74–76, 1976.

125. Bozian, R. C., and Shearer, C.: Copper, zinc, and manganese content of four amino acid and protein hydrolysate preparations. Am. J. Clin. Nutr., *29*:1331–1332, 1976.

126. Hauer, E. C., and Kaminski, M. V., Jr.: Trace metal profile of parenteral nutrition solutions. J. Parenteral Enteral Nutr., *1*:9A, 1977. (abstract)

127. Lowry, S. F., Goodgame, J. T., Smith, J. C., Sr., Maher, M. M., Makuch, R. W., Henkin, R. I., and Brennan, M. F.: Abnormalities of zinc and copper during total parenteral nutrition. Ann. Surg., *189*:120–128, 1979.

128. Davidson, I. W. F., and Secrest, W. L.: Determination of chromium in biological materials by atomic absorption spectrometry using a graphite furnace atomizer. Anal. Chem., *44*:1808–1813, 1972.

129. Kartinos, N. J.: Trace element formulations in intravenous feeding. *In* Johnston, I. D. A. (ed.): Advances in Parenteral Nutrition. Lancaster, England, Medical and Technical Publishing Co., Ltd., 1978, pp. 233–263.

130. Meret, S., and Henkin, R. I.: Simultaneous direct estimation by atomic absorption spectrophotometry of copper and zinc in serum, urine, and cerebral spinal fluid. Clin. Chem., *17*:369–373, 1971.

131. Sunderman, F. W., Jr., and Roszel, N. O.: Measurements of copper in biologic materials by atomic absorption spectrophotometry. Am. J. Clin. Pathol., *48*:286–294, 1967.

132. Davies, I. J. T., Musa, M., and Dormandy, T. L.: Measurements of plasma zinc. J. Clin. Pathol., *21*:359–365, 1968.

133. McNeely, M. D., Sunderman, F. W., Nechay, M. W., and Levine, H.: Abnormal concentrations of nickel in serum in cases of myocardial infarction, stroke, burns, hepatic cirrhosis, and uremia. Clin. Chem., *17*:1123–1128, 1971.

134. Davidson, S., Passmore, R., Brock, J. F., and Truswell, A. S.: Human Nutrition and Dietetics, 6th Edition, Edinburgh, Churchill Livingstone, 1975.

# *Chapter 11*

# VITAMIN REQUIREMENTS

At the end of the nineteenth century, nutritionists and biochemists began isolating organic substances called vitamins, which were essential components of normal metabolic processes. Subsequently, these substances were purified and many were produced synthetically. During the last 40 to 50 years, studies of healthy human volunteers have demonstrated that vitamins are intimately involved in the metabolism of carbohydrate, protein, and fat, and clinical symptoms of vitamin deficiencies have been described. Recommended daily dietary allowances for each vitamin have been established by the World Health Organization[1] and by the Dietary Allowances Committee and Food and Nutrition Board of the Research Council of the National Academy of Sciences[2] (Table 11–1). Despite extensive research, little is known of changes in vitamin requirements associated with disease and injury. Further, recommended daily allowances are based on oral intake, and intravenous requirements are uncertain. The situation is further complicated in that requirements for many vitamins vary with protein-calorie intake and catabolic rate. Finally, estimates of body vitamin stores by serologic or urinary measurements are often inaccurate, rendering determination of replacement therapy difficult.

In this chapter the biologic activities, recommended daily allowances, and deficiency syndromes of fat-soluble and water-soluble vitamins will be reviewed, with special attention directed toward proper vitamin support during intravenous nutrition. Tables 11–1 and 11–2 summarize this information and list available vitamin solutions.

## FAT-SOLUBLE VITAMINS

During early studies, it was convenient to divide the various vitamins into two groups, those soluble in fat and those soluble in water. The four fat-soluble vitamins are vitamins A, D, E, and K. There is little resemblance among them, except that they are lipid-soluble and derived from isoprene units. They play important roles in specialized functions of highly differentiated organisms and are not required by simple organisms such as bacteria. Because of their involvement in complex metabolic processes, the molecular mechanisms of their function are not fully understood. On the other hand, physiologic functions have been clearly defined for each of the vitamins.

The biologic half-life of fat-soluble vitamins in healthy man is variable but usually quite long. The biologic half-life of vitamin A, for example, has been reported to be as long as 600 days. Because of the long biologic half-lives, significant deficiencies of fat-soluble vitamins are infrequent. Patients requiring total parenteral nutrition, however, often have had inadequate intake of fat-soluble vitamins for prolonged periods and are often under significant stress, which alters vitamin metabolism. In addition, administration of high-quality protein to malnourished patients augments the release of fat-soluble vitamins from body stores and may precipitate acute deficiencies of fat-soluble vita-

**Table 11-1**   RECOMMENDED DAILY ALLOWANCES OF VITAMINS

| | FAT-SOLUBLE VITAMINS | | | | WATER-SOLUBLE VITAMINS | | | | | | | |
|---|---|---|---|---|---|---|---|---|---|---|---|---|
| | $A$ (IU) | $D$ (IU) | $E$ (IU) | $K$ (mg) | $B_1$ (mg) | $B_2$ (mg) | $B_3$ (mg) | $B_5$ (mg) | $B_6$ (mg) | $B_9$ ($\mu g$) | $B_{12}$ ($\mu g$) | $C$ (mg) |
| Oral | | | | | | | | | | | | |
| FAO/WHO[1] | 2500 | 100 | – | – | 0.9*/1.2 | 1.3/1.8 | – | 14.5/19.8 | – | 200 | 2.0 | 30 |
| NRC[2] | 5000 | 400 | 12/15 | – | 1.2/1.5 | 1.4/1.8 | 5 to 10 | 14/20 | 2.0 | 400 | 3.0 | 45 |
| Normal serum concentration per 100 ml[32] | 90 to 233 | 112 to 168 | 0.5 to 1.2 | – | 0.001 to 0.006 | – | 0.015 to 0.04 | 0.3 to 0.6 | 0.003 to 0.008 | 0.4 to 2.0 | 0.02 to 0.09 | 0.4 to 1.0 |
| Intravenous | | | | | | | | | | | | |
| STPN[97] | 8000 | 400 | 60 | 2.0 | 10 | 5 | 15 | 50 | 6.0 | 1000 | 10 | 200 |
| Jeejeebhoy[32] | 2500 | 250 | >52 | 0.71 | <16 | 7.5 | 29 | 150 | >5.5 | – | 12 | 500 |
| Blackburn[98] and AMA[99] | 3300 | 200 | 10 | – | 3 | 3.6 | 15 | 40 | 4.0 | 400 | 5 | 100 |
| Nichoalds[100] | 4200 | 420 | 2.1 | – | 21 | 4.2 | 10.5 | 42 | 6.3 | 600 | 15 | 210 |

*Top figure is daily allowance for females; bottom figure is for males.

**Table 11-2** VITAMIN SOLUTIONS AVAILABLE FOR INTRAVENOUS ADMINISTRATION (per 1.0 ml solution)

| PRODUCT AND MANUFACTURER | FAT-SOLUBLE | | | WATER-SOLUBLE | | | | | | | | | | |
|---|---|---|---|---|---|---|---|---|---|---|---|---|---|---|
| | A (IU) | D (IU) | E (IU) | $B_1$ (mg) | $B_2$ (mg) | $B_3$ (mg) | $B_5$ (mg) | $B_6$ (mg) | $B_7$ (mg) | $B_9$ (µg) | $B_{12}$ (µg) | C (mg) | Choline (mg) | Inositol (mg) |
| Pancebrin (Lilly) | 5000 | 500 | 1.1 | 5 | 1 | 1.5 | 10 | 1.5 | — | — | — | 30 | — | — |
| ViSyneral (Lisons) | 5000 | 500 | 1.0 | 5 | 0.5 | 2.5 | 10 | 1.5 | — | — | — | 25 | — | — |
| MVI (USV) (10 ml amp) | 1000 | 100 | 0.5 | 5 | 1 | 2.5 | 10 | 1.5 | — | — | — | 50 | — | — |
| Beject (Abbott) | — | — | — | 2 | 2 | 10 | 50 | 1 | — | — | 5 | 100 | — | — |
| Bejectal (Abbott) | — | — | — | 10 | 2 | 5 | 75 | 5 | — | — | — | — | — | — |
| Bejectal with C (Abbott) | — | — | — | 20 | 3 | 5 | 75 | 5 | — | — | 2 | 100 | — | — |
| Berocca C (Roche) | — | — | — | 5 | 5 | 10 | 40 | 10 | 0.1 | — | — | 50 | — | — |
| Berocca C 500 (Roche) | — | — | — | 2.5 | 2.5 | 5 | 20 | 5 | .05 | — | — | 125 | — | — |
| Betalin (Lilly) | — | — | — | 5 | 2 | 2.5 | 75 | 5 | — | — | 2.5 | — | — | — |
| Betalin F. C. (Lilly) | — | — | — | 125 | 3 | 2.5 | 50 | 5 | — | — | — | 75 | — | — |
| Bextral 100 (Central) | — | — | — | 100 | 2 | 2 | 100 | 2 | — | — | — | — | — | — |
| B-lase (Caser) | — | — | — | 100 | 2 | 2 | 100 | 2 | — | — | — | — | — | — |
| Folbesyn (Lederle) | — | — | — | 5 | 5 | 5 | 375 | 7.5 | — | 500 | 7.5 | 150 | — | — |
| Key-Plex with C (Hyrex-Key) | — | — | — | 5 | 5 | 11.5 | 40 | 10 | — | — | — | 50 | — | — |
| Kremplex (Kremers Urban) | — | — | — | 100 | 5 | 5 | 50 | 2 | — | — | 1000 | — | — | — |
| Kremplex-B (Kremers Urban) | — | — | — | 100 | 5 | 5 | 50 | 2 | — | — | — | — | — | — |
| Lyo-B-C with $B_{12}$ (Merck, Sharpe & Dohme) | — | — | — | 14.3 | 1.4 | 7 | 35.7 | 1.4 | — | — | 3.6 | 28.6 | — | — |
| Lyo-B-C Forte with $B_{12}$ (Merck, Sharpe & Dohme) | — | — | — | 14.3 | 1.4 | 7 | 71.4 | 1.4 | — | — | 3.6 | 71.4 | — | — |
| Minoplex (Savage) | — | — | — | 50 | 2 | 2 | 100 | 2 | — | — | — | — | 50 | — |
| Parlite (Lederle) | — | — | — | 2 | 2 | 2 | 30 | 1 | — | — | 5 | 100 | — | — |
| Plebex (Wyeth) | — | — | — | 10 | 2 | 5 | 100 | 5 | — | — | — | — | — | — |
| Savaplex (Savage) | — | — | — | 100 | 2 | 4 | 100 | 4 | — | — | — | — | — | — |
| Solu-B (Upjohn) | — | — | — | 2 | 2 | 10 | 50 | 1 | — | — | — | (100*) | — | — |
| Solu-B Forte (Upjohn) | — | — | — | 25 | 5 | 50 | 125 | 5 | — | — | — | 100 | — | — |
| Solu-B Mix-o-vial (Upjohn) | — | — | — | 5 | 5 | 25 | 125 | 2.5 | — | — | — | — | — | — |
| Surg-C (Saron) | — | — | — | 20 | 3 | 5 | 75 | 5 | — | — | — | 250 | — | — |
| Thex Forte (Ingram) | — | — | — | 100 | 5 | 5 | 100 | 2 | — | — | — | — | 10 | 10 |
| Vicam (Keene) | — | — | — | 50 | 2 | 2 | 50 | 5 | — | — | — | 50 | — | 50 |
| Vit-B Complex (Parke-Davis) | — | — | — | 10 | 2 | 10 | 50 | 5 | — | — | — | — | — | — |
| Vit-B Complex with C (Roche) | — | — | — | 10 | 2.5 | 2.5 | 50 | 2.5 | — | — | — | 75 | — | — |
| Vit-B Complex with $B_{12}$ (Wyeth) | — | — | — | 10 | 5 | 5 | 100 | 5 | — | — | 7.5 | — | — | — |

*Solu-B with C

mins. For these reasons, fat-soluble vitamin supplementation should be included in parenteral nutrition therapy. However, infusion of excessive amounts of fat-soluble vitamins should be avoided because of possible toxic side effects.

*Vitamin A.* Vitamin A is a colorless, highly unsaturated alcohol occurring in nature in several forms. The most common form is found in mammals and saltwater fish and is designated vitamin $A_1$ (retinol) (Fig. 11–1). Vitamin A is derived from carotenoid pigments found in green leaves of plants and in yellow tubers and fruits. The most common carotenoid is a hydrocarbon with the formula $C_{40}H_{56}$, beta-carotene. Vitamin A activity is measured in international units (IU), with one unit equal to 0.3 micrograms of crystalline vitamin A alcohol or 0.6 micrograms of beta-carotene. The decreased biologic activity of carotene is due to less efficient absorption from the intestine and to a low efficiency in converting carotene to vitamin A.

Orally ingested vitamin A is absorbed in the upper gastrointestinal tract, especially in the duodenum.[3] Likewise, the duodenum is the primary site where carotene is converted into vitamin A.[4] Marked inhibition of vitamin A and carotene absorption occurs when mineral oil is ingested simultaneously. Absorption is also inhibited in the presence of diarrhea, bile salt depletion, sprue, cystic fibrosis of the pancreas, and ileitis and in patients recovering from subtotal gastrectomy.[5] Absorbed vitamin A is transported by the lymphatic system to the bloodstream. Normal serum concentrations in the adult are 163 ± 53 IU per 100 ml.[6, 7] Vitamin A is picked up by the liver, where it is stored as an ester. The liver contains about 90 per cent of the vitamin A found in the body, representing about 600,000 IU. Assuming efficient utilization of these stores, this would be sufficient vitamin A for three months to a year or more. Hypo-

thermia, infection, and ingestion of liver poisons, however, result in rapid depletion of liver stores. For example, vitamin A stores are decreased 50 per cent by appendicitis, 70 per cent by pneumonia, and up to 89 per cent by chronic nephritis.[8] The depletion is thought to result from increased urinary losses of vitamin A.

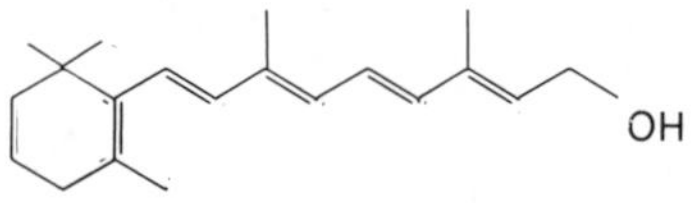

In depletion tests with animals and man, plasma vitamin A fell only after all stores were nearly exhausted. Consequently, serum levels of vitamin A are unreliable in estimating total body stores.[9] More accurate estimates can be obtained from measurements of vitamin A content in tissue, especially the liver, where 100 to 300 micrograms per gram of tissue is normal.[7]

The physiological functions of vitamin A are many. The vitamin is necessary for proper vision; for growth, especially in development and maintenance of epithelial tissues and bone; for reproduction, in which it is required for spermatogenesis in chicks but not in mammals; and for the development of the fetus. Deficiencies in man may arise because of interference with absorption or storage, inadequate dietary intake, interference with the conversion of carotene to vitamin A, or rapid loss of vitamin A from the body.[9] Interference with absorption or storage may occur in celiac syndrome, sprue, cystic fibrosis of the pancreas, ulcerative colitis, operations that bypass the duodenum, congenital partial obstruction of the jejunum, giardiasis, obstructions of the bile ducts, and cirrhosis of the liver. In addition, it has been observed in patients who have undergone operative procedures upon the pancreas. Diabetes and hypothyroidism have been associated with a failure to convert carotene to vitamin A. Infectious processes, such as pneumonia, scarlet fever, rheumatic fever, and mild respiratory infections, result in increased losses of vitamin A in the urine. A lack of vitamin A is associated with nyctalopia, xerophthalmia, phyrnoderma, decreased resistance to infection, retardation of growth, depressed production of corticosteroids, and mild leukopenia with a decrease in polymorphonuclear leukocytes and increase in juvenile forms.

**Figure 11–1**  Vitamin A.

Nyctalopia, or night blindness, may represent the earliest clinical manifestation of vitamin A deficiency. Yet its presence may be unrecognized if its onset is gradual. Initial complaints include inability to see at twilight or after exposure to bright lights. The molecular mechanism by which vitamin A contributes to night vision was first defined by Wald et al.[10] Vitamin A is oxidized to retinaldehyde by an alcohol dehydrogenase. In the rods of the retina the retinaldehyde, in turn, is part of a cyclic process that stimulates the visual nerves. Administration of vitamin A results in rapid reversal of night blindness in only one to three days.

Xerophthalmia is a manifestation of severe vitamin A deficiency during marked malnutrition. In xerophthalmia, metaplasia of the conjunctival membranes inhibits their secretions and produces consequent dryness. The earliest clinical signs are dryness, roughness, and a wrinkling of the conjunctiva, followed by swelling and redness of the lids, pain, and photophobia. Triangular, whitish, foamy patches, called Bitot's spots, may be seen at the canthi. The cornea loses its sensitivity and often becomes clouded. Ulcers of the cornea may occur and may be followed by softening and perhaps perforation of the cornea if the condition remains untreated. Prognosis in uncomplicated xerophthalmia is good if treatment is prompt and adequate. The luster may return to the cornea within five days, and Bitot's spots may become fragmented and disappear within five or six weeks. Other signs of vitamin A deficiency in the eye usually disappear within two months of vitamin A supplementation.

Phyrnoderma is a skin eruption that occurs over the entire body about hair follicles. The dry, firm, pigmented papules have central protruding carotenic plugs or spines situated below the follicle. Usually the lesions begin on the anterolateral surface of the thighs and the posterolateral surface of the upper forearms. Pustulation occurs in about a third of the cases. The dermatosis responds to moderate amounts of vitamin A and requires two to three months for complete resolution.

Vitamin A deficiency may affect other epithelial structures, especially mucus-secreting tissues, with carotinization of the respiratory, gastrointestinal, and genitourinary tracts, salivary and endocrine glands, and the vaginal epithelium. A variety of mechanisms have been suggested to account for the carotinization, but none has been proven.

Vitamin A deficiency is preventable with adequate maintenance therapy. The recommended oral intake of vitamin A is between 2500 and 5000 IU per day (see Table 11–1).

Up to 50 per cent of the vitamin A added to parenteral nutrition solutions may be bound to the glass or plastic of bags or infusion tubing within the first 24 hours.[11] In addition, vitamin A is susceptible to oxidation and is unstable in parenteral nutrition solutions, with none detectable after four weeks of storage.[12] These factors must be taken into consideration during parenteral nutrition, and suggestions for intravenous vitamin A infusion range between 2,500 and 8,000 IU per day (see Table 11–1).

A number of cases of hypervitaminosis A in human beings have been reported.[13-16] Symptoms include fatigue, malaise, lethargy, anorexia, irritability, severe headaches, hard, tender lumps in the extremities and cortical thickening of underlying bones, bone pain, and migratory arthralgia. Additional findings include increased intracranial pressure, dry skin, fissures of the skin and lips, loss of body hair, brittle nails, jaundice and hepatomegaly, and hypomenorrhea. In the reported cases, symptoms have become clinically evident after 6 to 15 months of excessive vitamin A intake ranging from 4000 to 25,000 IU per kilogram of body weight per day.[13, 17] All toxic symptoms appear to subside within three days after withdrawal of vitamin A, and blood levels return to normal within six weeks.

*Vitamin D.* There are more than ten substances that possess vitamin D activity. Two of the more important are vitamin $D_2$ (ergocalciferol) and vitamin $D_3$ (cholecalciferol) (Fig. 11–2). One milligram of vitamin D is equivalent to 40,000 IU. The D vita-

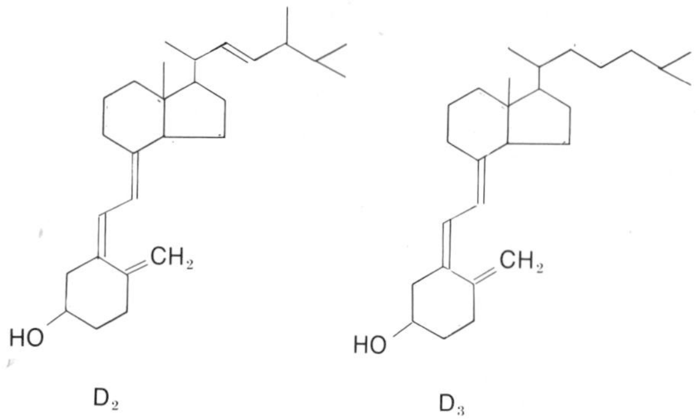

**Figure 11–2**   Vitamin D.

mins are white, odorless crystals soluble only in fats and organic solvents. When taken orally, they are absorbed mainly in the jejunum and ileum. Excess vitamin D is stored chiefly in the liver but is also found in the skin, brain, spleen, and bones.

Vitamin $D_3$, derived either from the diet or from the action of ultraviolet light on the skin, is transported to the liver by the bloodstream. There it is hydroxylated at the C-25 locus by the hepatocyte microsomes to form 25(OH)$D_3$. The vitamin is next acted upon by renal mitochondria to form the highly active molecule $1\alpha$, 25(OH)$_2D_3$. In this form, vitamin D regulates calcium and phosphorus homeostasis in conjunction with parathyroid hormone and thyrocalcitonin.[18] Vitamin D increases both absorption of calcium and phosphate from the intestine by separate active processes and also the rate of reabsorption of phosphate by the renal tubules. The vitamin appears to be necessary for mobilization of calcium and phosphate from bones by parathyroid hormone but not for that hormone's activity on the renal tubule.[19] In addition, there is some evidence that vitamin D may affect the absorption and serum concentration of magnesium.[20]

Deficiency of vitamin D in man is associated with osteomalacia, low serum calcium and phosphate levels, and elevated alkaline phosphatase concentrations. Tetany due to hypocalcemia may occur in the presence of relatively normal serum phosphate concentrations. The average recommended oral daily intake of vitamin D is between 100 and 400 IU. Estimated intravenous requirements are 200 to 420 IU daily (see Table 11–1). Vitamin D toxicity has been reported in adults taking 100,000 IU or more daily for several months.[21–23] Toxicity resembles hyperparathyroidism, with such symptoms as anorexia, nausea, vomiting, headache, drowsiness, diarrhea or constipation, polyuria and polydipsia, generalized weakness, stiffness, vague aches, and mild weight loss. Serum calcium and phosphorus concentrations are increased, and correspondingly high concentrations are found in the urine. Osteoporosis occurs with the simultaneous deposition of calcium in the heart, large blood vessels, lungs, renal tubules, and other soft tissues.[24] Anemia has been attributed to a high intake of vitamin D,[25] which may also contribute to increased absorption and urinary excretion of magnesium with a decrease in serum magnesium concentration.[26] Signs of renal failure and hypertension may also develop. Toxic effects of vitamin D are reversible if excessive administration is stopped in time.

*Vitamin K.*   Vitamin K occurs naturally in two forms — vitamin $K_1$ and $K_2$ — both of which are equally active (Fig. 11–3). Leafy vegetables contain high concentrations of vitamin $K_1$, while microorganisms contain mainly $K_2$. In the normal human, intestinal bacteria can synthesize adequate vitamin K to meet daily requirements. Absorption of orally ingested or bacterial vitamin K requires the presence of bile salts and pancreatic juice. Absorption is greatly decreased during obstructive jaundice, severe diarrhea, or administration of cholestyramine.[27] Prolonged antibiotic therapy may result in vitamin K deficiency by sup-

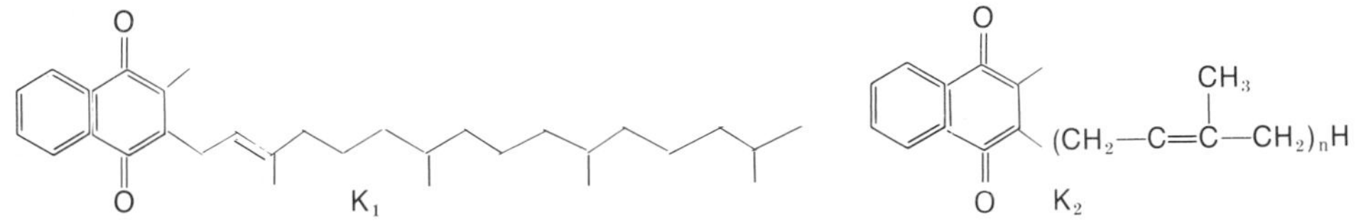

**Figure 11-3** Vitamin K.

**Figure 11-4** Vitamin E.

pression of vitamin K-producing bacteria.[28]

The role of vitamin K in blood coagulation was first proposed by Dam in 1935.[29] It is now known that vitamin K plays an essential role in the synthesis of clotting factors of both the intrinsic (Factors II, IV, IX, and X) and extrinsic (Factor VII) systems. The vitamin's role in synthesis of Factor II has been best defined.[30] Vitamin K enhances conversion of a liver precursor protein into prothrombin by carboxylation of the gamma carbon of 10-glutamic residues in the amino terminal region.[31]

Deficiency of vitamin K prolongs the prothrombin time. No recommended daily allowance has been established, but intake of 0.7 to 2.0 mg per day has been suggested (see Table 11-1). Jeejeebhoy et al.[32] advise giving 5 mg vitamin K intramuscularly once a week. Another alternative is to administer vitamin K when periodic measurements indicate prolonged prothrombin time. This method, however, maintains the patient in a state bordering on deficiency and may not be optimal.

Excessive administration of vitamin K has been associated with hyperbilirubinemia in newborn infants, which is possibly due to hemolysis or hepatocellular toxicity.[33] Porphyrinuria has also been observed in man following a 380 mg oral dose of vitamin K.[34] Vitamin K is available in a water-soluble form and, as such, can be added to the parenteral nutrition solutions. It is, however, relatively unstable when exposed to light and perhaps to amino acid solutions. It is best given orally or intramuscularly.

*Vitamin E.* Vitamin E was first isolated from wheat germ oil in 1936, and its chemical structure and synthesis were reported in 1938. It exists in nature as a series of closely related compounds that differ in the number and position of methyl groups attached to a chroman nucleus with a phytol side chain (Fig. 11-4). Vegetable oils are the richest natural source of vitamin E, with cereal products and eggs next in order. One milligram of *d*,l-alpha-tocopherol has been designated as one international unit.

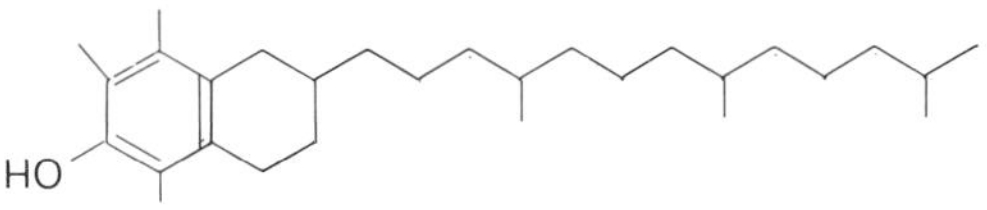

There is speculation as to the functioning of vitamin E in human nutrition. Its major activity may be as an antioxidant, inhibiting oxidation of unsaturated fatty acids by free radicals,[35] or its function may be more specific and unrelated to free radical protection.[36] Normal serum concentrations in adults with an adequate oral diet are greater than 0.5 mg per 100 ml.

Clinical symptoms of vitamin E deficiency in man have been well described. Early during vitamin E depletion, no physiological abnormalities are seen. With moderately severe depletion, however, there is an increase in erythrocyte hydrogen peroxide hemolysis, which may lead to a decrease in red cell survival and a mild anemia.[37-40] Iron supplementation, a potent free-radical generator, can greatly increase hemolysis in the presence of vitamin E deficiency and should be avoided. A decrease in blood creatine concentration due to excessive creatinuria may also occur with moderate vitamin E deficiency.[41] With prolonged and severe depletion, ceroid material is deposited in smooth muscle, and inclusion bodies, presumably derived from oxidized lipid, appear in reticuloendothelial cells of the bone marrow. Lesions in skeletal muscles resembling muscular dystrophy are also seen,[40] and anemia may become marked. Lake et al.[42] have recently documented increased platelet aggregation in patients with vitamin E deficiency. The finding may be important in treating bedridden patients, who are highly susceptible to thrombus formation. It is proposed that vitamin E may act to inhibit phospholipase A release, thereby decreasing release of the prostaglandin precursor arachidonic acid, or that it may inhibit activity of prostaglandin cyclo-oxygenase and decrease formation of thromboxane $A_2$. Until further data are available, it is advisable to maintain normal vitamin E levels in all patients at risk of thrombotic complications. The administration of large doses of vitamin E to patients with normal plasma vitamin E levels has not been shown to decrease platelet aggregation or inhibit platelet phospholipase release.

Patients likely to develop vitamin E deficiency include those with pancreatitis or cystic fibrosis of the pancreas with steatorrhea,[37, 43] adult patients with severe prolonged steatorrhea (e.g., those with short bowel syndrome or jejunoileal bypass), patients with severe malnutrition, and patients who have undergone gastric surgery.[44] Patients who were severely malnourished prior to initiation of parenteral nutrition and who require prolonged intravenous nutrition may also develop vitamin E deficiency, especially if supplemental vitamin E is not administered.

The recommended daily oral allowance for vitamin E is 12 to 15 IU. Suggestions for intravenous support range from 2.1 to 60 IU per day (see Table 11–1). The requirements for vitamin E are greatly increased by the presence of polyunsaturated fatty acids in the diet,[45] and additional vitamin E should be given when fat emulsions are administered during parenteral nutrition. To date, no toxic effects of vitamin E have been reported even after administration of large doses over a period of five months.[46]

## WATER-SOLUBLE VITAMINS

Water-soluble vitamins have less resemblance to each other chemically than do fat-soluble vitamins. The classification is useful from a nutritional viewpoint, however, in that deficiencies of water-soluble vitamins often have similar symptoms, and therapy is usually directed toward multiple replacement. Tissue stores of water-soluble vitamins are small, and deficiencies occur early with dietary restriction. Supplementation during parenteral nutrition is mandatory, not only because of small tissue stores but also because of the increased requirements associated with stress. Excess amounts of these vitamins are rapidly excreted in the urine, and toxic effects are rarely seen.

*Thiamine — Vitamin $B_1$.* Thiamine is a white crystalline compound readily soluble in water, only slightly soluble in ethyl alcohol, and insoluble in ether and chloroform. It is relatively stable in parenteral nutrition solutions unless heated to temperatures greater than 100°C or exposed to pH values higher than 7.0. It is present in whole grains, legumes, beef, pork, liver, nuts, and yeast. Its structure was first elucidated by Williams et al. in 1934,[47] and it has since been synthesized by coupling a pyrimidine with a thiazole molecule (Fig. 11–5).

Thiamine has important biochemical functions. When combined with two molecules of phosphoric acid to become thiamine pyrophosphate, it functions as a coenzyme for the enzyme transketolase. Transketolase, in turn, is important in the phosphogluconate pathway that carries out interconversions of 3-, 4-, 5-, 6-, and 7-carbon sugars. This pathway is an important source of reduced nicotinamide-adenine dinucleotide phosphate (NADP). Thiamine pyrophosphate participates as a coenzyme in the oxidative decarboxylation of alphaketoacids to aldehydes. Two important substrates for this reaction are pyruvate, which is metabolized to acetyl coen-

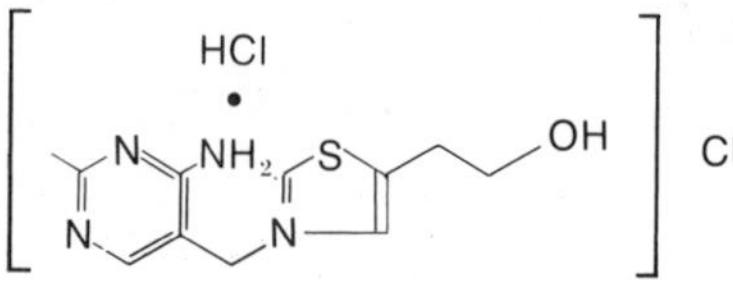

**Figure 11–5** Thiamine (Vitamin $B_1$).

zyme A, and alphaketoglutarate, which is metabolized to succinyl coenzyme A. Both these reactions require the participation of lipoic acid, nicotinamide-adenine dinucleotide (NAD), and coenzyme A. Thiamine is also believed to be a structural component of nervous system membranes.[48]

Nutritional deficiencies of thiamine are common. Owing to its limited distribution in foods, adequate thiamine may be lacking even in a fairly good diet and certainly in restricted diets. Patients with large urinary outputs may develop appreciable deficiencies because of renal losses. Prolonged antacid therapy may also lead to thiamine deficiency by destroying the ingested vitamin in the excessively alkaline bowel lumen.[49] Patients placed on parenteral nutrition are especially prone to developing thiamine deficiency: they are often malnourished and under significant stress with trauma or sepsis, they receive a thiamine-deficient diet if the substance is not added to the parenteral nutrition solution, and the provision of a high-carbohydrate diet increases greatly the requirements for thiamine.[50]

Thiamine deficiency causes beriberi in man. Mild deficiency is associated with a peripheral neuropathy characterized by paresthesia, hyperesthesia, anesthesia, and weakness. Initially, deep tendon reflexes are increased, but later they may be absent. Muscles become tender and may atrophy, with foot and wrist drop occurring. Fatigue, decreased attention span, and an impaired capacity for work are striking.

With increasing thiamine deficiency, neurological symptoms become more severe, and cardiovascular symptoms develop, leading to "wet beriberi." The heart becomes enlarged, particularly the right side. Mild effort results in significant tachycardia, and the patient may complain of palpitations and dull precordial or epigastric pain. Dependent edema develops. Arteriovenous shunting decreases circulation time, and venous pressure is often increased. These patients may develop digestive problems, anorexia, and constipation.

Acute pernicious beriberi may occur when patients are under physiological stress or when they receive high-

carbohydrate parenteral nutrition solutions without adequate thiamine supplementation. Cardiomegaly, generalized edema, and pleural effusions are often followed by pulmonary edema with a mortality rate of up to 50 per cent within several weeks. The cardiac failure caused by acute thiamine deficiency appears to be of the high-output variety and is thought to be due to interruption of pyruvate metabolism in cardiac muscle.[51] Loss of muscle striations and fatty degeneration with lymphocyte infiltration are typically found in the heart at autopsy.

Prolonged thiamine deficiency can lead to Wernicke's encephalopathy, which is characterized by disturbed consciousness ranging from mild confusion to coma, paralysis of the extraocular muscles, nystagmus, tremor, ataxia, and impaired vestibular function.[52, 53] Autopsies often reveal petechial hemorrhages into the gray matter around the third and fourth ventricles, and the aqueduct with the mamillary bodies is frequently involved. Microscopically, there is proliferation and dilatation of capillaries, proliferation of macroglia and microglia, and nerve cell degeneration, especially in the corpora mamillaria. At times, the inferior olives and optic nerves are also involved.

Early recognition of thiamine deficiency and adequate replacement result in rapid recovery from all impairments except the ataxia, which regresses more slowly and not always completely. In severe cases, damage to the cerebral cortex may result in Korsakoff's psychosis with impairment of memory and cognitive function.[54] Blennow[55] reported one case of Wernicke's encephalopathy during parenteral nutrition.

The requirements for thiamine in human nutrition vary with caloric intake. Oral intake of approximately 0.5 mg thiamine per 1000 calories is recommended.[56] Intravenous requirements are unknown, but 3 to 21 mg/day during parenteral nutrition have been recommended (see Table 11–1). The requirements for thiamine are further increased by fever, hyperthyroidism, and trauma. Thiamine is not stored in tissues to any great extent. Following excessive in-

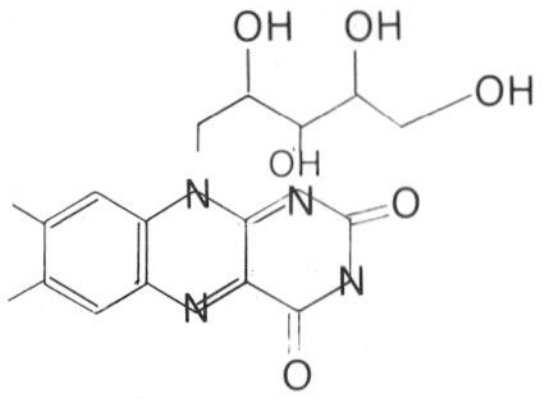

**Figure 11–6** Riboflavin (Vitamin B₂).

take, however, some tissue deposition occurs, affording temporary reserves capable of meeting the body's needs for a few weeks. The biologic half-life of thiamine has been estimated as 9 to 18 days.[57] Elimination of thiamine from the diet of healthy volunteers has resulted in significant thiamine depletion within 18 days. Deficiencies have been detected biochemically as early as seven days and clinical symptoms observed as early as nine days.[58] The major excretory route for thiamine is the kidneys. No toxic effects of thiamine have been reported in man, even after doses 200 times the daily maintenance dose. In rare cases, however, thiamine has caused reactions in man resembling anaphylactic shock. In these instances, large doses of thiamine had previously been given by injection, and the patients apparently had become sensitized.

*Riboflavin — Vitamin B₂.* Riboflavin is an orange-yellow crystalline compound that is only moderately soluble in water. It is heat stable, but readily decomposes when exposed to light or strong alkaline solutions. It is composed of a *d*-ribityl group and dimethylisoalloxazine (Fig. 11–6). Riboflavin occurs widely in nature, with milk, meats, and eggs being good sources.

Riboflavin is a constituent of two coenzymes, riboflavin-5'-phosphate and flavin adenine dinucleotide. These coenzymes are essential parts of a number of oxidative enzyme systems involved in electron transport, including amino acid oxidases, xanthine oxidase, succinic dehyrogenase complex, glutathione reductase, and many others.

There are apparently few tissue stores for riboflavin; normal patients placed on riboflavin-free diets demonstrate symptoms of riboflavin deficiency within as few

as seven days.[59] Symptoms include inflammation of the lips; fissures at the corners of the mouth; scaliness; greasiness; fissures in the folds of the ears and nose; seborrheic dermatitis about the nose and scrotum; and vascularization of the cornea. The symptom complex is called cheilosis. There may be ocular disturbances as well, with inflammation of the cornea; itching, burning, and dryness of the eyes; redness of the conjunctivae; photophobia; and dimness of vision.

The requirement for riboflavin appears to be related more to nitrogen balance than to caloric intake. The Food and Nutrition Board has recommended a daily oral riboflavin allowance of 0.07 mg per kilogram to the 0.75 power. According to this formula, adults require 1.3 to 1.7 mg riboflavin per day. Suggested intravenous requirements range from 3.6 to 7.5 mg per day (see Table 11–1). No toxic effects of riboflavin have been reported in man.

*Pantothenic Acid — Vitamin B₃.* Pantothenic acid is a water-soluble, yellow, viscous oil that is quite stable in the presence of oxidizing or reducing agents and moist heat. Structurally, it is a beta-alanine derivative containing a peptide linkage (Fig. 11–7). It is widely distributed in nature, with liver, meat, cereal, milk, egg yolks, and fresh vegetables being good dietary sources.

The only functional form of pantothenic acid is coenzyme A and, as such, it takes part in all acylation reactions. There is no firm evidence for a pantothenic acid deficiency syndrome in man. It has been suggested that deficiencies might result in malaise, headache, nausea, vomiting, and easy fatigability. There is some evidence that pantothenic acid acts as a stimulant to intestinal peristalsis and might, therefore, be useful in the treatment of postoperative ileus, but its efficacy remains to be proven.

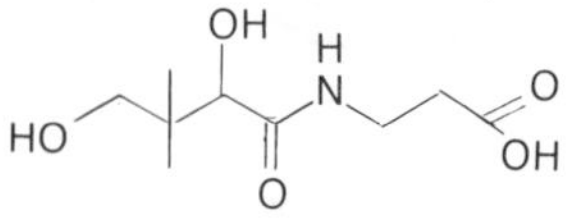

**Figure 11–7** Pantothenic acid (Vitamin B₃).

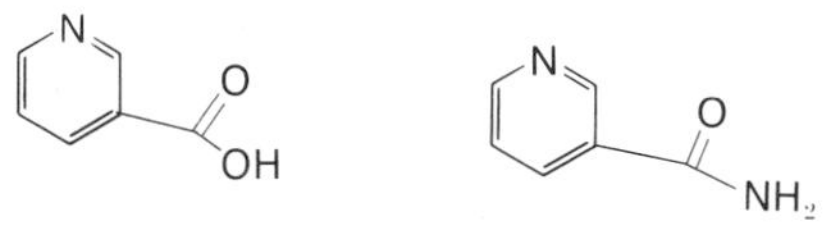

Nicotinic acid

Nicotinamide

**Figure 11–8**   Niacin (Vitamin B$_5$).

No daily allowance has been established by the Food and Nutrition Board, although a daily oral intake of 5 to 10 mg pantothenic acid is thought to be adequate for adults. The usual diet provides an average of 10 to 15 mg a day with a range of 9 to 20 mg.[60] Large doses of pantothenic acid, 10 to 20 grams, have been associated with diarrhea.[61] Few other toxic effects have been reported. Intravenous requirements during parenteral nutrition remain to be determined, but suggestions of 10 to 29 mg/day have been made (see Table 11–1).

*Niacin — Vitamin B$_5$.* Niacin is a stable white crystalline solid. Its structure is that of pyridine-3-carboxylic acid (Fig. 11–8). Niacin is found in large amounts in meats, fish, eggs, whole wheat, and polished rice.

The biologic function of nicotinic acid is related to its participation in the coenzymes NAD and NADP. These coenzymes participate in the intracellular respiratory mechanism of all cells by assisting in the stepwise transfer of hydrogen from products of glycolysis to the flavin mononucleotide. NAD and NADP can accept electrons from many biologic substrates. The reduced forms of the coenzymes play important roles in the microsomal system of biologic oxidations and in many biosynthetic reactions, such as the biosynthesis of fatty acids and various steroids.

Nicotinic acid deficiency leads to the disease pellagra. Early symptoms include weakness, lassitude, anorexia, and indigestion. With continued nicotinic acid deficiency, a characteristic dermatitis on the parts of the body exposed to sunlight, heat, or mild trauma occurs. The skin becomes thickened and pigmented. The pigmentation may persist for years after the dermatitis has healed. Diarrhea may also occur and may be severe, accompanied by vomiting

and dysphagia, with inflammation of the mouth. Achlorhydria may be present. Finally, the patient may become irritable and complain of headaches and sleepiness while exhibiting a loss of memory. Emotional instability may develop and progress to toxic confusional psychosis with acute delirium and catatonia.

The daily requirements for nicotinic acid are influenced by the total caloric intake. The minimum oral intake to prevent symptoms of pellagra is 4.4 mg niacin-equivalents per 1000 calories.[62] The daily allowance recommended by the Food and Nutrition Board is 14.5 to 19.8 mg niacin-equivalents. It should be noted that the amino acid tryptophan can be converted by the body to kynurenine, which is then converted in the liver and kidney to hydroxyanthranilic acid, a substitute for nicotinic acid. Various studies have indicated that an average of 60 mg tryptophan is equivalent to 1 mg niacin. When calculating dietary intake of niacin, therefore, it is necessary to think of niacin-equivalents. Intravenous requirements remain to be established, but it has been suggested that 40 to 150 mg niacin-equivalents be given daily (see Table 11–1).

*Pyridoxine — Vitamin B$_6$.* Pyridoxine hydrochloride, a pyridine derivative (Fig. 11–9), occurs as white platelets that are readily soluble in water. Pyridoxine is quite sensitive to light and ultraviolet irradiation, especially in alkaline solutions. It is found in egg yolk, meat, fish, milk, whole grains, cabbage, and legumes.

Pyridoxine functions as a coenzyme for transaminases. In addition, it functions as a coenzyme for the decarboxylases, which act on a number of amino acids, and also for two enzyme systems involved in metabolism of sulfur-containing amino acids. It aids in the conversion of tryptophan to nicotinamide, an important step in normal

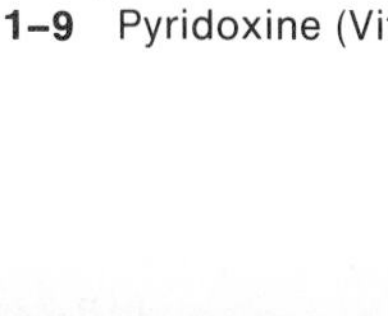

**Figure 11–9**   Pyridoxine (Vitamin B$_6$).

tryptophan metabolism. In the aldehyde form, vitamin $B_6$ enhances transport of amino acids and potassium into cells. The vitamin is also required for conversion of cysteine to pyruvic acid and oxalate to glycine and for synthesis of delta-aminolevulinic acid. It is essential for the function of phosphorylase, the enzyme that catalyzes breakdown of glycogen to form glucose-1-phosphate. It is a cofactor for a number of dehydratases, racemases, transferases, hydroxylases, synthetases, and many other enzymes.

A clinical syndrome associated with vitamin $B_6$ deficiency in man has been well described. Initially, patients develop personality changes, manifested by irritability, depression, and loss of a sense of responsibility. In addition, patients exhibit a filiform hypertrophy of the lingual papilla, stomatitis, seborrhea of the nasal labial folds, with acneiform papular rash of the forehead. Tryptophan metabolism is altered, leading to high urinary excretion of xanthurenic acid.[63] There also appears to be a strong tendency to develop infections, particularly of the genitourinary tract.[64] Serum glutamic-oxaloacetic transaminase and serum glutamic-pyruvic transaminase are lowered, and plasma and urinary levels of free amino acids may be altered.[65] Finally, a pyridoxine-responsive anemia, classified as sideroblastic anemia, may occur after prolonged pyridoxine deficiency.[66, 67] The likelihood of pyridoxine deficiency is increased in patients receiving antagonists to vitamin $B_6$, including isoniazid, penicillamine, semicarbozide, and cycloserine.[68]

The biologic half-life of pyridoxine ranges from 22 to 38 days.[69] A vitamin $B_6$-deficient diet has resulted in clinical symptoms in less than three weeks. The Food and Nutrition Board recommends 2.0 mg vitamin $B_6$ for adult men and 1.5 mg for adult women daily. Intravenous requirements have not been established, but recommendations of 4.0 to 6.3 mg a day have been made (see Table 11–1).

*Biotin — Vitamin $B_7$.* Biotin is soluble in water and is heat stable. It is a fairly simple organic ring compound (Fig. 11–10) and is widely distributed in food, including

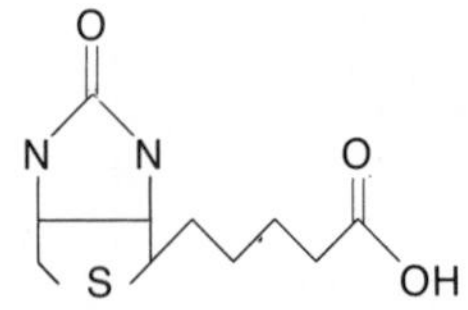

**Figure 11–10**   Biotin (Vitamin $B_7$).

liver, kidney, milk, and molasses. Much of the daily requirement for biotin is synthesized by intestinal flora,[70] thereby supplementing oral intake and making deficiency syndromes quite rare.

The main function of biotin is in carboxylation reactions, which proceed in two steps. The first is the binding of carbon dioxide to biotin with hydrolysis of ATP, and the second is the transfer of the "high energy" carbon dioxide to an acceptor.[71] It thus is active in the conversions of pyruvic to oxaloacetic acid, acetyl-CoA to malonyl-CoA, and propionyl-CoA to methylmalonyl-CoA. Biotin may also play a role in the conversion of folic acid to activated, reduced, and formylated forms and may participate in 1-carbon metabolism.[72]

Deficiencies of biotin have resulted in a fine-scale desquamation of the skin without pruritus. Other symptoms may include anemia, anorexia, nausea, lassitude, and muscle pain.

Adult requirements for biotin remain to be determined, although the average diet provides 150 to 300 micrograms per day.

*Folic Acid — Vitamin $B_9$.* Folic acid is a yellow, slightly water-soluble substance that is unstable in acidic solutions and upon exposure to sunlight. It consists of a pteridine moiety linked by a methylene bridge to para-aminobenzoic acid, which, in turn, is joined in peptide-like linkage to glutamic acid (Fig. 11–11). It is widely distributed in nature, particularly in the foliage of plants, as well as in yeast, cauliflower, liver, and kidney. Much of the folic

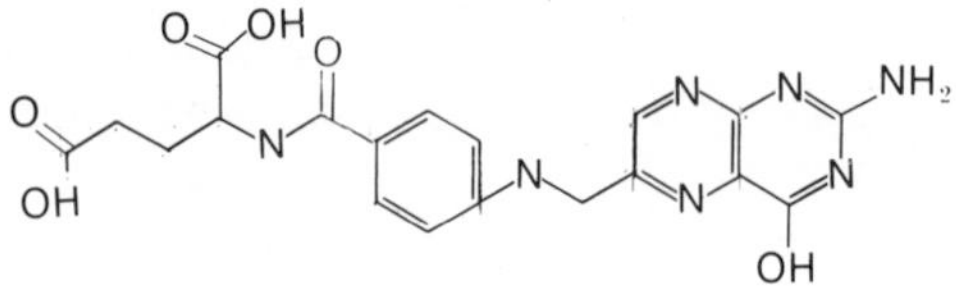

**Figure 11–11**   Folic acid (Vitamin $B_9$).

acid in foods is present as polyglutamates containing three to seven gamma-linked glutamate residues. The deconjugating enzymes in the duodenum and jejunum split off the glutamate residues to form monoglutamates, which are readily absorbed in the upper third of the small bowel. Normal human concentrations of serum folic acid range from 5 to 16 ng per milliliter.[73, 74] Body folate stores range from 5 to 10 mg, of which approximately half is in the liver.[75, 76] The serum concentration of folate does not accurately reflect tissue stores, as these stores are not readily mobilized.[77] Further, dietary folate markedly alters serum concentrations, accounting for as much as half of the basal level.[76] When serum folate concentration declines below 2 ng per milliliter, however, significant tissue store depletion can be assumed.

Folic acid participates in the uptake and transfer of 1-carbon fragments. It is thus involved in purine synthesis, pyrimidine nucleotide biosynthesis (methylation of deoxyuridylic acid to thymidylic acid), various 3-carbon amino acid conversions, including that of homocysteine to methionine, and the generation and utilization of formate.

Normally, folate stores can meet the body's needs for up to three to six months during complete folate restriction.[78, 79] More rapid depletion of body stores has been reported in chronic alcoholics, with symptoms of folate deficiency occurring within 5 to 10 weeks.[76] Symptoms may occur even earlier during severe stress or trauma if folate-free amino acid–ethanol solutions are infused intravenously to either healthy or malnourished patients.[80, 81] Folate deficiency during routine parenteral nutrition with folate-free amino acid–dextrose solutions has developed within 2 to 10 weeks in patients requiring nasogastric suction and having episodes of sepsis.[82, 83] The aspiration of gastric fluids contributes significantly to rapid folate depletion because of the high level of folic acid in bile.[84] Other clinical conditions leading to folate deficiency include inadequate ingestion associated with a poor diet; inadequate absorption, as with gluten-induced enteropathy;

various short gut syndromes; or the activity of competing drugs, such as diphenylhydantoin, barbiturates, cycloserine, and ethanol. Deficiencies may result from inadequate utilization of folate during administration of methotrexate, pyrimethamine, and triamterene, which block reduction of folic acid.[85, 86] Inadequate utilization may also occur with acquired or congenital enzyme deficiencies. Deficiency of vitamin $B_{12}$, which participates in the removal of a methyl group from methylfolate and the subsequent formation of the active compound tetrahydrofolic acid, may also result in clinical symptoms of folate deficiency.[87, 88] Finally, deficiencies may arise because of the increased requirements associated with pregnancy, malignancy (especially the lymphoproliferative disorders), sepsis, hyperthyroidism, and increased hematopoiesis, as with chronic blood loss or hemolytic anemia.

Symptoms of folic acid deficiency in man include megaloblastic anemia and occasionally diarrhea. The development of megaloblasts is apparently due to an arrest of the DNA synthesis during the S-phase of cellular growth. The earliest changes occur in bone marrow cells with nuclear defects in the late normoblasts, multiple Howell-Jolly bodies, and a shift to younger, larger cells of the erythroid series. Giant band cells are seen in the myeloid series. Progressive macrocytosis and hypersegmentation of polymorphonuclear leukocytes follow changes in bone marrow, with macrocytic anemia occurring relatively late.[76] Megaloblastosis is also present in other duplicating cells of the body, including the epithelial cells of the alimentary tract, where it produces glossitis and variable degrees of megaloblastosis along the entire tract.

Recommended oral dietary allowance for folic acid ranges from 200 to 400 micrograms per day, and suggested intravenous requirements range from 0.4 to 1.0 mg per day (see Table 11–1). The vitamin has low toxicity, with 10 to 30 mg intravenously or 200 mg orally being well tolerated.

*Cyanocobalamin — Vitamin $B_{12}$.* Cyanocobalamin is a dark red crystalline substance that is soluble in water and alcohol. It is stable in the presence of heat in neutral solutions but not in dilute acid or alkaline solutions. The main dietary source is liver, although it is also present in milk, meat, eggs, fish, oysters, and clams. In addition, enteric microorganisms, predominantly actinomyces, synthesize cyanocobalamin and contribute to dietary intake. Vitamin $B_{12}$ is formed by a corrin nucleus with a cobalt atom in the trivalent state linked to a nucleotide, 5,6-dimethyl-benzimidazole (Fig. 11–12). No other organic compound containing cobalt has been found in nature.

Absorption of ingested vitamin $B_{12}$ occurs by two mechanisms. One mechanism starts with gastric acid and intestinal enzymes separating ingested vitamin $B_{12}$ from polypeptide linkages to food. Vitamin $B_{12}$ subsequently attaches to gastric intrinsic factor. The vitamin $B_{12}$–intrinsic factor complex attaches to the mucosal cells

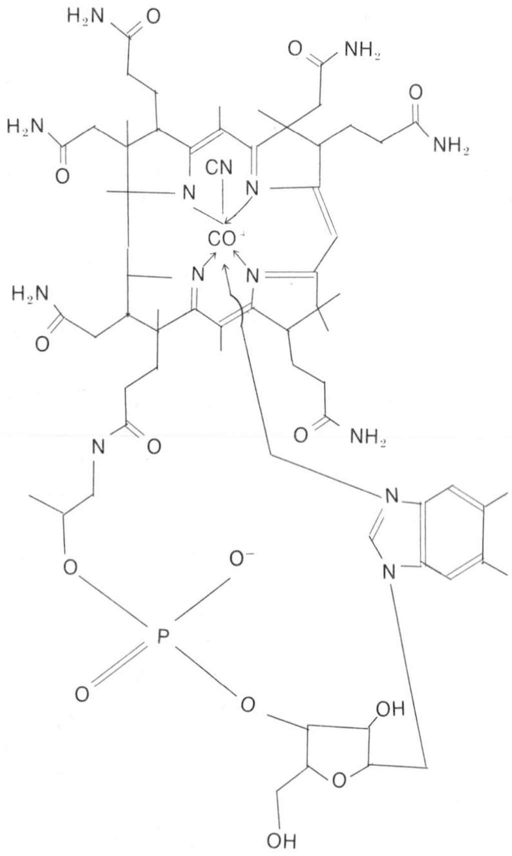

**Figure 11–12** Cyanocobalamine (Vitamin $B_{12}$).

throughout the entire small bowel but most efficiently in the terminal ileum in the presence of ionic calcium at a pH above 6.0. By an undetermined mechanism, the vitamin $B_{12}$ is released from its complex with intrinsic factor, traverses the intestinal cell, and enters the portal venous blood, where it is bound to a glycoprotein. The second mechanism of absorption is passive diffusion occurring along the entire small intestine. This latter mechanism accounts for only a small portion of total vitamin absorption.

Normal stores of vitamin $B_{12}$ are between 1 and 10 mg, with the liver containing 50 to 90 per cent of the total.[75, 89] Normal serum concentration ranges from 200 to 900 picogram per milliliter.[73, 90]

Vitamin $B_{12}$ plays many important roles in normal metabolism. Of primary importance is its ability to serve as a transmethylating agent. In this manner vitamin $B_{12}$ functions in the biosynthesis of thiamine, methionine, and possibly choline and plays a role in the metabolic pathways of glycine and serine. The vitamin transfers the methyl group from methyl folate to homocysteine, converting homocysteine to methionine and regenerating tetrahydrofolic acid. This process leads to synthesis of thymidylate and DNA. By a poorly understood mechanism, vitamin $B_{12}$ appears to assist in the movement of folate into cells. Vitamin $B_{12}$ deficiency, therefore, can lead to a megaloblastic anemia, even in the presence of adequate folate.[91] Vitamin $B_{12}$ appears to be involved in at least seven or eight different enzyme reactions as well. These include reduction of disulfide to sulfhydryl groups, activation of amino acids for protein synthesis, conversion of methylmalonyl-CoA to succinyl-CoA, conversion of beta-methylaspartic to glutamic acid, reduction of formate to methyl groups, reduction of ribonucleotides to deoxyribonucleotides by a ribonucleotide reductase, dismutation of vicinal diols to their corresponding aldehydes by means of a diol dehydrase reaction, and anaerobic degradation of lysine.[92] By these reactions vitamin $B_{12}$ plays an important role in fat and carbohydrate metabolism as well as in protein synthesis.

Because of the relatively large vitamin $B_{12}$ stores and a very efficient enterohepatic circulation system, deficiencies of vitamin $B_{12}$ are slow to develop and may require three to six years to become evident, even with no vitamin intake. Deficiencies may result from inadequate ingestion or inadequate absorption. Poor absorption may be due to the inadequacy or absence of secretion of gastric intrinsic factor or to diseases of the small intestine, especially those affecting the terminal ileum. Deficiencies may also result from poor utilization caused by vitamin $B_{12}$ antagonists, protein malnutrition, an abnormal $B_{12}$-binding protein in the serum, or congenital or acquired enzyme deficiencies or deletions. Increased requirements for vitamin $B_{12}$ are observed during hyperthyroidism and pregnancy. Increased excretion of vitamin $B_{12}$ occurs in patients with liver disease and may lead to deficiency states.

Vitamin $B_{12}$ deficiency is characterized by megaloblastosis similar to that seen in folate deficiency. Glossitis is common, and variable degrees of megaloblastosis may occur along the entire alimentary tract epithelium, which may lead to constipation. Patients may also develop megaloblastic anemia, termed pernicious anemia, associated with hypersegmented polymorphonuclear cells. The effect of vitamin $B_{12}$ deficiency on folic acid incorporation into red blood cells further accentuates the megaloblastic anemia. Vitamin $B_{12}$ is essential for myelin synthesis, and a deficiency may interfere with myelinization of peripheral nerves and posterior and lateral cords of the spinal column. Neurological symptoms of vitamin $B_{12}$ deficiency often begin insidiously with peripheral paresthesia, especially of the hands and feet. Diminution of vibration sense or position sense, unsteadiness, poor muscular coordination with ataxia, central scotomata due to optic nerve atrophy, moodiness, mental slowness, poor memory, confusion, agitation, delusions, hallucinations, and even overt psychosis may occur. Finally, a qualitative platelet defect may develop in severe vitamin $B_{12}$ deficiency and result in a total lack of aggregation and prolonged bleeding times.[93]

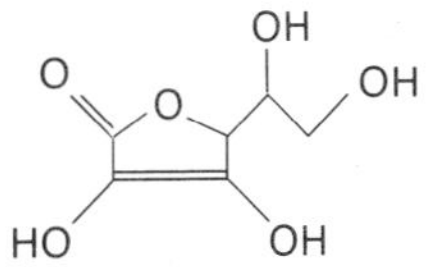

**Figure 11–13** Ascorbic acid (Vitamin C).

Recommended oral vitamin $B_{12}$ intake for adults is 2 to 3 micrograms daily. Suggested intravenous requirements range from 5 to 15 micrograms per day (see Table 11–1). Symptoms of vitamin $B_{12}$ deficiency may be treated with a single intramuscular injection of 100 micrograms or more of vitamin $B_{12}$. If the vitamin cannot be absorbed intestinally, a monthly injection of 100 to 500 micrograms is sufficient for prolonged maintenance. Doses up to 10,000 times maintenance levels have been shown to be non-toxic in man.

*Ascorbic Acid — Vitamin C.* Ascorbic acid is a simple compound (Fig. 11–13) that is highly soluble in water but quite insoluble in most lipid solvents. It is very sensitive to oxidation, particularly in the presence of copper, and is rapidly destroyed by alkaline solutions but fairly stable in weakly acid solutions.

Ascorbic acid has several important metabolic functions. Its primary role is in the formation of collagen. It appears to be essential for activity of proline hydroxylase and lysyl oxidase, which catalyze the conversion of proline to hydroxyproline and lysine to hydroxylysine. These two compounds are essential for maintenance of the tertiary structure of collagen. Ascorbic acid may also be involved in biologic oxidations and plays a part in the mitochrondrial electron transport chain with cytochrome C. Ascorbic acid is required in the metabolism of tyrosine, perhaps because of its protective action on the enzyme that oxidizes parahydroxyphenylpyruvic acid, a metabolic product of tyrosine. It further functions in the conversion of folic acid to tetrahydrofolic acid and in the hydroxylation of cholesterol to cholic acid. Finally, it may act to regulate cholesterol metabolism, as a deficiency is associated with a latent conversion of labeled acetate to cholesterol.

The essential role of vitamin C in the

prevention and cure of scurvy is now well established. Symptoms of scurvy include anemia, joint pain, and hemorrhage from mucous membranes of the mouth and gastrointestinal tract as well as from the skin, muscles, and subperiosteal tissues. The gums become swollen and tender with gingivitis and may ulcerate and even become gangrenous. Generalized weakness and emaciation are seen in later stages. The pathologic change leading to these symptoms is thought to be a reduction in intracellular substance with weakening of the capillary endothelial wall. Less severe deficiency of vitamin C is thought to be associated with slow healing of wounds, decreased ability to combat infections, and decreased ability to metabolize amino acids, especially tyrosine. Disease states that are often associated with vitamin C deficiency include infectious disorders, congestive heart failure, kidney and liver diseases, gastrointestinal disturbances, achlorhydria, diarrhea, purpura, endocrine disorders, and malignancies.

Daily oral requirements for ascorbic acid in man remain to be determined, although intake of 30 to 45 mg has been recommended (see Table 11–1). The biologic half-life of ascorbic acid is short. Symptoms of deficiency in normal volunteers on an ascorbic acid–free diet occurred as early as 29 days, and all patients were deficient after 90 days.[94] Vitamin C requirements may increase by as much as a hundredfold with major burns and extensive trauma, and if vitamin C is not supplied, normal body stores can be exhausted within 24 to 48 hours. Rapid infusion of vitamin C may result in a loss of up to 50 per cent in the urine if the renal threshold is exceeded. It is recommended, therefore, that infusions for replacement of deficiencies and maintenance be given intravenously at a steady rate. Suggested intravenous supplementation during parenteral nutrition ranges from 100 to 500 mg a day (see Table 11–1). Extremely large doses of vitamin C, in the range of 5,000 to 15,000 mg a day, may be associated with nausea and diarrhea. Some ascorbic acid is converted to oxalate, and large doses may lead to oxaluria and possible urinary stone formation. Finally, vita-min C interferes with the anticoagulant effects of heparin and Coumadin, with 2 mg ascorbic acid neutralizing 1 unit of heparin.[95, 96]

## SUMMARY

Requirements for fat-soluble and water-soluble vitamins must be recognized and met to assure optimal benefits of parenteral nutrition. Further research is necessary to determine more accurately the requirements for each vitamin as well as the effects of severe stress, trauma, infection, marked malnutrition, and intravenous administration of protein and large amounts of carbohydrates on those requirements. Deficiency syndromes, especially of the water-soluble vitamins, may occur rapidly during parenteral nutrition and may be difficult to detect because of the severity of the patient's illness. To avoid possible complications, only the recommended daily allowance of the fat-soluble vitamins should be given, while 2 to 15 times recommended allowances of water-soluble vitamins should be given. The large doses of water-soluble vitamins assure adequate support yet do not carry much risk of toxicity because of rapid urinary excretion of excesses.

Vitamin solutions currently available for intravenous administration are listed in Table 11–2. Comparison with proposed vitamin requirements in Table 11–1 indicates there is no available vitamin solution that is ideal for providing all necessary fat-soluble and water-soluble vitamins. Administration of several solutions is therefore necessary. One acceptable schedule is the following:

0.5 amp MVI.....................Q day

900 mg vitamin C.............Q day

600 to 900 micrograms
folic acid.........................Q day

100 to 200 micrograms
vitamin $B_{12}$ IM.................at start of parenteral nutrition and Q month

5.0 mg vitamin K IM.........Q week

# REFERENCES

1. Passmore, R., Nicol, B. M., Rao, M. N., et al.: Handbook on human nutritional requirements. W.H.O. Monog. Ser., *0*(61):1–66, 1974.
2. Dietary Allowances Committee and Food and Nutrition Board: Recommended Dietary Allowances, 8th Edition. Washington, D.C., National Academy of Sciences, 1974.
3. Loran, M. R., Althausen, T. L., Spicer, F. W., and Godstein, W. I.: Transport of vitamin A across human intestine in vitro. J. Lab. Clin. Med., *58*:622–626, 1961.
4. Patel, S. M., Mehl, J. W., and Deuel, H. J., Jr.: Studies on carotenoid metabolism; site of conversion of cryptoxanthin to vitamin A in the rat. Arch. Biochem. Biophys., *30*:103–109, 1951.
5. Adams, J. F., Johnstone, J. M., and Hunter, R. D.: Vitamin-A deficiency following total gastrectomy. Lancet, *1*:415–417, 1960.
6. Adlersberg, D., Kann, S., Maurer, A. P., Newerly, K., Winternitz, W., and Sobotka, H.: Vitamin A metabolism in liver disease. Gastroenterology, *10*:822–830, 1948.
7. Underwood, B. A., Siegel, H., Weisell, R. C., and Dolinski, M.: Liver stores of vitamin A in a normal population dying suddenly or rapidly from unnatural causes in New York City. Am. J. Clin. Nutr., *23*:1037–1042, 1970.
8. Moore, T.: Vitamin A. Amsterdam, Elsevier/North Holland Biomedical Press, 1957. pp. 355–374.
9. Roels, O. A., and Lui, N. S. T.: The vitamins. Vitamin A and carotene. *In* Goodheart, R. S., and Shils, M. E. (eds.): Modern Nutrition in Health and Disease, 5th Edition. Philadelphia, Lea & Febiger, 1973, pp. 142–157.
10. Wald, G., and Hubbard, R.: The synthesis of rhodopsin from vitamin A. Proc. Natl. Acad. Sci. U.S.A., *36*:92–102, 1950.
11. Hartline, J. V., and Zachman, R. D.: Vitamin A delivery in total parenteral nutrition solution. Pediatrics, *58*:448–451, 1976.
12. Howard, L., Chu, R., Feman, S., and Wolf, B.: Vitamin A deficiency in a patient with long term intravenous nutrition. J. Parenteral Enteral Nutr., *1*:10A, 1977.
13. Bergen, S. S., Jr., and Roels, O. A.: Hypervitaminosis A: Report of a case. Am. J. Clin. Nutr., *16*:265–269, 1965.
14. Elliott, R. A., Jr., and Dryer, R. L.: Hypervitaminosis A: Report of a case in an adult. J.A.M.A., *161*:1157–1159, 1956.
15. Soler-Bechara, J., and Soscia, J. L.: Chronic hypervitaminosis A. Arch. Intern. Med., *112*:462–466, 1963.
16. Di Benedetto, R. J.: Chronic hypervitaminosis A in an adult. J.A.M.A., *201*:700–702, 1967.
17. Vitamin A intoxication in infancy. Nutr. Rev., *23*:263–265, 1965.
18. Omdahl, J. L., and Deluca, H. F.: Vitamin D. *In* Goodheart, R. S., and Shils, M. E. (eds.): Modern Nutrition in Health and Disease, 5th Edition. Philadelphia, Lea & Febiger, 1973, pp. 158–165.
19. Lifshitz, F., Harrison, H. C., and Harrison, H. E.: Influence of parathyroid function upon the in vitro transport of calcium and phosphate by the rat intestine. Endocrinology, *84*:912–917, 1969.
20. George, W. K., George, W. D., Jr., Haan, C. L., and Fisher, R. G.: Vitamin D and magnesium. Lancet, *1*:1300–1301, 1962.
21. Donegan, C. K., Messer, A. L., and Orgain, E. S.: Vitamin D intoxication due to Ertron: Report of 2 cases. Ann. Intern. Med., *30*:429–435, 1949.
22. Covey, G. W., and Whitlock, H. H.: Intoxication resulting from administration of massive doses of vitamin D, with report of 5 cases. Ann. Intern. Med., *25*:508–515, 1946.
23. Anderson, D. C., Cooper, A. F., and Nayler, G. J.: Vitamin D intoxication with hypernatremia, potassium and water depletion and mental depression. Br. Med. J., *4*:744–746, 1968.
24. Bauer, J. M., and Freyberg, R. H.: Vitamin D intoxication with metastatic calcification. J.A.M.A., *130*:1208–1215, 1946.
25. Scharfman, W. B., and Propp, S.: Anemia associated with Vitamin D intoxication. N. Engl. J. Med., *255*:1207–1212, 1956.
26. George, W. K., George, W. D., Jr., Haan, C. L., and Fisher, R. G.: Vitamin D and magnesium. Lancet, *1*:1300–1301, 1962.
27. Gross, L., and Brotman, M.: Hypoprothrombinemia and hemorrhage associated with cholestyramine therapy. Ann. Intern. Med., *72*:95–96, 1970.
28. Haden, H. T.: Vitamin K deficiency associated with prolonged antibiotic administration. Arch. Intern. Med., *100*:986–988, 1957.
29. Dam, H.: The antihemorrhagic vitamin of the chick. Occurrence and chemical nature. Nature, *135*:652–653, 1935.
30. Suttie, J. W.: Mechanism of action of vitamin K: Demonstration of a liver precursor of prothrombin. Science, *179*:192–194, 1973.
31. Stenflo, J., Fernlund, P., Egan, W., and Roepstorff, P.: Vitamin K dependent modifications of glutamic acid residues in prothrombin. Proc. Natl. Acad. Sci. U.S.A., *71*:2730–2733, 1974.
32. Jeejeebhoy, K. N., Langer, B., Tsallas, G., Chu, R. C., Kuksis, A., and Anderson, G. H.: Total parenteral nutrition at home: Studies in patients surviving 4 months to 5 years. Gastroenterology, *71*:943–953, 1976.
33. Lawrence, B.: Danger of vitamin K analogues to newborn. Lancet, *1*:819, 1955.
34. Rosenberg, H. R.: Chemistry and Physiology of the Vitamins. New York, Interscience Publishers Inc., 1945, p. 509.
35. Tappel, A. L.: Free-radical lipid peroxidation damage and its inhibition by vitamin E and selenium. Fed. Proc., *24*:73–78, 1965.
36. Schwarz, K.: Role of vitamin E, selenium and related factors in experimental nutritional liver diseases. Fed. Proc., *20*:58–67, 1965.
37. Gordon, H. H., Nitowsky, H. M., and Cornblath, M.: Studies in tocopherol deficiency in infants and children. Am. J. Dis. Child., *90*:669–681, 1955.
38. Horwitt, M. K., Harvey, C. C., Duncan, G. D., and Wilson, W. C.: Symposium on the role of some of the newer vitamins in human metabolism and nutrition; effects of limited tocopherol intake in man with relationships

to erythrocyte hemolysis and lipid oxidations. Am. J. Clin. Nutr., 4:408–419, 1956.

39. Horwitt, M. K., Century, B., and Zeman, A. A.: Erythrocyte survival time and reticulocyte levels after tocopherol depletion in man. Am. J. Clin. Nutr., 12:99–106, 1963.

40. Binder, H. J., Herting, D. C., Hurst, V., Finch, S. C., and Spiro, H. M.: Tocopherol deficiency in man. N. Engl. J. Med., 273:1289–1297, 1965.

41. Nitowsky, H. M., Tildon, J. T., Levin, S., and Gordon, H. H.: Studies of tocopherol deficiency in infants and children. VII. The effect of tocopherol on urinary, plasma and muscle creatine. Am. J. Clin. Nutr., 10:368–378, 1962.

42. Lake, A. M., Stuart, M. J., and Oski, F. A.: Vitamin E deficiency and enhanced platelet function. Reversal following E supplementation. J. Pediatr., 90:722–725, 1977.

43. Braunstein, H.: Tocopherol deficiency in adults with chronic pancreatitis. Gastroenterology, 40:224–231, 1961.

44. Losowsky, M. S., Leonard, P. J., Kelleher, J., and Pulvertaft, C. N.: Vitamin E deficiency after gastric surgery. Am. J. Clin. Nutr., 20:366, 1967. (abstract)

45. Roels, O. A.: Present knowledge of vitamin E. In Present Knowledge in Nutrition, 3rd Edition. New York, Nutrition Foundation, 1967, pp. 86–88.

46. AMA Drug Evaluations: Vitamins and Sources of Vitamins, 1st Edition. Chicago, American Medical Association, 1971, pp. 102–106.

47. Williams, R. R., Waterman, R. E., and Keresztesy, J. C.: Crystalline antineuritic vitamin. J. Am. Chem. Soc., 56:1187–1191, 1934.

48. Itokawa, Y., Schulz, R. A., and Cooper, J. R.: Thiamine in nerve membranes. Biochim. Biophys. Acta, 266:293–299, 1972.

49. Christakis, G., and Miridjanian, A.: Diets, drugs, and their interrelationships. J. Am. Diet. Assoc., 52:21–24, 1968.

50. Nadel, A. M., and Burger, P. C.: Wernicke encephalopathy following prolonged intravenous therapy. J.A.M.A., 235:2403–2405, 1976.

51. Olson, R. E.: Proceedings of a conference on beriberi. Fed. Proc., 17(Suppl. 2): 24–27, 1958.

52. Victor, M., Adams, R. D., and Collins, G. H.: The Wernicke-Korsakoff syndrome. A clinical and pathological study of 245 patients, 82 with post-mortem examinations. Contemp. Neurol. Ser., 7:1–206, 1971.

53. Ghez, C.: Vestibular paresis: A clinical feature of Wernicke's disease. J. Neurol. Neurosurg. Psychiatry, 32:134–139, 1969.

54. Victor, M., and Adams, R. D.: On the etiology of the alcoholic neurologic diseases with special reference to the role of nutrition. Am. J. Clin. Nutr., 9:379–397, 1961.

55. Blennow, G.: Wernicke's encephalopathy following prolonged artificial nutrition. Am. J. Dis. Child., 129:1456, 1975.

56. Sauberlich, H. E., Herman, Y. F., and Stevens, C. O.: Thiamine requirements of the adult human. Am. J. Clin. Nutr., 23:671–672, 1970.

57. Ariaey-Nejad, M. R., Balaghi, M., Baker, E. M., and Sauberlich, H. E.: Thiamine metabolism in man. Am. J. Clin. Nutr., 23:764–778, 1970.

58. Ziporin, Z. Z., Nunes, W. T., Powel, R. C., Waring, P. P., and Sauberlich, H. E.: Excretion of thiamine and its metabolites in the urine of young adult males receiving restricted intakes of the vitamin. J. Nutr., 85:287–296, 1965.

59. Tillotson, J. A., and Baker, E. M.: An enzymatic measurement of the riboflavin status in man. Am. J. Clin. Nutr., 25:425–431, 1972.

60. Chung, A. S. M., Pearson, W. N., Darby, W. J., Miller, O. N., and Goldsmith, G. A.: Folic acid, vitamin B_6, pantothenic acid and vitamin B_12 in human dietaries. Am. J. Clin. Nutr., 9:573–582, 1961.

61. Gershberg, H., and Kuhl, W. J., Jr.: Acetylation studies in human subjects with metabolic disorders. J. Clin. Invest., 29:1625–1632, 1950.

62. Goldsmith, G. A., Sarett, H. P., Register, V. D., and Gibbons, J.: Studies of niacin requirement in man; experimental pellagra in subjects on corn diets low in niacin and tryptophan. J. Clin. Invest., 31:533–542, 1952.

63. Sauberlich, H. E., Canham, J. E., Baker, E. M., Raica, N., Jr., and Herman, Y. F.: Human vitamin B_6 nutriture. J. Sci. Ind. Res., 29(8):S28–S37, 1970.

64. Wayne, L., Will, J. J., Friedman, B. I., Becker, L. S., and Vilter, R. W.: Vitamin B_6 in internal medicine. Arch. Intern. Med., 101:143–155, 1958.

65. Aly, H. E., Donald, E. A., and Simpson, M. H.: Oral contraceptives and vitamin B_6 metabolism. Am. J. Clin. Nutr., 24:297–303, 1971.

66. Weintraub, L. R., Conrad, M. E., and Crosby, W. H.: Iron-loading anemia. Treatment with repeated phlebotomies and pyridoxine. N. Engl. J. Med., 275:169–176, 1966.

67. Hines, J. D., and Harris, J. W.: Pyridoxine-responsive anemia. Description of three patients with megaloblastic erythropoiesis. Am. J. Clin. Nutr., 14:137–146, 1964.

68. Kilsell, M. E. (ed.): Vitamin B_6 in metabolism of the nervous system. Ann. N.Y. Acad. Sci., 166:1–364, 1969.

69. Tillotson, J. A., Sauberlich, H. E., and Canham, J. E.: Use of carbon-14-labeled vitamins in human nutrition studies: Pyridoxine. Proceedings of the Seventh International Congress of Nutrition. Vol. 5, Physiology and Biochemistry of Food Components. Elmsford, N.Y., Pergamon Press, Inc., 1966, p. 556.

70. Oppel, T. W.: Studies of biotin metabolism in man; excretion of biotin in human urine; relationship between biotin content of diet and its output in urine and feces; excretion of 2 biotin-like substances in urine. Am. J. Med. Sci., 204:856–875, 1942.

71. Mechanism of action of biotin-enzymes. Nutr. Rev., 21:310–313, 1963.

72. Bridgers, W. F.: Present knowledge of biotin. Nutr. Rev., 25:65–68, 1967.

73. Hall, C. A., Bardwell, S. A., Allen, E. S., and Rappazzo, M. E.: Variation in plasma folate levels among groups of healthy persons. Am. J. Clin. Nutr., 28:854–857, 1975.

74. Rothenberg, S. P., daCosta, M., and Rosenberg, Z.: A radioassay for serum folate: Use of a two-phase sequential-incubation, ligand-binding system. N. Engl. J. Med., *286*:1335–1339, 1972.

75. FAO–WHO Expert Group: Requirements of ascorbic acid, vitamin D, vitamin $B_{12}$, folate, and iron. W.H.O. Tech. Rep. Ser., *452*:1–75, 1970.

76. Eichner, E. R., Pierce, H. I., and Hillman, R. S.: Folate balance in dietary-induced megaloblastic anemia. N. Engl. J. Med., *284*:933–938, 1971.

77. Whitehead, V. M., Comty, C. H., Posen, G. A., and Kaye, M.: Homeostasis of folic acid in patients undergoing maintenance hemodialysis. N. Engl. J. Med., *279*:970–974, 1968.

78. Herbert, V.: Experimental nutritional folate deficiency in man. Trans. Assoc. Am. Physicians, *75*:307–320, 1962.

79. Herbert, V.: A palatable diet for producing experimental folate deficiency in man. Am. J. Clin. Nutr., *12*:17–20, 1963.

80. Ibbotson, R. M., Colvin, B. T., and Colvin, M. P.: Folic acid deficiency during intensive therapy. Br. Med. J., *4*:145, 1975.

81. Wardrop, C. A. J., Heatley, R. V., Tennant, G. B., and Hughes, L. E.: Acute folate deficiency in surgical patients on aminoacid/ethanol intravenous nutrition. Lancet, *2*:640–642, 1975.

82. Ballard, H. S., and Lindenbaum, J.: Megaloblastic anemia complicating hyperalimentation therapy. Am. J. Med., *56*:740–742, 1974.

83. Steinberg, D.: Folic acid deficiency: Early onset of megaloblastosis. J.A.M.A., *222*:490, 1972.

84. Baker, S. J., Kumar, S., and Swaminathan, S. P.: Excretion of folic acid in bile. Lancet, *1*:685, 1965.

85. Waxman, S., Corcino, J. J., and Herbert, V.: Drugs, toxins, and dietary amino acids affecting vitamin B-12 or folic acid absorption or utilization. Am. J. Med., *48*:599–608, 1970.

86. Reilly, M. J.: Folic acid U.S.P. Am. J. Hosp. Pharm., *27*:494–495, 1970.

87. Hall, C. A.: Vitamin $B_{12}$-binding proteins of man. Ann. Intern. Med., *75*:297–301, 1971.

88. Herbert, V., and Zalusky, R.: Interrelations of vitamin $B_{12}$ and folic acid metabolism: Folic acid clearance studies. J. Clin. Invest., *41*:1263–1276, 1962.

89. Rappazzo, M. E., Salmi, H. A., and Hall, C. A.: The content of vitamin $B_{12}$ in adult and foetal tissue: A comparative study. Br. J. Haematol., *18*:425–433, 1970.

90. Herbert, V.: Folic acid and vitamin $B_{12}$. *In* Goodhart, R. S., and Shils, M. E. (eds.): Modern Nutrition in Health and Disease, 5th Edition. Philadelphia, Lea & Febiger, 1973, pp. 221–244.

91. Cooper, B. A., and Lowenstein, L.: Relative folate deficiency of erythrocytes in pernicious anemia and its correction with cyanocobalamin. Blood, *24*:502–521, 1964.

92. Silber, R., and Moldow, C. F.: The biochemistry of $B_{12}$-mediated reactions in man. Am. J. Med., *48*:549–554, 1970.

93. Levin, P. H.: A qualitative platelet defect in severe vitamin $B_{12}$ deficiency. Response, hyperresponse, and thrombosis after vitamin $B_{12}$ therapy. Ann. Intern. Med., *78*:533–539, 1973.

94. Hodges, R. E., Hood, J., Canham, J. E., Sauberlich, H. E., and Baker, E. M.: Clinical manifestations of ascorbic acid deficiency in man. Am. J. Clin. Nutr., *24*:432–443, 1971.

95. Owen, C. A., Jr., Tyce, G. M., Flock, E. V., and McCall, J. T.: Heparin–ascorbic acid antagonism. Mayo Clin. Proc., *45*:140–145, 1970.

96. Rosenthal, G.: Interaction of ascorbic acid and warfarin. J.A.M.A., *215*:1671, 1971.

97. Report on Workshop on Vitamins and Minerals. Symposium on Total Parenteral Nutrition, American Medical Association, Nashville, Tenn., Jan., 1972.

98. Blackburn, G. L., and Bistrian, B. R.: Nutritional care of the injured and/or septic patient. Surg. Clin. North Am., *56*:1195–1224, 1977.

99. Department of Food and Nutrition: Guidelines for Multivitamin Preparations for Parenteral Use. Chicago, American Medical Association, 1975.

100. Nichoalds, G. E., Meng, H. C., and Caldwell, M. D.: Vitamin requirements in patients receiving total parenteral nutrition. Arch. Surg., *112*:1061–1064, 1977.

# INDEX